D0091594

A Physician's Guide to Pain and Symptom Management in Cancer Patients

A Physician's Guide to Pain and Symptom Management in Cancer Patients

Second Edition

Janet L. Abrahm, M.D.

The Johns Hopkins University Press
Baltimore & London

Drug dosage: The author and publisher have made reasonable efforts to deter-mine that the selection and dosage of drugs discussed in this text conform to the practices of the general medical community. The medications described do not necessarily have specific approval by the U.S. Food and Drug Administra-tion for use in the diseases and dosages for which they are recommended. In view of ongoing research, changes in governmental regulations, and the con-stant flow of information relating to drug therapy and drug reactions, the reader is urged to check the package insert of each drug for any change in indications and dosage and for warnings and precautions. This is particularly important when the recommended agent is a new and/or infrequently used drug.

© 2000, 2005 The Johns Hopkins University Press
All rights reserved. Published 2005
Printed in the United States of America on acid-free paper
9 8 7 6 5 4 3 2 1

The Johns Hopkins University Press
2715 North Charles Street
Baltimore, Maryland 21218-4363
www.press.jhu.edu

Library of Congress Cataloging-in-Publication Data

Abrahm, J. (Janet)
    A physician's guide to pain and symptom management in cancer
patients / Janet L. Abrahm.—2nd ed.
        p. ;   cm.
    Includes bibliographical references and index.
    ISBN 0-8018-8100-5 (hardcover : alk. paper)—ISBN 0-8018-8101-3 (pbk. :
alk. paper)
        1. Cancer—Palliative treatment. 2. Cancer pain.
    [DNLM: 1. Neoplasms—therapy. 2. Pain—prevention & control.
3. Palliative Care—methods. QZ 266 A159p 2005] I. Title
RC271.P33A27 2005
616.99'406—dc22

                                                          2004022318

A catalog record for this book is available from the British Library.

To my parents, Helen and Paul Abrahm;
my brothers, Stanley and Donald Abrahm;
and my aunt, Ruth Garner

Contents

Figures and Tables

Acknowledgments

There are many people to whom I am indebted and for whose help I am very grateful. *A Physician's Guide to Pain and Symptom Management in Cancer Patients* was inspired by my patients and their families, who have taught me much and whose wisdom, I felt, should be shared. I owed it to them and to their memories to help other clinicians reduce the suffering of patients with cancer and minimize the pain of their survivors.

I have also learned a great deal from the medical, nursing, pharmacy, and clinical psychology students with whom I have worked, and the medical interns, residents, fellows, nursing personnel, social workers, pastoral counselors, and ward clerks who have helped me care for my patients. Some of the most important insights I have gained over the years came from interactions with them.

I am grateful to a number of colleagues and teachers whose example sustained me as I worked to relieve the distress of cancer patients and the bereaved families they left behind. First among these are Elizabeth Quinlan-Bohn, certified Physician Assistant, and Mary Cooley, Ph.D., O.C.N., C.R.N.P. Elizabeth embodies the spirit of hospice and commitment to patient care. Her gentle good nature, extraordinary compassion and professionalism, and attention to the physical and spiritual comfort of her patients set a standard that all who work with her seek to emulate. Mary shared with me her office and her insights into grief, bereavement, and the needs of cancer patients and their families; and for a number of years she has supported me in my clinical and educational efforts in palliative care. I must also include the former members of the Philadelphia Veterans Administration Hospice Consultation Team: Jule Callahan, R.N., M.P.H.; Debi Selm, M.S.N., O.C.N., C.R.N.P.; Kathy Rossetti, M.S.W.; Lucy Pierre, M.Div., C.P.E.; Lisa Davis, Pharm.D.; Motria M. Krawczeniuk, Pharm.D.; and Denise Daily, R.D.

Others who have been very generous with their time, information, and support include Priscilla Kissick, former Executive Director of Wissahickon Hospice; Marian Wheeler and Katherine Washburn, who repeatedly suggested that I "write all this down"; the Board of the Project on Death in America, Faculty Scholars Program; Mary Calloway; and Drs. William Breitbart, Nathan Cherny, Malcolm Cox, Kathleen Foley, Robert Kaiser, Michael Levy, Ruth McCorkle, Russell Portenoy, Marcelle Shapiro, David Weissman, and Charles Von Gunten.

For editorial advice and unwavering support for this project, I thank my husband, David R. Slavitt, and my editor, Jacqueline Wehmueller.

ACKNOWLEDGMENTS FOR THE SECOND EDITION

One year after the first publication of this book, in January 2001, I joined the Division of Psychosocial Oncology and Palliative Care at the Dana-Farber Cancer Institute and moved into new digs in Cambridge, Massachusetts. For both my new job and my move to Cambridge, and for many of the new insights you will find in this revised and updated edition, I want to thank Dr. Susan Block. Susan is our Division Chief, and her vision and leadership make the work we do possible. I also would like to acknowledge the support and guidance of the members of our Pain and Palliative Care Team: Maureen Lynch, M.S., A.P.R.N., B.C.P.C.M., A.O.C.N.; Mary Jane Ott, M.N., M.A., R.N.C.S.; Bridget Fowler, Pharm.D.; Sarah Murphy, L.I.C.S.W.; David Giansiracusa, M.D.; our fellows past and present: Vicki Jackson, M.D., M.P.H.; Lauren Dias, M.D.; Alexie Cintron, M.D., M.P.H.; Mary Buss, M.D.; and Jacob Roth, M.D.; our program assistants and managers, past and present: Cheryl Adamick, Shawn Curtis, Kristen Morda, Nina Gadmer, and Don Cornuet; and our collaborators in Chaplaincy, Katherine Mitchell; in Ethics, Dr. Martha Jurchak; and in the Anesthesia Pain Service, whose chief is Dr. Edgar Ross.

I have had a great deal of assistance from other colleagues at Dana-Farber and at the Brigham and Women's Hospital. I am very lucky that Dr. Mary Cooley, whose help I acknowledged in the first edition, has relocated to Dana-Farber, and we continue our close collaboration. For their reviews of portions of the new edition, I would like to thank Dr. Edgar Ross, Dr. Laurie Rosenblatt, Ilene Fleischer, R.N., and Diane Bryant, R.N. For their support of our Pain and Palliative Care Program, I would like to thank the leadership at Dana-Farber, including Dr. Edward Benz, Dr. Lawrence Shulman, Dr. Jim Griffin, Dr. Lee Nadler,

Dr. Robert Mayer, Dr. Philip Kantoff, James Conway, and Dr. Patricia Reid Ponte.

I would not have embarked on this second edition if it were not for the readers of the first, who found it very useful and to whom I promised corrections of several errors they discovered! Finally, I need to acknowledge the physicians, nurse practitioners, nurses, and social workers at Dana-Farber who have so generously welcomed our team as collaborators in the care of patients and their families. The work with them is what sustains me, and it is what I have learned from them that I hope to share with the readers of this book.

For their encouragement, patience, and valuable editorial assistance, I again thank my husband, David R. Slavitt, and my editor, Jacqueline Wehmueller.

Introduction

Despite extensive efforts to prevent cancer and find its cure, each year cancer causes hundreds of thousands of men and women to suffer. Many are cured, but along the way they may have undergone devastating physical, psychological, and financial injuries. Less fortunate patients, whose cancer is resistant to curative therapies, are often told, "I'm sorry. There is nothing more we can do for you." But this is not true. Suffering can be prevented or treated whenever it occurs, whether at diagnosis or during curative therapy, or if the cancer recurs.

In addition to disease-oriented treatments, cancer patients need comprehensive treatment for the physical, psychological, social, and spiritual disorders brought on by the disease or by the therapies directed against it. They will benefit from clinicians (physicians, nurses, nurse practitioners, physician assistants) who are expert at relieving their pain or other troubling symptoms, who will make the patient, not the disease, the focus of their attention, and who can anticipate patients' hidden concerns, answer their unasked questions, and help them deal with their fears.

There are a number of oncology texts that focus on the details of disease-oriented treatment. *A Physician's Guide to Pain and Symptom Management in Cancer Patients* complements such texts, concentrating on symptom-oriented, patient-focused treatment. Designed for a busy practicing clinician, it is more thorough than a handbook but less comprehensive than a textbook.

A Physician's Guide will be particularly useful to clinicians who wish to enhance their relationships with patients and their families and expand the focus of their care. Physicians, nurse practitioners, and physician assistants who work in primary care, general internal medicine, family practice, geriatrics, or oncology (medical, radiation, or surgical), or with hospice or palliative care programs, will find information that spans the cancer trajectory from diagnosis to death. I offer help with communication challenges that occur at each stage, address the issues of most concern to patients and their loved ones, describe how to assess and manage the most troubling symptoms, and review how clinicians can provide expert, compassionate care for the dying and their bereaved families.

In writing this book, I relied on the work of experts in the field whose remarkable research and untiring efforts have delineated regimens that have revolutionized symptom management and palliative care. This work is referenced in the bibliography at the end of each chapter. I drew also from the lessons I learned from my patients and their families during my twenty-five years as a teacher and clinician, as a relative and friend of people who have had cancer, and from my colleagues. The clinical stories that appear in the book were crafted from these experiences.

Both superior communication skills and technical expertise are required if we are to succeed in relieving the distress of cancer patients, and the organization of the book reflects these dual requirements. In Part I, Hidden Concerns, Unasked Questions, I discuss the unique issues that need to be addressed if we are to provide optimal care to cancer patients and their families; suggestions for how to address these issues are included. Part II, Pain Control and Symptom Management, is a detailed presentation of the technical aspects of symptom assessment and management; it includes therapeutic protocols for the most common problems, including those that occur in the patient's final days. In both Part I and Part II, clinical scenarios illustrate many of the dilemmas presented by patients and their families. Important practice points are highlighted throughout the text and in numerous tables.

PART I. HIDDEN CONCERNS, UNASKED QUESTIONS

"What is wrong with me? Am I dying?"

The questions begin even before the official cancer diagnosis is made, and they continue throughout the course of treatment, whether the patient is cured or enters the cycle of relapse and retreatment that ultimately leads to death. In this way, of course, cancer patients are not unlike any other patients, who deliver the most surprising replies to, "What brought you here today?" My father, a general internist who was

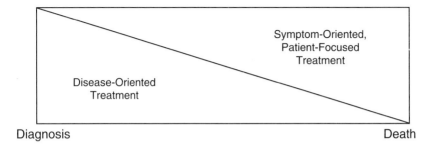

Diagnosis   Death

I.1. Comprehensive Management of Patients with Cancer. Comprehensive management of patients with cancer includes both disease-oriented and symptom-oriented patient-focused treatments. At diagnosis, disease-oriented therapies predominate, but some attention to symptoms is required. As the disease progresses and becomes irreversible, treatments designed to maximize the patient's quality of life and further his or her goals predominate.

in private practice for more than fifty years, cautioned me that it is usually more important to listen carefully for what patients don't say than to what they do.

This is certainly true for patients with cancer, whose concerns often differ in significant ways from those of patients without cancer. The proximity of death and the specter of helplessness, grief, suffering, and loss of dignity demand their attention. Most often, however, patients and their families do not openly share with their physicians their fears about the disease, the problems it produces, or the agents used to treat them.

Mrs. Ventimilio,* for example, who had been cured of a small, localized breast cancer for over ten years, unexpectedly appeared at my office one day for a "full check-up." During the course of the evaluation, she admitted that she had gone to a funeral the previous day and had begun to wonder whether she was really cured or whether the breast cancer was lying undetected inside her. Had I failed to discover that fear, I would not have been able to eliminate it or the stress it was causing.

Another patient, Mr. Ashton, with metastatic lung cancer, asked me for pills so he could commit suicide "when the time is right." As we discussed his request further, it appeared that he was concerned not for himself but for his elderly wife: he feared that she might ruin her health

---

*All names of patients and their physicians are pseudonyms.

trying to care for him as he died. As he came to understand about hospice programs and how hospice personnel and his friends and family could work together, he, too, was reassured. In both these cases, it was the hidden concerns, the unasked questions, that were the real source of distress.

Part I addresses the unique concerns of cancer patients and their families and offers ways of dealing with the unasked questions. Over the years, I have discussed many difficult issues with patients and their families, and some of these talks went much better than others. I include a number of sample dialogues that demonstrate what I have learned about how to communicate concern, elicit useful responses from patients and their families, and satisfy their needs.

Chapter 1. Early Days

This chapter may be especially helpful for clinicians who are just starting to take responsibility for telling patients bad news, initiating advance care planning, and discussing a prognosis that may be limited to a few more months of life. It begins with a review of what makes a conversation difficult, and offers techniques to analyze what about our own experiences, feelings, and identities contributes to our unease as we prepare for the meeting. By understanding what we are bringing to the conversation, we can better address the concerns of patients and their families. A particularly difficult discussion, especially for a beginner, is telling a patient that he or she has cancer or that the cancer has recurred. Early Days includes a review of techniques for breaking bad news and for dealing with the patient's response. Of interest to more experienced clinicians may be the discussion of why physicians can be reluctant to raise the subjects of advance directives and resuscitation or of prognosis, and the methods I offer for presenting these issues to patients and their families. I also review the role of ethics consultation teams.

Chapter 2. Helping Patients Accept Opioid Pain Medication

A major source of hidden concerns and unasked questions is the need of some patients to take opioids for the relief of their pain. Unless a number of barriers are overcome, patients won't take their medication and will continue to suffer severe pain. Chapter 2 addresses the misconceptions of patients and their families about the use of opioids: becoming addicted, having no effective medication later if the pain worsens, becoming constipated or "doped up," or going against the teachings of their religion. This chapter provides examples of patients and families with such concerns, as well as suggestions for anticipating and overcoming them. I also review other impediments to compliance, including patients' reluctance to admit how much pain they are experiencing and the role of hidden agendas in impairing your ability to relieve their pain. Here, we may expect to confront guilt, denial, and anger, all of which I discuss. Finally, I explain how educating colleagues can enhance patients' compliance.

CHAPTER 3. APPROACHING THE END

As death approaches, other communication problems surface. Chapter 3 deals with the most common of these. Many difficulties arise from misunderstandings among the clinician, the patient, and the family about the true extent of the disease, the goals of treatment, and the expected outcomes of whatever therapy is chosen. Others, as this chapter will explain, are the consequence of differences in the priorities that patients, families, and physicians place on the various symptoms the patient is experiencing and the remedies that are reasonable to relieve them.

Another challenge is helping patients and their families make the transition to comfort care. I explain how the rigors of the chemotherapy schedule have caused most patients and their family caregivers to stop being involved in work, their community, and even their family. If patients and their families reintegrate important activities into their lives, their days can be full without chemotherapy, and it will be easier to accept that the patient no longer will benefit from it. I also suggest how to readdress the issues of resuscitation, and review the concerns of two groups of patients who, despite very advanced cancer, still want to be resuscitated: dying parents who have young children, and families and patients who are waiting for a miracle. Once the patient and family have accepted comfort care, hospice programs can help clinicians and their office staff alleviate family insecurities. I detail hospice eligibility criteria for patients who do not have cancer and the levels of clinical care that hospice programs provide (a detailed description of hospice services is given in Chapters 7 and 8).

House staff who help us care for dying patients frequently ask us, "How do we know when it's time to stop what we normally do?" I answer their question in this chapter and also review our experience with the grief rounds we hold for house staff. Despite these efforts at providing the best of care, some patients with advanced disease ask us to assist them in committing suicide. I review the hidden concerns underlying these requests and offer sample dialogues and information that will be useful in addressing them. Finally, I offer strategies for self-preservation for the clinicians who do this very tough work.

PART II. PAIN CONTROL AND SYMPTOM MANAGEMENT

Part II is a symptom assessment and management handbook. Its five chapters review how to assess pain and treat it by pharmacologic and nonpharmacologic means, how to detect, assess, and address distressing problems other than pain, and how to care for patients in their final days and for their bereaved families.

CHAPTER 4. ASSESSING THE PATIENT IN PAIN

A thorough pain assessment reveals both the cause or causes of the pain and the factors that exacerbate the experience of pain for each patient. It is the foundation on which both pharmacologic and nonpharmacologic therapies rest. Chapter 4 reviews the components of a comprehensive pain assessment, provides examples of a number of measurement tools available for this purpose, defines the characteristics of the various types of pain, and describes in detail a number of cancer-related pain syndromes that occur only rarely in patients without cancer. At the end of the chapter, I discuss how to determine whether the patient is suffering from anxiety, depression, delirium, or social or spiritual distress. These can exacerbate the experience of pain and can in themselves adversely affect the quality of life of patients and their families.

CHAPTER 5. PHARMACOLOGIC MANAGEMENT OF CANCER PAIN

This chapter reviews pharmacologic therapy, the cornerstone of cancer pain treatment. I discuss the use of nonsteroidal anti-inflammatory drugs and opioids, delivered by the oral, transmucosal, topical, transdermal, rectal, intravenous, subcutaneous, or spinal routes, and how to choose among these agents and routes. I include a specific discussion of the use of methadone for cancer pain. I also discuss treatment of the common opioid-induced side effects: constipation, nausea, sedation, delirium, and respiratory depression. Adjuvant pain relievers are then reviewed, including adjuvants for nerve pain (such as corticosteroids, anticonvulsants, tricyclic antidepressants, baclofen, clonidine, and ket-amine), agents for bone pain (such as NSAIDs, corticosteroids, external beam radiation and radiopharmaceuticals, bisphosphonates, calcitonin, vertebroplasty and kyphoplasty, and radiofrequency ablation), neu-roleptics, and skeletal muscle relaxants. Also included are anesthetic methods, such as topical and oral agents, neural blockade, and neu-roablation. Special mention is made of the considerations needed in treating older patients, including those who are cognitively impaired, and patients with active or past histories of substance abuse.

Several tables detail the NSAID and opioid drugs available, their formulations, the doses recommended, and caveats about their use; other tables list the same information for laxatives, antiemetics, psycho-stimulants, agents that treat delirium, adjuvant agents for neuropathic pain, antidepressants, adjuvants for bone pain, and topical and oral anesthetics.

Very practical suggestions for common clinical situations are offered: how to start a patient on opioids; how to change the opioid dose, route, or agent safely; and how to relieve excruciating pain rapidly.

CHAPTER 6. NONPHARMACOLOGIC STRATEGIES FOR PAIN AND SYMPTOM MANAGEMENT

The National Center for Complementary and Alternative Medicine has defined five domains of complementary and alternative therapies: (1) alternative medical systems, (2) manipulative and body-based meth-ods, (3) mind-body interventions, (4) biologically based therapies, and (5) energy therapies. In this book, I do *not* review the biologically based therapies, which include special diets, such as the Atkins or Ornish di-ets, herbal treatments, megadose vitamin therapy, or use of particular substances not proven effective by conventional medical studies, such as laetrile. I also do not review energy therapies such as qi gong, Thera-peutic Touch, Reiki, and healing touch, but I do provide references for those who are interested in these areas.

I discuss what I consider to be those nonpharmacologic techniques for which there is the most evidence supporting their effectiveness in relieving pain and other sources of distress in cancer patients. These include acupuncture/acupressure and yoga, two of the alternative medical systems that include philosophies and practices that are com-pletely independent of the usual medical approach. I also discuss ma-nipulative and body-based methods, including cutaneous interventions, massage and vibration, transcutaneous electrical nerve stimulation (TENS), and positioning and exercise. Finally, I review the mind-body interventions that include education, cognitive and behavioral interventions such as diversion of attention, relaxation and breathing, mindfulness meditation, hypnosis, biofeedback, and spiritual counseling. As a hypnosis practitioner, I am more familiar with the use of this technique and therefore am able to provide a discussion of some misconceptions that have limited its use, along with a sample relaxation exercise that cancer patients may find useful. I also review art therapy, music therapy, and speech and language therapy.

CHAPTER 7. MANAGING OTHER DISTRESSING PROBLEMS

This chapter continues the symptom assessment and management handbook. The discussion includes anxiety and depression, oral complications (candida, xerostomia), gastrointestinal problems (ascites, diarrhea, and nausea and vomiting, including treatment-induced nausea and vomiting), respiratory problems (dyspnea, cough, hemoptysis, and hiccups), skin disorders (fungating lesions, pressure sores, and pruritus), and insomnia. I also include the common treatable causes of weakness and fatigue: Eaton-Lambert syndrome, anemia, metabolic abnormalities, anorexia, and malnutrition. Patients and their families commonly believe that enteral or parenteral nutrition will restore patients' strength and prolong their lives. I explain why this is not always the case and why enteral and parenteral feeding are not usually indicated for people with advanced cancer. I also offer coping strategies to help patients suffering from weakness or fatigue modify their activities to maximize what they can achieve despite their diminishing capacity.

The material in the text is supplemented by tables detailing the drugs and their recommended doses for the problems reviewed. The chapter includes a discussion of hospice: its philosophy, the team members, the services they provide, and what is included in the Medicare Hospice benefit. Finally, I review the role of palliative care consultation teams.

CHAPTER 8. THE LAST DAYS . . . AND THE BEREAVED

Here I review the art and science of helping the dying and the bereaved. I describe the various aspects of a comprehensive program for care of the dying and support for their families, and further explore the role of the hospice team in ensuring that all the important pieces are in place, including bereavement care. Families often want to know when the patient is approaching the end. I provide the clues that will help in recognizing when patients are making the transition and have only weeks remaining. I revisit families' ethical concerns about pain management and review the doctrine of double effect. I also mention the importance of supporting the inpatient ward team, who care for the bulk of dying patients in the United States. The first part of the chapter, The Dying Patient, includes an outline of the symptom complex of dying patients and some treatment recommendations, including a table of pharmacologic therapies for the most common problems: pain, death rattle, terminal restlessness, dyspnea, delirium, dehydration, massive hemoptysis, nausea, vomiting, and myoclonus. I also provide an algorithm for agitation in the last days. For clinicians who have not been present when one of their patients died, I end this first part of the chapter with some thoughts on how to continue to comfort the newly bereaved.

The second half of the chapter deals with the survivors: how we can continue to help the bereaved family and friends. I discuss the manifestations of loss, grief, and mourning, and the differentiation between grief and depression. I also describe a typical bereavement program through which we can support survivors and educate them about what they can expect to feel, and indicate how to identify those who would benefit from formal counseling or informal support groups. The chapter also includes the bereavement materials our team uses in our program.

Finally, I review complicated mourning—survivors who delay mourning or who never recover from their losses. I discuss the factors that predispose to this syndrome, provide a screening tool that identifies people at greatest risk, and offer suggestions for identifying and providing ongoing support and treatment for them.

At the end of the book you will find two annotated listings of additional materials. The first contains materials of interest to clinicians, and includes information on books, handbooks, journals, patient education materials, videos, websites, CDs, and organizations. The second provides listings of books, organizations, support groups, videotapes, websites, and CDs that you may wish to recommend to your patients and to families who have no special medical training. I have often been asked to provide such resources, and those I include have been particularly useful for my patients and their families and friends.

PART I

Hidden Concerns,
Unasked Questions

EARLY DAYS

The foundation of our relationships with patients and their families is profoundly affected both by how we first tell them they have cancer and by how we deal with their response to the news. The nonverbal clues we provide during these crucial interactions reveal a great deal about how willing we are to discuss their fears and how certain they can be of our ongoing emotional support.

Patients and their families need to know we will help them throughout the course of their illness, especially if it eventually causes their death. We must make it clear that we will not abandon them if the medical treatments lose their effectiveness and will use our expertise to help them achieve the best possible quality of life at every stage of their illness.

Part of our responsibility, then, is to communicate clearly our interest in understanding patients' values, hopes, and goals so that we can choose the most appropriate treatments for them and carry out their wishes regarding resuscitation or prolonged support by a ventilator or feeding tube.

In this first chapter, therefore, I review the components of difficult conversations, how we should "break the bad news," and how we can best respond to the reactions of patients and their families. I also consider how to begin discussions of resuscitation and other extraordinary support (advance care planning), and what is known about why such discussions are so difficult for us to undertake; I include several examples of phrases that work, as well as some examples of phrases that only confuse patients further.

DIFFICULT CONVERSATIONS: THE THREE CONVERSATIONS

To be able to deliver bad news with skill and compassion, we must prepare ourselves emotionally for what is likely to be a very difficult conversation. In rehearsing what we are going to say, we need to be aware of our feelings about the impending meeting and to analyze carefully all the elements that make this a "room we would rather not enter." What makes a conversation difficult? Members of the Harvard Negotiation Project (the people who brought us the very useful book *Getting to Yes*) lay out the key elements in *Difficult Conversations: How to Discuss What Matters Most* (Stone et al. 1999). The book is designed for businesspeople, but the principles apply equally well to clinicians.

Stone and colleagues suggest that within any difficult conversation lie three conversations: (1) the "What Happened?" conversation, (2) the "Feelings" conversation, and (3) the "Identity" conversation.

THE THREE CONVERSATIONS

The "What Happened?" conversation
Given the same set of "facts," does your story differ from theirs?
Can you move from certainty to curiosity?

The "Feelings" conversation
What are you feeling: Sadness? Anger? Guilt? Frustration?

The "Identity" conversation
Is your sense of who you are being challenged?
Have you lost your balance?

(Adapted from Stone et al. 1999)

These conversations can be illustrated by an encounter I had with Yu Hsin and his wife, Jenny.

Yu Hsin, a 33-year-old man, had non-Hodgkin's lymphoma of the small bowel. He had been married to Jenny for ten years and they had three children, 8, 6, and 4 years old. Surgical resection of his tumor was not possible. I had tried several chemotherapy regimens, after each of which the tumor responded. However, the manifestation of each response was severe gastrointestinal bleeding. I went to visit Yu in the hospital on the day he was going to be transferred to a rehabilitation facility. This had been his third hospitalization for bleeding and near perforation of the intestine because of tumor necrosis. I knew that Yu's bowel would surely perforate if we tried chemotherapy again. The surgeons thought surgery would not be helpful. As I prepared to enter the room, I steeled myself to tell Yu and Jenny that we could not risk any more treatment.

We chatted for a while about the planned transfer, which they both looked forward to. Jenny asked when Yu would be coming back for his next treatment, and I replied that, as sorry as I was to say it, I thought there was nothing else I could do for him, that he would bleed to death or his bowel would perforate if I continued the therapy. Yu took the news stoically, but Jenny asked angrily how I could stop treating him if his lymphoma was responding to the treatment. She accused me of abandoning them and giving up on Yu. I could barely look at them. I felt numb and distant, as though observing all of us from far away. I reassured Jenny that we would find something to help Yu, hoping that my saying it would make it so. I told Yu that I was glad he was feeling so much better and that we'd talk about next steps when he came to the office. I could not wait to leave.

THE "WHAT HAPPENED?" CONVERSATION

I remember very clearly how I felt as I left the room. I had given other patients bad news that had elicited anger from both the patients and their families, but rarely had I felt so distraught. I did not understand then what was different about this conversation.

Later, using the framework of Stone and colleagues, I was finally able to realize what had happened. As Stone and colleagues put it, there are a number of interpretations of the same "facts." So what were the "facts" here? As I saw it, I had given Yu state-of-the-art treatment that was placing him in danger of bleeding to death or dying from a bowel perforation. It was unfortunate, but certainly it was not fair for them to blame me for the location of the lymphoma. Jenny, I surmised, was in denial about Yu's true condition and the danger further therapy would bring.

As Stone and colleagues caution, however, "You only know your own story." In shutting down in response to their anger, I was not able to ask Jenny to tell me more about her reaction to my news. To this day, I don't know why she thought we could continue his treatments. Maybe she thought the bleeding was a good sign: that the tumor was being flushed out of his system, and the blood transfusions were bringing in clean, safe blood to replace the cancerous tissue. Maybe as a woman she did not think Yu's bleeding was any more dangerous than the monthly bleeding she experienced.

How much more helpful I would have been had I explored why she was so angry and her interpretation of Yu's response to his treatments. How I wish I at least had not said, "There is nothing more I can do for him," even as a part of my explanation of why I wasn't offering ongoing chemotherapy. Was that why she felt I was abandoning her and giving up on Yu? I'll never know.

Stone and colleagues would suggest that instead of my "certainty," I should have allowed my natural "curiosity" about the reasons for her response to emerge. I should have made more of an effort to hear what she was trying to tell me. So why didn't I do that? Why did I withdraw emotionally?

The "Feelings" Conversation

I think the key is in my feelings about Yu, not in Jenny's anger. And that gets us to the "Feelings" conversation, which refers to the emotions that are welling up within us that we don't allow to come to the surface and be named. I am sure I felt very sad, not only for Yu but for Jenny and their children. I think I was also feeling guilty, inadequate, and helpless, and these emotions were contributing to my emotional disconnection from Yu and Jenny.

If, before our meeting, I had reflected on how I was feeling, I could have shared at least my sadness with them, rather than presenting a false cheerfulness. I am sure my body language was giving me away anyway, and the dissociation between what they could see and what I was saying must have contributed to their distrust.

Later, I could have shared my guilt, inadequacy, and helplessness with colleagues. I eventually did seek consolation from a wonderful third-year fellow after he told us of the success he was having with one of his patients. "Your patients always seem to do so well," I said. "I must be doing something terribly wrong with mine." He laughed, put an arm around my shoulder, and said, "Janet, I only talk about the ones who are doing well. There are plenty who don't." He took me to the cafeteria for coffee, helped me explore my feelings, and gave me some strategies for coping with the emotions raised by the work we both did.

The "Identity" Conversation

I probably could have dealt with my feelings, if that was all that was going on. But what shut me down was that Jenny's accusations echoed the doubts I was feeling about myself as a physician. As Stone and colleagues say, "'The Identity Conversation' looks inward: it's all about who we are and how we see ourselves. How does what happened affect my self-esteem, my self-image, my sense of who I am in the world? What impact will it have on my future? What self-doubts do I harbor? In short: before, during, and after the difficult conversation, the Identity Conversation is about what I am saying to myself about me."

What happened to me, Stone and colleagues suggest, was that I lost my "balance." My sense of competence, trustworthiness, loyalty, professionalism all were under attack. I reeled not from the blows inflicted by Yu's sadness or Jenny's anger, but from my own doubts that her anger and his despair had triggered. Unaware as I was of this disequilibrium, I shut down and used only my "executive functions" for the rest of the conversation, going through the motions, and reinforcing Yu and Jenny's sense of abandonment and betrayal. Had I recognized that I was losing my balance, I could have remained present intellectually and emotionally.

MOST CONVERSATIONS I HAD with my patients were much less emotional, even when I had bad news to impart. A discussion of recurrent hypercalcemia, for example, would not have been a "difficult conversation." There is nothing about hypercalcemia that triggers feelings in me of sadness, inadequacy, helplessness, or guilt, and nothing that triggers questions about my competence as a physician. But as a first-year oncology fellow, the dilemma Yu presented triggered all these feelings in me. And that is probably why I dreaded having the conversation in that hospital room.

Now, I'm better at recognizing these "loaded" conversations ahead of time. I ask patients and their families how they interpret the "facts" I give them, and explore how the case affects my own feelings and my sense of who I am. Now, before the encounter, I can prepare myself by talking over the facts and the feelings with colleagues or our staff.

The alternative, it seems to me, is simply to avoid the conversations that are just too painful for us. Or we may, unconsciously, strictly limit our emotional involvement with our patients. This lack of personal exploration into what makes a conversation difficult for us is likely to contribute to our reluctance to share bad prognoses with patients who really need to know them. We need to recognize what telling a patient that she has only weeks or months to live does to our emotional equilibrium, and need to understand how it can challenge our identity as physicians. Otherwise, the pain we experience at the thought of having these conversations may lead us to abandon our patients when they need us most.

HOW TO BREAK BAD NEWS

There is another early experience I will never forget: the first time I had to tell someone I'd just met that she had acute leukemia. I was a first-year fellow in Hematology/Oncology when I was called to the emergency room one evening to see Miss Etta Brown.

"I'm All Right, Dear. Are You?"

Miss Brown was a 56-year-old woman who presented with a two-week history of profound weakness and the onset that day of a rash. The laboratory called me to review her peripheral blood smear, and I agreed that it contained the blast cells typically seen in patients with acute leukemia. Her rash was petechial, and she had no other symptoms or remarkable physical findings; but analysis of her marrow aspirate confirmed that she had acute myelogenous leukemia.

I was severely shaken by the implications of her diagnosis. But I composed myself, put on what I thought was my most cheerful face, then went into her hospital room and sat on her bed. I took her hand in mine and in my most encouraging manner said, *"I'm sorry, but your bone marrow test shows that you have a cancer in your bloodstream; we call it acute leukemia. It is causing your rash and your weakness. We have good treatment for it, though, and there is every chance you will go into a remission."*

My face must have belied my words, however, because she replied, with evident concern, *"I'm all right, dear. Are you?"*

Miss Brown had been sick for some time, she later told me. She was frightened because she could no longer walk to church without becoming very weak and short of breath. When the rash appeared, she was certain she was about to die, but she did not share her fear with me until *after* I had told her about the leukemia. My news actually came as a reprieve from an immediate death sentence, and she was greatly relieved. She now understood what was wrong and could prepare herself to fight it. She felt better that night, she said, than she had felt in a long time.

The reverse situation is probably more common—and more distressing. Mr. Alessio, for example, was a patient who had been admitted for pneumonia. I was called to consult when the team discovered that the infection was caused by an obstructing lung cancer. The reaction I got when I told him of his cancer was disbelief, denial, and intense anger.

At the time, I ascribed the difference in the two responses to the personalities of the patients. But subsequently, I found a more likely explanation in the book *How to Break Bad News: A Guide for Health Care Professionals*, by Dr. Robert Buckman, a medical oncologist (Buckman 1992). As he states, "The reactions of patients often depend on the gap between their expectations and what the physicians tell them." Miss Brown's expectations were, if anything, worse than the news I had given her, and she expressed relief. For Mr. Alessio, however, the gap was enormous, and his reaction was commensurate with his shock.

How to Break Bad News, as the title suggests, describes how to convey distressing information to patients and how to cope with their reactions. It delineates the principles that underlie these discussions and includes a step-by-step procedure to ensure that all important elements are detailed.

Dr. Buckman relates that he wrote the book after witnessing the following exchange (which I continue to hope is apocryphal). A urologist stood at the door of a hospital room, talking to two of his patients within. He said that both men could be discharged that day and that the results of their prostate biopsies were available. He told one man that his biopsy showed only inflammation. He then informed the other that his biopsy had shown cancer and suggested that he make an appointment to talk with him about it later that week. Then he left.

PRACTICE POINTS: BREAKING BAD NEWS
- Make yourself, the patient, and the family comfortable.
- Find out what they know.
- Find out what they want to know.
- Tell them in words they can understand, and in small chunks.
- Let them know this is only the first of many discussions.
- Respond to their feelings.
- Ask them to summarize what you told them; ask whether they have further questions.
- Provide psychological support.

I can't remember ever being quite that callous, but I am sure there were times when I did not plan the encounter carefully enough to minimize the impact of my news on the patient or his family.

ASSEMBLING THE TEAM

How should we deliver bad news, and whom should we bring to the encounter with us? Suppose the roles were reversed: you just had a colon polyp removed. How would you want to get the pathology report? On the phone? In the office? Who would you want to have there with you? A family member? A trusted friend? Or, let's say you've just had restaging CT (computerized tomography) scans after a course of chemotherapy for ovarian cancer. Would you like the office nurse who has been giving your chemotherapy to be there when the physician tells you the results? The social worker who has been counseling you and your husband? Each of us is likely to answer in a different way.

That is why it is so important to be sure the patient has a chance to think about this before the meeting takes place. With a little planning time, patients can usually arrange to have the right people with them. Whenever we schedule tests, we can ask patients to bring someone with them when they return for the results, so that when those results are problematic, patients will have the support they need. If we know the test results are bad, we can ask the relevant office personnel to free up time to be with us when we meet with the family, both to support us and to counsel the family when we need to move on to the next patient.

In the inpatient setting, we can ask the social worker to schedule the meeting at a time convenient for everyone who needs to be there, and to include whomever has been involved in the patient's care (e.g., the primary nurse, the chaplain). Be sure to ask the social worker to find a room in which everyone can be seated comfortably, rather than allowing the family and the rest of the team to stand while you and the patient are seated.

For the conversation itself, Dr. Buckman's book contains a number of very useful, often commonsense suggestions, which I review in the sections that follow.*

MAKE YOURSELF, THE PATIENT, AND THE FAMILY COMFORTABLE

With the team, the patient, and the family waiting for you at the meeting place, take a moment before you enter. Rehearse to yourself what it is you are about to say; try to dispel any feelings of guilt (which are almost always unwarranted), take a deep breath or two, and bring your

---

*Adapted from R. Buckman, *How to Break Bad News: A Guide for Health Care Professionals,* Baltimore: Johns Hopkins University Press, 1992.

full focus onto how you can be of most help to this patient and her family.

As you begin your encounter, use body language that indicates you have all the time in the world. This I learned from my brother, a gastroenterologist in private practice and a very busy guy. When accompanying him on follow-up visits, I noticed that he stretched out in a chair near the patient's bed or chair, looking as if he were camped out for the afternoon. He asked the questions he needed to ask, including open-ended ones, let the patients ask all they wanted, examined them, and then left. None of the encounters took more than about fifteen minutes, but as we left the patients seemed satisfied with the time my brother had spent with them.

FIND OUT WHAT THEY KNOW

After you and the family are comfortably settled, with a box of tissues close by, explore what the patient understands about what is wrong. You may know what the patient has been told by the house staff or by the surgeon who did the operation, but you need to determine what the patient remembers from those discussions and whether he or she understands the implications. You might say, *"The results of your tests finally came back, and I thought I would let you know what they are and what we're going to do about them. Of course, I will be answering any questions you have. But before I begin, it would help me to know what you already know and what you think is wrong with you."*

Someone has usually told the patient that he has cancer and has explained its type, stage, and location before I, an oncologist, am asked to see him. Some of these patients, when I ask what they think is wrong with them, repeat for me what they have been told, word for word. They also seem to understand the implications of their diagnosis. Others, given the same information by their own physicians, have said, *"They told me I have a tumor. You don't think that could be cancer, do you?"* This patient either hasn't understood what he was told (and was too embarrassed to admit this to his physician) or finds the implications too overwhelming. He may be in a state of denial, unable to accept that he could possibly have cancer. The discussion you have with him will be very different from the one you can have with the first type of patient. For this second type I usually ask what he thinks a tumor is and what it means to him to have cancer. I follow his lead and try to allay any fears or correct any misconceptions that he reveals. But I also make it clear that he does have cancer and that I will be there to help him with all that is to come because of it.

Find Out What They Want to Know

Dr. Buckman counsels that we should next find out how patients want you to deliver the news and what they want to know. Dr. Diane Meier, professor of geriatrics and director of the Center to Advance Palliative Care at Mt. Sinai Medical Center, New York, suggests we try the following: *"In my experience, I have found that some patients want to know all the details each time I speak with them, while others would rather I described the big picture, leaving them free to ask for more details when they felt they needed them. In general, which would you prefer?"*

Next, having some idea of how broad or fine the strokes should be, we need to find out more about the picture we've been commissioned to paint. Miss Brown, for example, asked me how long she had to live. This sounds like a fairly straightforward question—but so, on the face of it, does a child's question, "Where do I come from?" Many parents have responded to this by launching into a discussion of the birds and the bees, only to be met with perplexed looks and the complaint, "I have to do a report for school on the city I come from. I just need to know if we come from Philadelphia or San Francisco."

Miss Brown, it turned out, had tickets for a cruise in three months, and she wanted to know whether she was likely to be able to go on that cruise. She did not want to discuss her ultimate outcome. To approach patients' or family members' questions, therefore, I usually ask them to be a little more specific about what they want to know and why they want to know it. I find that I'm more likely, that way, to answer the correct question.

Tell Them in Words They Can Understand, and in Small Chunks

Once you have a handle on the question, the next steps are similar to those you would use in any routine form of patient education. If you were explaining an operation, a colonoscopy, or the fact that someone had an ulcer and needed to take certain medications, you would use words patients could understand and, when appropriate, visual aids.

When you are breaking bad news, however, you need to divide the information into smaller chunks. After the news that she has cancer has sunk in, a patient is unlikely to remember much else from that first talk.

Some oncologists even advise giving patients an audiotape of the first meeting, which they can review later, at their leisure.

HOW TO DEAL WITH THE RESPONSE

THE ROLE OF SILENCE

At this point, I stop talking and wait for a response. As I mentioned above, patients' reactions are likely to reflect the difference between their expectations and what I have just told them. Those who have been very ill or in pain, yet have previously been told there is nothing wrong with them, may, like Miss Brown, express relief that the source of their suffering has been identified. It is, naturally, much harder for those who have had no hint about the cancer.

The first minute, until the patient or a family member says something, seems endless. But my silence is very important. Patients who have just heard bad news are numb and shocked. It can take thirty to forty seconds for the information to sink in, for patients to replay internally what you've just said, and then to voice a thought or a feeling. The longer you let the silence last, the greater is the chance that they will have the time they need to process what you've told them. You can sit there with your hands in your lap, or you can lightly touch their hand or arm. Be alert to a withdrawal of the hand or arm, as the contact may not be welcome at that time.

RESPOND TO THEIR FEELINGS

Their first response may be verbal or nonverbal. Some reply with disbelief: *"You must be mistaken. The tests must have been mixed up in the lab. I feel fine. There can't be anything wrong with me."* Others may look up at you in great pain, may cry, or be totally silent. To the mute-stricken patient, rather than ask, *"How can we help?"* I would say, *"What do you need us to do right now?"* which calls for a more limited response. A patient might reply, *"Schedule the next tests you have to do as soon as possible. I can't wait much longer to find out how far this thing has spread."* Or, *"Call my husband. He said he wanted to come with me, but I was sure everything would be fine, so I told him not to bother."*

When the patient or family member is angry, I wait out the storm. Families may express their anger at other physicians who have "missed the diagnosis," even if it was not apparent at the time of the consultation.

Patients can be angry at me, or angry at their family for making them come to the doctor, or at God for allowing this to happen. Some patients turn the anger inward. They may not seem angry right after you tell them the news, but at later visits they may appear depressed or withdrawn. Some are blaming themselves for sins of omission or commission that they feel caused the cancer or delayed its diagnosis.

I have tissues within reach for the tearful patient, and I try to offer some form of nonverbal support such as putting my hand on the patient's arm or shoulder, as I mentioned above. I speak reassuringly, make no attempt to stop the initial flow of tears, and, by making no effort to leave, indicate my willingness to be present no matter how emotional the patient becomes. The tears usually subside quickly, and I find I have established trust and a personal bond that will be helpful in what I hope will be the months and years to come.

To provide what Dr. Buckman would call an "empathic response" to a patient who is angry or crying, I would first identify the emotion, then ask questions that would help me in identifying its source, and then say something to indicate I had made the connection between the emotion and its source.

Jason, a patient with prostate cancer, seemed to be blaming himself for developing the cancer. I said to him, *"I can really feel how angry you are. What is your understanding of how you became ill?"* He responded, "Well, I smoked didn't I? And everyone knows that smoking causes cancer." I was tempted to correct Jason's misconception right away, and to reassure him. But if I contradicted him, our conversation would come to a close prematurely. Instead, I pursued the questioning, so that I could learn about all his sources of concern: *"And what else do you think contributed to your illness?"*

I didn't know what he was going to say. He might tell me he hadn't gone to the doctor for years despite his wife's multiple urgings that he do so. He might report lapses in attendance at church services, failure to eat right, drinking too much alcohol—the list could go on and on. I never know what I'm going to hear. As I listened expectantly, Jason said that he had been having an affair and was furious with himself for being unfaithful to his wife, and that his cancer was a just punishment. He finished with, *"I guess that's about it."*

I was totally floored! But I replied, *"As I understand it, you're angry at yourself, and you're angry both because you feel your smoking caused your cancer and because you had an affair, for which you feel you deserve to be pun-*

ished by getting prostate cancer. Is that right?" I settled down, as did he. I felt I could now correct his misunderstanding about the relationship between smoking and prostate cancer. But I could also, if I had the time and the comfort level to do so, begin exploring with Jason issues of forgiveness and punishment. If not, I could express my sincere concern for his pain and explore whether he might seek help from a spiritual counselor.

Tell Them the Plan

Once patients have assimilated both the news and its implications for them, have had time to react, and have shared their underlying concerns, you can move on to the plan, which usually includes further testing, referrals, or a chemotherapy regimen. I tell patients that this is only the first of many discussions, and that our whole team will continue to answer their questions and provide or arrange for the support and counseling they or their family need. I often suggest that patients record all their questions in a notebook or keep a tape recorder nearby so they won't forget to ask them at the next visit. I encourage them to include questions from family or friends who are not at the meeting, but who are likely to raise a number of additional concerns.

Ask Them to Summarize What You Told Them; Ask Whether They Have Further Questions

To bring this first encounter to a close, I usually say, *"I know we have gone over a lot of ground today. Since I may have used some technical terms that were unclear, it would help me if you would summarize for me what we've discussed."* Patients' answers, like their answers to the first questions about what they knew about their disease, provide me with important information for our next visit. Despite my best efforts, I find that some people are still unclear whether or not they have cancer. I usually just reiterate their diagnosis, tell them what tests or treatment I have scheduled, and urge them to write down any questions that occur to them during the interval until our next meeting.

Most patients understand at least their diagnosis and the need for further tests. I remind them that I am available to answer their questions and those of their family or friends and that we will be talking again later, as new information appears. While it may seem longer, these talks usually take no more than fifteen to twenty minutes, though I usually plan for a thirty-minute session.

Provide Psychological Support

Often, the first time I meet patients is after they have been told they have cancer. They are sometimes frightened, or numb, anxious to find out what will come next, or optimistic that they will be cured. Our first interview offers an excellent opportunity to begin psychological support, even during the limited time of an office visit.

We do this by expanding the routine history of the disease, adding questions that reveal how the cancer was found and explore the emotional impact of the experience. We use the questions suggested by Faulkner and Maguire (1994), British experts in communicating with patients with cancer.

PRACTICE POINTS: ASSESSMENT OF NEW PATIENT
- Medical history
- Seeking advice
- Impact of treatment
- Current state of the patient's disease and its impact
- Current psychological state
- Current mood state
- Overall level of functioning
- Other important life events

(From Faulkner and Maguire 1994)

Consider Joe Palermo, a 65-year-old man who has experienced symptoms of benign prostatic hypertrophy (BPH) for several years. Prostate specific antigen (PSA) levels were borderline during that time and are not elevated now. On routine digital rectal exam, however, Joe's internist found a nodule that on biopsy proved to be cancer. Further studies have indicated that the cancer has not spread beyond the prostate. Joe's internist referred him to Dr. Kew, the radiation oncologist, because Joe is interested in receiving radiation therapy rather than surgery.

In the course of a normal medical history, Dr. Kew would ask Joe how long he had had the symptoms of BPH, how troublesome they were, and when the nodule was discovered, and then would review the biopsy and staging studies with him. She would then explain the risks and benefits of the proposed treatment.

This typical history, however, provides Dr. Kew with only the sketchiest view of Joe as a person who has to cope with this new diagnosis and plan of treatment. She knows nothing of Joe's psychological state: how is he dealing with the diagnosis and the staging procedures? What are his fears and hopes? Does he need more intensive psychosocial support during the planned therapy? To get to know the patient better, Faulkner and Maguire (1994) suggest that in addition to the medical history we should explore a number of other areas.

SEEKING ADVICE.   After the medical history, Dr. Kew should next review with Joe his experiences as he sought advice from physicians about his cancer. She asks Joe whether he feels there were any delays in getting to the diagnosis (e.g., did he regret not having earlier studies done to evaluate his borderline PSA? Were they offered? Did he refuse them? How does he feel about refusing them?). Dr. Kew can also explore how Joe felt when his internist found the nodule, how he felt about the staging procedures, and what his concerns and hopes are now, as he anticipates the radiation treatment. What led him to the radiation therapist rather than back to the urologist who did the biopsy? Has anyone he knows ever gone through treatment for prostate cancer? What happened to them, and how does Joe feel about that?

Faulkner and Maguire suggest that, after the treatment begins, follow-up visits can be used to question more than just the physical side effects of the treatment. For example, Dr. Kew would normally question Joe about diarrhea, dysuria, skin changes, rectal pain, and fatigue, and do a complete review of systems. But in addition, consider how much more Dr. Kew will know if she also asks questions in the other areas (Faulkner and Maguire 1994, pp. 36–42).

IMPACT OF TREATMENT; CURRENT STATE OF THE PATIENT'S DISEASE AND ITS IMPACT.   Typical questions to explore the impact of Joe's treatment would be (p. 36): "*How has the treatment been affecting you? What has the impact been on your day-to-day life? Has it had any effect on your ability to continue working, and to maintain your normal social life, hobbies and interests?*" Faulkner and Maguire also recommend asking questions that explore Joe's relationship with his partner (including their sexual relationship), his mood, and his ability to concentrate. Checking in on how the patient thinks things are going can help Dr. Kew dispel Joe's misconceptions and clarify the goals of the treatment.

Dr. Kew asks Joe and his wife, Bonnie, about how he is coping. Bonnie tells her that after three weeks of daily therapy, the reality of his cancer diagnosis has just

begun to sink in, and she thinks he has been having a great deal of difficulty dealing with the feelings that have begun to emerge. Joe reports that he has developed
insomnia and a poor appetite, and he no longer looks forward to things he used to
enjoy, like playing poker with his friends.

CURRENT PSYCHOLOGICAL STATE; CURRENT MOOD STATE.   What is
wrong? Joe may have just begun to face the psychological hurdles presented to patients newly diagnosed with cancer (pp. 1–6):

1. Uncertainty about the future: Will I be cured? How do I plan if I don't
   know how much time I will have?
2. The search for meaning: How do I make sense of what I have done
   during my life? Did I leave a mark? Will I be remembered?
3. Loss of control: Is there anything I can do to increase my chance of
   cure? What if there isn't?
4. The need for openness: Who should I tell? What will they think?
5. The need for emotional support: I don't want to be a burden. Do I
   have enough support from my friends or my family?
6. The need for medical support: Can I count on my oncologist? My primary care physician? What if there's nothing more they can offer?

If these questions remain unresolved, patients can develop chronic
anxiety or depression. In fact, as I will discuss in Chapter 7, the symptoms Joe is reporting are typical manifestations of depression and are
often reversible with appropriate treatment. By including in her assessment the questions that can reveal psychological distress, Dr. Kew will
be able to refer Joe for the help he needs.

**PRACTICE POINTS: PSYCHOLOGICAL HURDLES OF THE NEWLY
DIAGNOSED CANCER PATIENT**

- Uncertainty about the future
- The search for meaning
- Loss of control
- The need for openness
- The need for emotional support
- The need for medical support

(Adapted from Faulkner and Maguire 1994)

OVERALL LEVEL OF FUNCTIONING; OTHER IMPORTANT LIFE EVENTS. Receiving radiation therapy for prostate cancer can cause a number of physical discomforts that might seriously interfere with Joe's ability to lead a normal life.

Joe began to need to defecate so frequently that at first he limited his trips away from home to places within two minutes of a restroom. A few weeks later, Bonnie says, he just stopped trying to leave home, giving up his poker group because he didn't want to explain to his friends why he wanted them to move the game permanently to his house. Bonnie is afraid that even if Joe is cured, the price he has paid will have been much too high. "What use is living if it's going to be like this?"

Dr. Kew could never have discovered Joe and Bonnie's misunderstanding about the permanence of the treatment-related changes if she hadn't explored how Joe's work was going and whether he had been keeping up with social activities. She now can offer treatment and help them make plans for when the side effects are likely to abate. Joe is less likely to be depressed if he believes he will soon return to his normal life.

Faulkner and Maguire caution, however, that the changes people report in their moods may be unrelated to their treatments. The real cause may be an unrelated problem, such as losing a job, or the serious illness or death of a close friend or relative. By pursuing the etiology of what you perceive as a significant personality or mood change, you are able to detect the true cause of the distress.

As was true for Joe, Selina Basset's response to some bad news was delayed. It didn't occur during our first encounter, but later, at home and at work. Her distress was difficult to diagnose, because her delayed response manifested as signs and symptoms that are also found with known metabolic or other complications of her malignancy.

Delayed Presentation of Psychological Distress

Selina Basset was then a 41-year-old corporate lawyer who had visited her gynecologist on a Friday for her routine yearly physical exam. Her doctor found a small (1.5 cm) lump in her right breast. His attempts to aspirate fluid from it were unsuccessful, and he therefore recommended immediate surgery. Mrs. Basset requested a consultation with a medical oncologist before agreeing to the surgery, and I was able to see her later that same day.

After examining her, I reiterated her gynecologist's concern that the mass might be cancerous and that it needed to be removed. She seemed to accept what I considered to be quite distressing news in a matter-of-fact way. She said she would arrange for the surgical consultation, and she called later to inform me that a lumpectomy was scheduled for the following Thursday, as she had important work pending that she did not want to postpone.

The following Tuesday, however, I received a call from her husband, concerned because his wife was acting strangely: *"Selina asks the same questions over and over and seems to be disorganized and distracted. What do you think is the matter?"*

I first wondered whether she could be hypercalcemic or have brain metastases, but dismissed both as unlikely. After all, her tumor was very small and as recently as four days before she'd had no other abnormal physical or laboratory findings. Also, her husband did not report any other symptoms or signs that would support these diagnoses.

It was more likely that Mrs. Basset was experiencing an acute anxiety reaction or an agitated depression. The lump in her breast, if cancer, would suddenly transform her from an independent, healthy, successful career woman into a "patient" with a possibly *fatal* condition. While she had not discussed this fear with me, her gynecologist, or her husband, it may well have precipitated her psychological distress, which would explain the behavior her husband described.

Patients like Mrs. Basset may respond to an anxiolytic agent such as Xanax (alprazolam) in the short term, but if they have not coped well with bad news in the past or do not have other sources of psychological support, they often benefit from working with a psychotherapist or a psychiatrist.

Therapists have a variety of important roles to play in helping patients and their families deal with the disease and its treatment. These roles include providing continuity of caring, being a knowledgeable advisor, and teaching valuable skills.

Therapists can provide the support a patient needs not only at the time of diagnosis but throughout the course of treatment. Many patients feel uncomfortable complaining to their physicians. They do not want to seem to be "bad" patients; they cannot risk alienating our affections. It is OK to complain to a therapist, however, who is someone with whom the patient can share disappointments and fears. The therapist can provide the continuity of caring many patients need to deal with the stresses of the disease and its treatment.

Therapists can also help a patient understand about the cancer, its treatment, or the expected range of emotional and psychological responses. And they are often more aware than are patients, their families, or their friends of how effectively physicians can manage symptoms such as pain or nausea. They can convince patients that it is safe (and important) to reveal their symptoms to us so that we can relieve them.

Finally, therapists can teach patients important skills to help them cope with cancer. Many therapists are trained in cognitive therapies such as relaxation, imaging, or hypnotic techniques that help patients deal with depression, anxiety, and pain. They can also teach patients a variety of coping strategies that will help them to reestablish a sense of control or to become more comfortable sharing that control with their physicians or their families.

Mrs. Basset benefited from the Xanax and welcomed the referral to a psychologist. She was found to have localized breast cancer, and she continued to see her therapist after the surgery and throughout the adjuvant radiation therapy. She told me that the therapist had been an important source of support and information while she was making her decision whether or not to undergo adjuvant chemohormonal therapy. Mrs. Basset said she felt freer to share with him certain concerns, rather than "bother" me, her husband, or her friends with such things. "My idea of appropriate table talk," she said, "doesn't extend to speculating about how my sex life will change if I go on chemotherapy."

HOW TO RAISE THE SUBJECT OF ADVANCE CARE PLANNING

YOU NEED TO USE THE "D" WORD

Mrs. Basset decided to take the adjuvant therapy. As she later told me, she had wanted to be sure that if the cancer ever came back, she would know that she'd done everything she could to prevent it. If she didn't take the treatments and the cancer later recurred, she thought her family would be thinking, "Why didn't Mom just tough it out? Didn't she care enough about us to fight?"

She discussed her decision not just with her family and her therapist but also with Monica Sloan, the nurse practitioner who co-practiced with her gynecologist. Monica called me later to recount their conversation. Monica's father had undergone chemotherapy for lung cancer and during the treatment, when his resistance to infection was at its lowest, had developed such a severe pneumonia that he needed to be intubated and have his breathing supported by a respirator for several days. There-fore, although this was not a usual part of her job, when Mrs. Basset told her she had decided to undergo chemotherapy Monica broached the subject of advance care planning. Monica explained what advance directives were and how a power of attorney for health care could speak for Mrs. Basset if she was unable to express her own wishes.

Monica asked Mrs. Basset what her wishes were concerning resuscitation: *"I realized she is going to be in for a rough time, so I thought I should find out what her wishes are regarding resuscitation and being maintained on life support. Mrs. Basset seems to like to be in control, so I assumed she would want us to document her preferences, in case the chemotherapy caused a life-threatening complication. But I couldn't seem to get her to give me a straight answer."*

I asked Monica what, exactly, she had asked Mrs. Basset. She replied, *"I asked her, 'Do you want everything done?' and she said, 'Of course.' So then I described the details of resuscitation and the various life-support measures, and Mrs. Basset said, 'I don't want any of that. My mother had a stroke, and our family was terribly traumatized watching her die. I don't want my own family to suffer like that.' I was confused, so I asked again, 'But you want everything done?' and she repeated 'Yes.' Mrs. Basset is usually so clear. How can she want two totally contradictory things?"*

She didn't. She simply didn't interpret Monica's questions in the same way Monica did. When asked if she wanted "everything done," Mrs. Basset probably thought she was being asked whether she wanted all possible measures taken to cure her of her cancer. What Mrs. Basset didn't understand was that she was being asked what she wanted done if she *died.* So I asked Monica, *"Did you use the 'D' word? Did you say, 'If you die, do you want us to resuscitate you? Once we have, do you understand that we will have to keep you on life support machines for days or even weeks to preserve your life?'"*

Monica seemed rather shocked with the words I used, but admitted she hadn't mentioned dying. I suggested that, rather than asking "Do you want everything done?" which has a number of interpretations, she should use the "D" word. Mrs. Basset could then focus on what she wanted done if she *died.* Even if she didn't want to be resuscitated, she might find it acceptable to use life support for a period of time to recover from a complication. If, like Monica's father, she developed pneumonia, she might let us use ventilatory support for a week or two.

When I saw Mrs. Basset, I was able to clarify her wishes. She did want everything done to cure her cancer, and she also wanted us to do whatever was necessary to *prevent* her from dying. She was even willing to allow intubation for a reversible condition. But if she died, she was *not* willing to be resuscitated, and she was not willing to have her life prolonged by extraordinary measures. Given her experiences with her mother, I was not surprised by her decision. But I was surprised by her next remark, and at the time I didn't recognize the concern from which it arose: *"I guess I won't be going to heaven, but at least I won't be putting my family through hell."*

THE PATIENT WITH SPIRITUAL CONCERNS

Years later, a Jesuit priest leading an ethics seminar explained the moral dilemma many Catholics like Mrs. Basset thought they faced if they refused to have their life maintained by artificial means: they assumed they were committing the moral equivalent of suicide and expected to be punished for this mortal sin. This hidden moral dilemma has caused many patients unnecessary anxiety.

The Catholic Church is, in fact, much more compassionate than that. In 1957, and reaffirmed in the latest Catechism in 1994, the Church expressed its understanding that people are not expected to accept extreme measures to prolong their lives. Refusing to be resuscitated or to be kept alive by artificial means is acceptable to the Church; it is not a sin and is not considered suicide. As written in the Catechism, "Discontinuing medical procedures that are burdensome, dangerous, extraordinary, or disproportionate to the expected outcome can be legitimate; it is the refusal of 'overzealous' treatment. Here one does not will to cause death; one's inability to impede it is merely accepted" (*Catechism of the Catholic Church* 1994, Subheading I, Respect for Human Life, 2278, 2279).

I wish I had known this when I was counseling Mrs. Basset. I could have answered her unasked question, eliminated the guilt she was feeling, and diminished her suffering. In fact, the teachings of Islam and of many Orthodox Jewish rabbis affirm the same principle: people with terminal illnesses are not required to endure unrelieved pain or suffering or to allow their lives to be prolonged by technological means. Some Orthodox rabbis and fundamentalist Islamic teachers, however, do not agree. Since all life is a gift from God, they reason, diminishing it by even one breath is morally unacceptable. For Buddhists, the question hinges more on the quality of the dying than of the death itself: the mind must be alert to do the work that needs to be done to prepare the soul for death and eventual rebirth. Therefore, the maintenance of life at all costs is not a priority.

WHY ADVANCE CARE PLANNING IS SO DIFFICULT FOR MANY PHYSICIANS

I was pleased that Monica had questioned Mrs. Basset about advance directives. Such discussions with people beginning intensive chemo-therapy, or even with those having far-advanced cancer, are by no means routine. Though I am now more comfortable with them, initially I had these discussions only to avoid being in the position of having an intu-bated patient look up at me accusingly and write on his Magic Slate, *"I never wanted to live like this. You told me about the other side effects of the chemotherapy, but you left this one out. Why didn't you ever ask me what I wanted?"*

WHY ARE PHYSICIANS RELUCTANT TO DISCUSS ADVANCE CARE PLANNING?

- Physicians are forced to face their own feelings about mortality.
- Physicians are loath to cause pain.
- Physicians feel guilty or are afraid of being blamed.
- Physicians perceive that death equals failure; they feel impotent.
- Physicians assume they do not need to ask: they know their pa-tients' wishes.

Luckily, that has never actually happened to me. But the question re-mains: why is it so hard to bring up the subject? What feelings do these difficult conversations evoke? What effect do they have on our sense of self? According to the literature, this reluctance to discuss advance care planning has many components, as discussed in the sections that follow.

PHYSICIANS ARE FORCED TO FACE THEIR OWN FEELINGS
ABOUT MORTALITY

Discussions about advance directives force us to ask ourselves how *we* would answer these questions, and many of us are not ready to face our own mortality. In my own case, I did not complete an advance directive or a document naming my power of attorney for health care until about ten years ago. What prompted me was the combination of frequent travels from Philadelphia to New York City, the perils of the New Jersey Turnpike, and the New York law requiring clear, written documentation of my wishes should I become incapacitated. Since making my own arrangements, however, I have noticed that it seems easier to discuss advance planning with patients.

PHYSICIANS ARE LOATH TO CAUSE PAIN

Physicians are loath to cause pain, and discussions of mortality are at the least awkward and at the worst terrifying for patients and their families. The stress on the patient and on me is something I still have to brace myself for, every time.

PHYSICIANS FEEL GUILTY OR ARE AFRAID OF BEING BLAMED

By raising the possibility that a patient might die, physicians place themselves in what seem to be two contradictory positions—on the one hand assuring people that we will make them well, and on the other reminding them that, after all, they are mortal. Patients who don't want to hear this may blame us for their vulnerability to death, and their anger at their disease may be transferred to us as the bearers of bad news. This fear of blame is one of the major impediments, Dr. Buckman says, to physicians' discussing advance directives with their patients.

Alternatively, even when patients don't blame us we may feel guilty, that it is our fault that they are at risk of dying. I would wager that many physicians share with me an experience I had when I entered medical school: we were told that one in three of us would cause someone to come to harm because we had not worked hard in medical school and didn't know enough. Our errors of commission or omission might even kill someone. It is not surprising, then, that we are reluctant to bring up the subject of death.

Dr. Jerome Groopman, who cares for many patients dying of AIDS or cancer, states in his book *The Measure of Our Days*, what I fear is a sentiment shared by many physicians: "Although I knew that Matt was going to die, that everything had been done for him that could be done, *I still felt a deep sense of failure, of guilt.* We, his doctors, had failed Matt, unable to save his young life [italics mine]" (Groopman 1997). Daniel Callahan, the director of the Hastings Center for Medical Ethics, explains that, as physicians, we are suffering from a delusion: that advances in medical technology will indefinitely postpone death. Any death, in that context, must be one for which we must accept the blame and the guilt (Callahan 1993).

PHYSICIANS PERCEIVE THAT DEATH EQUALS FAILURE; THEY FEEL IMPOTENT

Advance directive discussions may make physicians feel impotent; we are admitting that at some point there will be nothing more we can do to prolong the patient's life. During my first week as an intern, as I vividly recall, I encountered a physician who felt just this way. During sign-out rounds, the resident explained to us that one of the patients was expected to die. If that happened, the intern was to call and inform the family. When the resident left, I heard my colleague who was on call that night mutter to himself, *"No one is going to die on my shift!"* And no one did; he kept the patient alive until the next morning, when he would no longer be "responsible."

In their zeal to inspire us to study, our teachers told us that death is the enemy and that when someone dies we have lost the battle. "What patient," they implied, "would choose a losing general to lead his army?"

In my experience, however, most patients don't want any kind of general caring for them. They want someone who is knowledgeable, experienced, and confident, but who also can be approached with questions and fears. They want physicians who know their own and medicine's limitations.

In fact, many patients are disturbed by the knowledge that, in this technological age, they can be kept alive in ways that are not acceptable to them. This knowledge is one of the underlying motivations for the movement toward legalizing assisted suicide. It is unlikely, then, that patients will lose faith in us or in medicine simply because we ask them to state their preferences about being resuscitated or being kept alive by artificial means.

PHYSICIANS ASSUME THEY DO NOT NEED TO ASK; THEY KNOW THEIR PATIENTS' WISHES

Lastly, some doctors may feel the discussion is unnecessary, that they know their patients well enough to be able to act on their wishes without ever directly asking them to complete an advance directive. Studies have indicated, however, that this assumption is incorrect. In these studies, both physicians and patients' families inaccurately predicted the patient's perceived quality of life. They thought the patient would choose a much lower quality-of-life score than he or she in fact reported. Physicians and families similarly could not predict patients' wishes about treatments that would prolong life. Doctors chose for the patient what they would want for themselves, not what the patients, in separate questioning, said they preferred.

WHEN TO INITIATE THE DISCUSSION; WHAT TO SAY

Clearly, each discussion must be tailored to the needs of the patient and family in question. But there are several general principles that can aid in generating from the discussion the information you need, while maintaining the confidence of patients and their families. These are reviewed in the following sections.

DISCUSSING RESUSCITATION
The "Near Miss"

The timing of the DNR discussion depends, of course, on a number of factors. For example, in the office one morning I met two new patients: Harry Bennett, a 65-year-old man with metastatic non–small cell lung cancer, and Mabel Reeves, a 65-year-old woman coming for adjuvant therapy for breast cancer. I felt much more pressure to have the talk with Harry than I did with Mabel, because I was less worried that something would happen to her before we had a chance to explore her goals and values.

As it happened, however, I neglected to have the discussion with Harry on that visit. Before his second visit with me, he was admitted to the intensive care unit (ICU) for a post-obstructive pneumonia. Although he was not intubated, he did require noninvasive positive pressure ventilation (BiPAP). While he recovered in the hospital, I decided to discuss with Harry and his wife, Selma, his wishes regarding advance directives. I suggested, and they agreed, that he had had a "near miss." While I was hopeful that the radiation therapy would prevent a recurrence of this problem, we needed to talk about what would have happened had his respiratory status not improved. The "near miss" had made clear to both of them how near Harry was to another respiratory decompensation, and they now understood much more clearly what life in the ICU entails. Both Harry and Selma were glad to review their options with me in the aftermath of the experience. Harry put it this way: "That felt like a ride through the rapids and I was lucky to make it. I need to have a better plan if this river is going to shoot me through them again."

But how do you explain what you are offering and what the outcome is likely to be to someone who has never experienced either a resuscitation or how it feels to be in an ICU? I don't think it makes sense to list for patients all the procedures we can perform, even if we explain them in terms that patients and their families can understand. Dr. Stephen Pantilat, a hospitalist, an assistant professor of medicine at the University of California, San Francisco, and a faculty scholar of the Project on Death in America, shared with me a very useful analogy that illustrates the problems with that approach.

He asked me to imagine that I was going to buy a computer for the first time, and that I encountered two different salespeople. He asked me to decide which person was more likely to be able to help me buy the computer that would best fit my needs.

> Salesperson 1: "How much memory and RAM do you need? How many scuzzy ports? Do you use a modem or a wireless system? Is the computer going to be networked?"
>
> Salesperson 2: "What do you want to use the computer for? Do you need to use the Internet? Do you make presentations for talks and use videos or materials from other documents in the talks? Do you want to be able to check your e-mail while you are working on other projects?"

Clearly, I hope we would all resemble Salesperson 2. We, too, have specialized knowledge and experiences that our patients are unlikely to share. But advance care planning entails much more than simply determining whether patients want cardiopulmonary resuscitation (CPR) if they die. It includes what is important to patients in their lives, what makes their lives worth living, and what would be unacceptable to them. We know, as they cannot, what life on a ventilator, in a coma, or as a quadriplegic might entail, and we need to help them make choices to ensure that their lives, even if limited by illness or injury, will have quality for them.

When I start advance care planning with a patient who is going to begin chemotherapy, therefore, I explain that to be an effective advocate, I need to know the patient's values and the outcomes that are acceptable to him. I reassure him that just because I have raised the possibility of a serious complication, I am not suggesting that the treatment will not work. I might initiate the discussion by saying something like this, stopping to respond to the patient's or family's replies:

PRACTICE POINTS: DISCUSSING ADVANCE CARE PLANNING

- Initiate the discussion with the patient early in the relationship.
- Anticipate and address unasked questions.
- Find out what makes this patient's life worthwhile, as well as what would be completely unacceptable.
- Reassure the patient that having this discussion does not mean that you think the treatment will not work.
- Clarify the difference between taking measures to prevent death and taking measures to restart and sustain life once a cardiac or respiratory arrest has occurred.
- Ask specifically about the patient's wishes regarding resuscitation should he or she die, and the expectations about what life would be like after the resuscitation attempt.
- Correct unrealistic expectations and misconceptions about the process and likely sequelae of resuscitation and about the experience of being kept alive by a respirator.
- Discuss the utility and limitations of a durable power of attorney for health care, living wills, and other written advance directives for health care.
- Encourage patients who are undecided at the initial encounter to discuss the subject with you again at later visits.

Now that you will be beginning treatment, I know you are aware of the possible complications the chemotherapy can cause. As we discussed, they might even cause you to become so desperately sick for a time that you would die if we didn't use machines to do the work that your own body is unable to do. You might need to be connected by a tube in your nose or throat to a respirator to help you breathe.

Do you know anyone to whom that happened? How did it make you feel? How do you think you would cope with something like that? How would you feel about not being able to talk with us? How would you feel about being dependent on that kind of a machine, in a bed in an intensive care type of setting? Do you know anyone who was in an intensive care unit? Did you visit him? How did it make you feel?

If you needed that done to preserve your life, do you think you could live like that? For a while? For how long? Would there be something we could do to ease the experience for you, if you needed that machine to help you breathe?

I usually discuss some of the other areas involved in advance directives at another visit. If the patient is so ill or the chemotherapy so toxic that I feel I need to know the patient's wishes at this visit, however (as is the case for some patients with lymphomas or lung cancer), I continue with the discussion. Depending on the patient's answers, I say some or all of the following:

Before you go today, I was hoping you could share with me your feelings about a particularly aggressive kind of treatment, the kind you would need if, suddenly, your heart should stop beating, or you stopped breathing, or you were in a coma and couldn't eat or drink or tell us what you wanted us to do. Have you completed a living will, in which you indicate what you want us to do if you can't tell us yourself? Have you asked anyone to make these decisions for you, someone who would know what you wanted if you couldn't tell us yourself?

If the patient responds yes, I ask for a copy of the living will and record the name of the person who has the durable power of attorney for health care. If the patient does not have either of these, I resume the discussion, suggesting it would be very normal for her to begin thinking about it. I also remind her that she may have some experiences that can help her make a decision. I continue,

I know it may seem to be a strange time to be talking about this, just after we've discussed the therapy for your cancer, but that's just why we're talking about it now. I always talk about this with people before I begin treatment. Many have thought a lot about this already and want the chance to discuss it with me, but are afraid to bring it up; they often have had a relative who was kept alive for a time on machines and have formed clear views on this topic. For many others, it is the first time they've been asked to think about it. They want to take their time and discuss it with their families. Do you have any views about what you would like done?

If the patient's answer is no, then I continue:

Have you heard about CPR, or seen someone being brought back to life, perhaps on TV? Have you seen emergency-room doctors shock the heart back to life and give medications to keep its beat regular, or use a tube to feed a person, or a machine to help a person breathe, as we just discussed?

Has that happened to anyone you know? What happened? Did it make you think about what you would want if that happened to you? What did you decide? Could I help you understand more about the process? Would you like to talk a bit about how you might feel if you woke up in an ICU connected to a breathing machine and unable to talk? Should we be including [your spouse] in this discussion?

Would you like more information on how to fill out a document that would instruct us in your wishes, or one that shows how to appoint someone to make the choices for you, who would be given your power of attorney for health care?

If the reply is yes, I give the patient the standard forms and, when possible, have someone on my staff go over them with her. Another common form, "Five Wishes," is available from Aging with Dignity (P.O. Box 1661, Tallahassee, FL 32302-1661; website: www.agingwithdignity.org; the cost is $5 per copy).

If the reply to my question is no, I continue:

You know that I have every hope that the treatment will work. And it's really very unlikely that something this serious will happen. But if it does, what kind of treatments seem reasonable to you?

This approach helps patients know that they can discuss their concerns with me. I have given them some examples of situations with which they may or may not be able to identify, and they know it's important to me that they give me some guidance.

In the above scenarios, you will have recognized that I use the side effects expected from chemotherapy as a springboard for the discussion. Those of you who care for patients with equally dismal prognoses (e.g., end-stage lung disease, heart failure, cirrhosis, AIDS, or metastatic cancer), with whom it is equally important to do advance care planning, might use the seriousness of these diseases for your springboard:

Mrs. Elliot, you know we have discussed on many occasions how far advanced your lung disease is. I am glad that you feel so well today, and I plan to continue this regimen as it seems very effective. However, given the seriousness of your underlying condition, there is something important we need to discuss.

Discussing Prognosis

Studies suggest that it is especially important to ascertain the wishes of patients who have metastatic cancer. But our patients and their families can't really engage in a meaningful discussion of resuscitation and mechanical life support until they have a realistic understanding of the prognosis. Prognosis, however, is shrouded in uncertainty, and the natural tendency when confronted with uncertainty about such an important subject is to avoid the discussion altogether (Levy 1999). Further, the cultural "norms" of medicine dictate that we be optimistic rather than accurate (Christakis 1999).

We may assume that patients who want to know their prognosis will ask us about it. There are no data, however, on how often patients with cancer do ask about their prognosis. In fact, our patients are known to withhold other concerns from us because they want to be "good patients" and "fighters," not "quitters." As I will discuss in Chapter 4, they don't tell us about their unrelieved pain, and only about 15 percent of them volunteer the information that they have completed an advance directive (thereby saving us the pain of this talk, altogether!) (Lamont and Siegler 2000).

Clearly, discussing prognosis does not fit easily into a standard office visit and requires skills that our medical training, for those of us who are not family physicians, geriatricians, or psychiatrists, was unlikely to develop. Only when I began to practice palliative medicine did I learn how to run a family meeting, counsel patients in psychological distress, and help people cope with their grief and anger (Tulsky 1995; von Gunten et al. 2000). Those of us who have not been adequately prepared for these tasks may decide not to mention prognosis for fear of harming patients or family members through our lack of expertise.

It is useful, however, to have a discussion of prognosis with a patient who is in relatively good health but who you think has only months left to live. For example, studies show that patients' preferences for resuscitation are affected both by the likely outcome of treatment, especially a bad functional or cognitive outcome (Fried et al. 2002), and by their understanding of their prognosis.

The data overwhelmingly suggest that resuscitation of inpatients with cancer usually has a terrible outcome. The most optimistic result on the effect of resuscitation was in a study of patients hospitalized at MD Anderson Cancer Center. Of 244 patients who had a cardiac arrest, none of the 171 patients who had an anticipated arrest were discharged from the hospital, and only 16 of the 73 patients who had an unanticipated arrest were discharged. So of these 244 patients with cancer, only 16 (6 percent) survived to discharge. The paper did not report whether any of these patients ever returned home (Ewer et al. 2000). Other studies have suggested that although as many as 60 percent of these patients can be successfully resuscitated in the hospital, *almost no one with metastatic cancer who has a cardiac arrest goes home.* It doesn't matter whether the patient is receiving cancer-directed therapy or palliative care only—patients with metastatic cancer who suffer cardiac arrest do not do well (in fact, only 13 percent of patients with any stage of cancer who are resuscitated in a hospital are able to return home) (Faber-Langendoen 1991; Rubenfeld and Crawford 1996; Schapira et al. 1993). Sharing this information with patients is likely to help them make more informed decisions about being resuscitated, especially if their idea of what is likely to happen to them if they're resuscitated is based on what they have seen on television.

Looking at it another way, patients will elect to be resuscitated unless they think their disease is so far advanced that they have a very small chance of surviving a year. Patients who thought they had a more than 10 percent chance of surviving six months, for example, usually wanted to be resuscitated. Only patients who thought they had a less than 10 percent chance of surviving six months overwhelmingly chose comfort care and did not want to be resuscitated (Weeks et al 1998). If patients are to make rational choices in their advance care plans, we need to make clear the likely outcome of resuscitation and give patients an accurate prognosis.

When patients or their families seem unrealistic about the prognosis, I try very hard to integrate information about their prognosis into our discussion about advance directives. Patients who have been resuscitated for an uncomplicated cardiac arrhythmia in the past and have gone home with no sequelae, or who have a close relative or friend who has been resuscitated, are particularly likely to want resuscitation. It is much harder for them to understand that having metastatic cancer greatly reduces their chances of being successfully resuscitated and being able to return home from the hospital after a cardiac arrest.

You might say something like the following, stopping to deal with the patient's comments as they occur:

As we discussed before, your cancer has spread. We will be doing every-thing we can to help you maintain an active and fulfilling life for as long as possible. As we go along, you'll decide, as you always have, which treatments are worth the trouble. And I will let you know, as I always have, what the chances are that the treatment will be of benefit to you.

I will, however, need you to tell me soon how you feel about some extreme treatments, like restarting your heart should it stop or keeping you alive on breathing machines. I feel fairly confident that you or your family have thought about this a little already; you might even have discussed it among yourselves—or you may have been afraid to bring it up because you didn't want to hurt each other.

It's important for you to take into account, while you're making your de-cision, what the outcome is likely to be if we do resuscitate you. I would imag-ine that you're thinking, "Well, if I die in the hospital, of course I want to be resuscitated so that I can go back home." Unfortunately, while there is a very good chance we could restart your heart, there is really almost no chance that you would get well enough to go home. I know that seems hard to believe, but it's true, and I knew you would want to know this to help you decide.

IT IS ALSO VERY IMPORTANT to clarify patients' wishes about being intu-bated, not as part of a resuscitation but to prevent them from dying. As was true in Mrs. Basset's case, many people who do not want to be re-suscitated if they die would be willing to receive respiratory support for a time to allow them to recover from a reversible process. I therefore include a discussion such as this:

I also need to understand how you feel about being kept alive on a breath-ing machine. The treatments are very likely to decrease your resistance to in-fection, and you might develop a serious pneumonia. While you were recov-ering you might need a breathing tube and a machine called a respirator to help you breathe. You wouldn't be able to eat or to talk, but you'd be able to communicate with us in other ways. Would that be OK with you?

Because many patients are worried about having their lives pro-longed by these machines, I also add, "*I would never use a breathing ma-chine to prolong your suffering, though. If it looked as if you were so seriously ill that the respirator were no longer helping you, we would help you to die nat-urally and peacefully.*"

Even if you have not been able to discuss this with a patient before she is in an ICU, studies indicate that it is still useful to have the discussion with her there. Patients' preferences about life-sustaining treatments are likely to remain the same over time even if their general medical or psychological conditions have markedly improved.

Over half the patients I talk to about this have an answer ready the first time I ask, and the others know I'm available to talk with them further when they do decide. Many patients stop me before I get very far into the discussion, saying that if their time has come they want to be left in peace. In fact, patients seem much less reticent to discuss these issues than I had ever imagined. When I have had such conversations in the hospital with a newly referred patient, the patient in the next bed has often volunteered his own wishes about resuscitation. A number have even asked, *"Would you tell my doc for me, doc? She seems to change the subject every time I try to bring it up."*

The more I do it, the easier it gets. Nowadays, I find that I'm more comfortable asking people whether they want me to resuscitate them if they die than I am taking their sexual histories!

HOW TO DISCUSS ADVANCE CARE PLANNING WITH THE PATIENT'S FAMILY: WHAT WORKS AND WHAT DOESN'T

An even more difficult situation arises with patients on life support who have given you no advance directives indicating their wishes about resuscitation or artificial life support. You are then forced to discuss these issues with their families. The experiences I had with the families of Mr. Madison and Mr. Jordan illustrate many of the problems that arise in such situations, and the techniques for addressing them.

The Role of the Pre-Meeting

A pre-meeting was the key to resolving the dilemma of how to proceed with the care of John Madison, a patient I had cared for over several months before his admission to the ICU. A pre-meeting helped the care team come to a consensus and decide how to communicate their concerns to Mr. Madison's wife, Alana.

John Madison was a 56-year-old man with refractory progressive pancreatic cancer. He had spent six weeks recuperating from a series of infectious complications related to his chemotherapy and was stable enough for discharge to a rehabilitation facility, when he developed a pulmonary embolus and was intubated.

His wife had brought him more than a thousand miles from their home in Barbados, hoping that he was eligible for an experimental treatment. He had made her promise, however, that she would not let him die in this strange city, that she would bring him home if he got worse.

We had met the Madisons weeks before the intubation, when we were asked to help with his pain management. We had spent many hours talking with Alana. During these talks, Alana described John as the love of her life, and the man who had rescued her from terrible social and financial circumstances (the details of which she declined to share).

The ICU attending physician, Dr. Bush, and the social worker, Nancy Lopez, asked us to participate in a family meeting that was being held because Alana was distraught. John could communicate with her by writing her notes, and he repeatedly begged her to take him home. Alana was asking everyone she could find to help her locate and pay for a medical flight so John could die at home, as she had promised him. Our palliative care team asked Dr. Bush, Nancy, and John's nurses to have a short (a 15 minute) pre-meeting with us before we all met with Alana.

A pre-meeting ideally includes the attending physician, key consultants, and the social worker, nurses, and chaplain who know the family well. During this meeting, the group members review what they know about the patient's medical condition and likely prognosis, and what they know of his values and goals, either from direct communications with him or from his family. They also discuss what they know about his family's goals and values, especially those of his health proxy, and determine whether there are key differences between these values and the patient's. If there is no health proxy, they try to identify the best surrogate decision-maker for the patient.

Finally, at the pre-meeting the team members discuss their own agendas and how well or badly they match the priorities of the patient and his family. The group then determines what information is missing that the patient's family can supply. If the group members feel they know enough, they can come to a consensus on a plan of care to offer during the family meeting.

In our pre-meeting, however, it became clear that the ICU team members did not agree on what the meeting with Alana should accomplish. For us to reach a consensus, we caregivers first had to identify what each of us thought was most important to Mr. Madison's care. Nancy's priority was Alana and John's relationship and the work that needed to be done before he died. She wanted to focus on the futility of Alana's quest and on counseling her to use the time they had left discussing the things they needed to say to each other. Mr. Madison's nurses wanted most of all for the team to respect John's wishes by supporting Alana's efforts to get them home. Dr. Bush, however, was focused on his professional duty to Mr. Madison. He felt he could not send John anywhere that could not deliver care comparable to the care John was receiving in our ICU.

Before we talked this through, Nancy and the nurses had not understood why Dr. Bush did not want to send John home. They now agreed that Dr. Bush's concerns should be a main focus of the family meeting. And Dr. Bush realized that he had found the words that would convey to Alana how seriously he took his obligation to John. We all decided that Nancy would first offer her thoughts to Alana, and then Dr. Bush would explain why he needed to transfer John to a comparable facility in his home country.

We were now ready to meet with Alana. Alana listened to Nancy's concerns, but told her that their "good time" had occurred when John was recuperating; what was happening now was a nightmare. Alana repeated her request that we help her take John home by financing the plane ride and contacting the appropriate home services. It was only when Dr. Bush talked to Alana about their shared ideas of duty to Mr. Madison that Alana was finally able to understand our reluctance to send him home. *"Alana, you have very eloquently explained to us the duty you owe John. You promised you would not let him die here, and you are doing everything you can to keep that promise. But I have a duty to him, too. I cannot send him somewhere that cannot give him the level of comfort we can give him here. If you can find a physician back home who agrees to accept him for care in a local ICU, and I satisfy myself that John can get the care he needs there, I would be happy to help him get a flight home."*

For the first time since Mr. Madison was admitted to the ICU, Alana seemed to sense the team's compassion for her and her husband. She understood the concern that prompted Dr. Bush's resistance to the transfer, and agreed that she wouldn't take John home unless it could be to an ICU. The pre-planning meeting, therefore, was crucial to our successful meeting with Alana. We aligned our goals and helped Dr. Bush find the words Alana needed to hear.

While our palliative care team had known Alana and John Madison for some time before his admission to the ICU, we had never met Mr. Jordan's family. They did not even know that Mr. Jordan had cancer and had been undergoing chemotherapy treatments.

The Dilemmas Posed by an Uninformed Family

Mr. Jordan had just begun treatment for an aggressive large cell lymphoma. He was the 70-year-old patriarch of a large family, with many children, grandchildren, and great-grandchildren, but he had never let me speak with any of his family members. He said that he did not want his family to treat him any differently because of his illness, and he felt that this would inevitably occur if I spoke with his wife or anyone in his family. He had also not given clear answers to my questions about resuscitation or being maintained by artificial means. He said he would think about it and let me know at our next meeting, but by our next meeting he was intubated, suffering from neutropenic sepsis and pneumonia.

Now his family members were the only ones who might be able to help me determine what he would have wanted. These discussions are hard enough, but they are often made even more difficult by the house officers caring for the patient, who often have asked the family, *"What do you want us to do?"* That was what had happened here—when I first met the Jordans they were having an anguished family meeting with the chaplain, trying to decide what they should tell the doctors to do. After I introduced myself to the family and told them what was wrong with Mr. Jordan, I explained that the house officers had misled them. I did not need them to tell me what they wanted me to do; I needed them to tell me *"What* Mr. Jordan *would have wanted."*

"What do *you* want us to do?" not only is the wrong question, it also unnecessarily burdens the family and adds to their distress. This burden is one that physicians should more appropriately shoulder. It is our responsibility to carry out the patient's wishes, and we are in the best position to know what is in his best interest. By focusing on *what the patient would have wanted*, we maintain the ethical principles of Autonomy and Beneficence. *Autonomy* affirms that patients have an absolute right to refuse or accept any offered treatment. If we can discern their wishes, we will be acting as a *Surrogate* for them, expressing these wishes since they no longer can. *Beneficence* means that we should act in the best interest of the patient. With our knowledge of both the long-term and short-term prognoses, we are clearly in a better position than is the family to know what this best interest is. If the family can help us understand the patient's wishes, we can offer the most beneficial plan. Even when family members are not able to give us guidance, we will at least have assured them that we are the ones who will decide, and this is usually comforting.

I therefore never ask families what *they* want me to do. For a moment, let down your guard and imagine yourself in the position of a family member being asked, *"Do you want us to take your mother off the ventilator?"* Now try to answer it—experience the tremendous burden—and you will understand immediately why I avoid it. It's overwhelming, as though I just threw you a 30-pound medicine ball. You can also understand the answers that families give to house officers who ask such a question: *"I can't take the responsibility of turning off the machines"*; or *"We can't decide right now. We have to wait until [so-and-so] comes and we discuss it with [him]."*

So how can you conduct an effective family meeting? First, be sure everyone is comfortably seated in a room in which everyone can be heard. Addressing each family member in turn, ask them how they think the patient is doing and what they think the likely outcome will be. Ask them what is of most concern to them, and what questions they have. Only after you have heard from everyone should you begin to answer questions, correct misconceptions, and provide what you think are realistic goals of care.

PRACTICE POINTS FOR A FAMILY MEETING

- Hold a pre-meeting with all the patient's health care providers to establish consensus on "best choices" and identify family decision-maker(s).
- Find a site and seats for all participants.
- Ask the family to review with you how they think the patient is doing and what they see as the problems.
- Ask the family what they think is likely to happen.
- Ask the family what they hope/fear will happen.
- Let each person in the family who wishes to speak do so.
- Delineate any key differences in priorities among the patient, health proxy, and care team.
- Explain to the family what is possible and what is likely.
- Work to achieve consensus.

To begin the discussion about prolonging the patient's life using extraordinary measures, you might say:

Unfortunately, your [parent, child, spouse, sibling, etc.] never told me directly what he wanted me to do if the only way he could be kept alive was by being connected to these machines. He never even told me what to do if he died—whether I should let him be brought back to life or direct that he be left in peace. I am his physician, and carrying out his wishes is an important part of my responsibility to him, which I am happy to do. I do need your help, though, to determine what he would have wanted.

If he were sitting here with us, what do you think he would say? Did he ever let any of you know how he felt, possibly while you were all watching one of those medical TV programs like ER? Did he ever comment on relatives or friends who were resuscitated, or needed machines to keep them alive? Sometimes people say things like, "I would never want to be kept alive if I were a vegetable" or "If I go, just let me be. At least I'd have my dignity, not like [so-and-so], who was on those machines for months before he finally died."

PRACTICE POINTS: ADVANCE CARE PLANNING WITH FAMILIES

- When you don't know the patient's wishes, hold a family meeting. When it is culturally appropriate, ask them to help you determine what the patient would have wanted. Do not ask families, "What do you want me to do?"
- When you know the patient's wishes, ask the family whether the patient told them the same information. If all are in agreement, assure the family members that you will honor these wishes.
- If the family disagrees with what you know to be the stated wishes of the patient, determine whether the treatment team (including the chaplain, social worker, and nurses) feel they can help resolve the disagreement.
- If it cannot be resolved in this way, or if there is a disagreement among the treatment team members, obtain an ethics consultation.

This is the kind of conversation I had with the Jordans. The family members, unburdened and visibly relieved, turned to one another and tried to remember any comments Mr. Jordan had made that could possibly help me. Finally, one of the grandchildren said, *"Yeah, I remember when Aunt Sadie had the stroke, and Grandpa said he never wanted to be kept alive on those machines."* Many of his family echoed these sentiments, adding supporting evidence from comments they had heard him make. I was able then to be sure that I carried out his wishes.

With the help of Mr. Jordan's family, I was serving as his surrogate decisionmaker. Some patients, however, express their autonomy through their families. In these families, individuals do not make decisions in isolation; important matters are decided by family consensus, informed either by knowledgeable or powerful family members or by those thought to have the most right to guide the family. Only by carefully questioning the patient (if possible) or the family and by seeking advice from those familiar with the usual ethical norms of the culture in question—or from clergy or other, knowledgeable clinicians who have come to know the family well—will the family decision-making process reveal itself.

Of course, there are instances where a family tells me they don't care if the patient didn't want life support, they want everything done anyway. This response usually occurs early after the resuscitation, when the patient has not been on life support long and the family cannot imagine any outcome other than a quick and complete recovery.

Engaging clergy, social workers, and other counselors can often provide support for these families and help them understand that letting go is the last gift they can give the patient. If under such circumstances a family is still reluctant to allow you to honor the patient's wishes, these professionals can both support the family and help you reach a mutually agreeable plan with them.

ETHICS CONSULTATIONS

When there is conflict in the family, or between the caregivers and the family, or between caregivers (such as nurses and physicians), an ethics consultation may be needed. Many hospitals have an ethics committee that develops administrative policies in such areas as advance care directives, withholding/withdrawing life-sustaining treatment, consent from patients with limited decision-making capacity, medical futility in care at the end of life, and disclosure of adverse events. Some hospitals also have individuals specially trained in medical ethics who are able to provide consultation services to help the dissenting parties come to a consensus about the path to take.

Dr. Albert Jonsen, a pioneer in the field of bioethics, offers a very useful framework for using ethical principles to approach clinical problems (Jonsen et al. 1992). When approaching problematic cases, he suggests reviewing (1) the medical indications, (2) patient preferences, (3) quality of life, and (4) contextual features.

To obtain this information, both the medical caregivers (including all members of the medical team) and the patient and family are interviewed. An ethics consultant (who can be a physician, nurse, or nonclinician specializing in medical ethics) initially interviews the hospital caregivers to clarify the medical history and hospital course of the patient, the facts of the situation in dispute, the values that are in conflict, the medical options that are available, and the reasons for the disagreement. If the dispute is between groups of caregivers (e.g., the nursing staff versus the doctors), the consultant will interview each group separately. If the conflict is between the caregivers and the patient or family, the consultant will interview all the caregivers together.

After the caregiver interviews, the ethics consultant interviews the patient and family, including the health care proxy, first to review the history leading up to the present conflict, and then to determine what they understand to be the facts, what they feel their options are, what they hope/fear will happen, what they feel would be the patient's wishes and values as they apply to this situation, and what they believe are the reasons for the disagreement with the caregivers.

When the consultant has concluded these two meetings, he or she facilitates a meeting between the two groups to try to resolve the conflict by reaching a consensus between the two. References at the end of this chapter provide more information about ethics consultations.

SUMMARY

As this chapter illustrates, the early days after a diagnosis of a serious illness hold many challenges for patients and their clinicians. We must learn to recognize which conversations we find difficult, and why. We need to prepare ourselves to tell patients bad news and then do so, clearly and compassionately, accepting whatever reaction ensues, be it despair, anger, or silence. There is no better way to demonstrate at the outset our commitment to being there to help. As we begin to understand why physicians can be reluctant to raise the subject of advance directives, resuscitation, and prognosis, we will be better able to initiate advance care planning and to discuss a prognosis that may be very limited. Knowing patients' priorities and goals, we can honor these when the patients are no longer able to communicate their choices. When goals differ, ethics consultation teams can help broker a solution. Innovative programs that train oncology fellows in these communication skills may create practitioners who are as well prepared to conduct these discussions as they are to give chemotherapy and treat its side effects.

Bibliography

Back AL, Arnold RM, Tulsky JA, et al. 2003. Teaching communication skills to medical oncology fellows. *J Clin Oncol* 21:2433–2436.

Breitbart W, Payne D, Passik SD. 2004. Psychological and psychiatric interventions in pain control. In *Oxford Textbook of Palliative Medicine*, 3rd ed, Cherny NI, Calman K (eds). Oxford: Oxford University Press.

Buckman R. 1992. *How to Break Bad News: A Guide for Health Care Professionals*. Baltimore: Johns Hopkins University Press.

Callahan D. 1993. *The Troubled Dream of Life*. New York: Simon & Schuster.

Catechism of the Catholic Church. 1994. Part Three, Life in Christ, Section 2, Chapter 2, Article 5. Pauline, St. Paul Books and Media.

Danis M, Garrett J, Harris R, Patrick DL. 1994. Stability of choices about life-sustaining treatments. *Ann Intern Med* 120:567–573.

Emanuel LL, Danis M, Pearlman RA, Singer PA. 1995. Advance care planning as a process: structuring the discussions in practice. *J Am Geriatr Soc* 43:440–446.

Everhart MA, Pearlman RA. 1990. Stability of patient preferences regarding life-sustaining treatments. *Chest* 97:159–164.

Faulkner A, Maguire P. 1994. *Talking to Cancer Patients and Their Relatives*. Oxford: Oxford Medical Publications.

Fischer GS, Tulsky JA, Rose MR, Arnold RM. 1996. Opening the black box: an analysis of outpatient discussions about advance directives. *J Gen Intern Med* 11(suppl 1):115.

Groopman J. 1997. *The Measure of Our Days: New Beginnings at Life's End*. New York: Viking Penguin.

Hanson LC, Tulsky JA, Danis M. 1997. Can clinical interventions change care at the end of life? *Ann Intern Med* 126:381–388.

Lamont EB, Siegler M. 2000. Paradoxes in cancer patients' advance care planning. *J. Palliat Med* 3:27–35.

Lesko LM. 1997. Psychological issues. In *Principles and Practice of Oncology*, 5th ed, DeVita VT, Hellman S, Rosenberg SA (eds). Philadelphia: Lippincott-Raven.

Morrison RS, Morrison FW, Glickman DF. 1994. Physician reluctance to discuss advance directives. *Arch Intern Med* 154:2311–2318.

National Comprehensive Cancer Network (NCCN). 2003. NCCN Clinical Practice Guideline: Palliative Care (Version 1.2003). *JNCCN* 1:394–420.

Quill TE, Brody H. 1996. Physician recommendations and patient autonomy: finding a balance between physician power and patient choice. *Ann Intern Med* 125:763–769.

Responsa of Rav Moshe Feinstein, Volume 1, Care of the Critically Ill. 1996. Translated and annotated by Moshe Dovid Tendler. Hoboken, N.J.: KTAV Publishing House.

Rinpoche S. 1993. *The Tibetan Book of Living and Dying*, Gaffney P, Harvey A (eds). New York: Harper San Francisco.

Schneiderman LJ, Kaplan RM, Pearlman RA, Teetzel H. 1993. Do physicians' own preferences for life-sustaining treatment influence their perceptions of patients' preferences? *J Clin Ethics* 4:28–33.

Stone D, Patton B, Heen S. 1999. *Difficult Conversations: How to Discuss What Matters Most*. New York: Viking.

HOW PROGNOSIS AFFECTS THE DNR TALK

Christakis N. 1999. *Death Foretold: Prophecy and Prognosis in Medical Care*. Chicago: University of Chicago Press.

Ewer MS, Kish SK, Martin CG, et al. 2000. Characteristics of cardiac arrest in cancer patients as a predictor of survival after cardiopulmonary resuscitation. *Cancer* 92:1905–1912.

Faber-Langendoen K. 1991. Resuscitation of patients with metastatic cancer: is transient benefit still futile? [see comments]. *Arch Intern Med* 151:235–239.

Fried TR, Bradley EH, Towle VR, Allore H. 2002. Understanding the treatment preferences of seriously ill patients. *N Engl J Med* 346:1061–1066.

Levy MM. 1999. Making a personal relationship with death. In *Managing Death in the Intensive Care Unit*, Curtis JR, Rubenfeld GD (eds). Oxford: Oxford University Press.

Rubenfeld GD, Crawford SW. 1996. Withdrawing life support from mechanically ventilated recipients of bone marrow transplants: a case for evidence-based guidelines. *Ann Intern Med* 125:625–633.

Schapira DV, Studnicki J, Bradham DD, et al. 1993. Intensive care, survival, and expense of treating critically ill cancer patients. *JAMA* 269:783–786.

Tulsky JA, Chesny MA, Lo B. 1995. How do medical residents discuss resuscitation with patients? *J Gen Intern Med* 10:436–442.

von Gunten CF, Ferris F, Emanuel LL. 2000. Ensuring competency in end-of-life skills: communication and relational skills. *JAMA* 284:3051–3057.

Weeks JC, Cook EF, O'Day SSJ, et al. 1998. Relationship between cancer patients' predictions of prognosis and their treatment preferences [see comments]. *JAMA* 279:1709–1714.

ETHICS CONSULTATIONS

Dubler NN, Liebman CB. 2004. *Bioethics Mediation: A Guide to Shaping Shared Solutions*. New York: United Hospital Fund of New York.

Jonsen AR, Siegler M, Winslade WW. 1992. *Clinical Ethics*, 3rd ed. New York: McGraw-Hill.

Helping Patients Accept Opioid Pain Medication

ADDRESSING HIDDEN CONCERNS

As physicians, one of our hardest tasks is convincing patients to accept our advice. This is especially difficult when we want them to take medications for a disease that is not bothering them—hypertension, for example. But I have found an equally strong reluctance on the part of many patients, even those in severe pain, to accept my prescriptions for opioids.

Studies have indicated that patients, families, and physicians share a number of fears and misconceptions about opioids that contribute to these drugs being underprescribed and infrequently used. In my experience, patients and their families rarely initiate discussions of such concerns when I recommend opioids. Their *unasked* questions can prevent them from accepting the relief that is available, however. I therefore assume that patients and families have all these fears and that I need to dispel the fears if I am to have any chance of getting cooperation with a prescribed medication regimen. These hidden concerns about opioids and ways to address them are discussed in the following paragraphs.

Fear of Addiction

Some physicians continue to resist prescribing opioids to their patients with cancer pain because they mistakenly believe that the risk of addiction is between 5 and 10 percent. Data indicate that the risk is far lower, however—fewer than 2 in 10,000 cancer patients with pain will develop addiction to an opioid drug.

PATIENTS' AND CAREGIVERS' FEARS ABOUT OPIOIDS

- Fear of becoming addicted to opioids
- Fear of exhausting effective pain medication, leaving themselves with untreatable severe pain later in the course of their disease
- Misconceptions about health care providers' ability to prevent side effects
- Misunderstandings about religious teachings on the therapeutic use of opioid drugs

---

Patients taking opioids for prolonged periods *will* become *physically dependent* on them: if the drug is abruptly stopped, they will experience a withdrawal syndrome. But addiction is not simply physical dependence; patients who are *addicted* want to use the drugs for their psychological effects—they *want to "get high."* They seek drugs for the escape they provide, and in their efforts "to get out of life" they continue to use drugs even when the drugs are harming themselves or others.

Patients with pain, on the other hand, simply want "to get back into" their lives. When the pain is gone, they no longer ask for pain-relieving medication. By prescribing opioids incorrectly, however, physicians can cause patients with pain to exhibit what looks like drug-seeking behavior, a condition called *opioid pseudo-addiction.* Someone with severe pain from breast cancer metastatic to bone may exhibit such behavior, for example, if prescribed Percocet every 6 hours as needed for pain. The pain relief provided by oxycodone, the opioid in Percocet, lasts 3 to 4 hours at most, leaving the patient with 2 hours of unrelieved pain. Such a patient might appear to be "addicted" because she asks the nurse for medication "2 hours early," but she is simply in severe pain.

Most patients, rather than developing drug-seeking behavior, strongly resist taking opioids because they share the physician's concern about the risks of addiction. The Just Say No! campaign of the 1980s, together with media portrayals of people who take drugs, are powerful disincentives for patients considering the use of opioids to relieve their pain. And if a son or daughter is or has been addicted to opioids, the patient may be reluctant to accept opioids even to control excruciating pain. These patients have expressed to me their fear that if they take the medication, they will experience the same disintegration they saw in their child.

PRACTICE POINTS: OVERCOMING FEAR OF ADDICTION

- Assume that the patient or family has concerns about opioids.
- Reassure them that the patient will not become a drug addict: cite studies showing that fewer than 2 in 10,000 cancer-pain patients who take opioids become "addicts."
- Reassure the patient and family that if the source of the pain disappears, the patient will no longer wish to take the opioid.
- Tell them that addicts use drugs to get out of their lives; patients need opioids to get back into their lives.
- Draw analogies between the need for opioids and the need for other medications.

Earlier in my career, I was unaware of patients' reluctance to take opioids (and their families' uneasiness about administering them). I first became aware of this when I was faced with a patient whose pain seemed unaccountably resistant to therapy.

Opioids Don't Equal "Dope"

Mr. Pugh was a 68-year-old man with metastatic prostate cancer; his wife always accompanied him on his visits to my office. He was now bedridden by his pain. I had increased his opioid dosage several times, but the pain seemed undiminished. I was mystified until the visiting nurse called me from Mr. Pugh's home to report that none of the medication bottles had even been opened. When the nurse asked why, his wife replied, "What makes you think I would give him any of that dope!?"

Neither the patient nor his wife, of course, had ever told me of their concerns about the opioids. In fact, as I noted earlier, I have never had a patient or family member voluntarily disclose such fears when I first recommended opioid therapy. I suggest, therefore, that you proceed under the assumption that these concerns are present, even if not articulated. To break the ice, you might adopt an opening I have used successfully: *"If you take this medicine, you know, you won't start stealing TV sets."*

I usually get a laugh but, along with it, an admission of a worry that is not entirely a joke. What can follow is a valuable opportunity for a frank discussion of the source and nature of the fears of this particular family. They are usually surprised that you have "guessed" their state of mind, and your ability to understand them so well may help them listen more closely to what else you have to say. It's important to explain that the patient won't "turn into an addict"—won't begin taking drugs for fun. Citing the findings I mentioned above (that fewer than 2 in 10,000 cancer-pain patients taking opioids become addicts) will often provide additional reassurance.

Many perfectly reasonable people will have trouble understanding that taking a drug that causes physical dependence does not mean they are "addicted" to it. Addiction carries with it dramatic negative connotations (stealing that TV set!), and it is particularly important that patients taking opioids not be locked into that word *addiction*. They need not label themselves as addicts.

To help patients understand the distinction, I use as an example someone in their family who may be receiving digoxin or insulin and draw attention to the similarities by saying,

Your aunt takes insulin every day for her diabetes. If she didn't, you know how sick she would get. These opioids are as important to your health as the insulin is to hers. Yes, your body is dependent on them, just as hers is on the insulin—in the sense that neither of you can stop the medicine suddenly, or you'll get sick. But that doesn't mean you're an addict. You don't consider her "addicted" to insulin shots; you shouldn't consider yourself addicted because you need an opioid to relieve your pain.

I realize that the medications aren't really comparable and that people are dependent on opioids and on insulin in different ways, but I find that this comparison helps demystify the drugs and makes it easier for patients to imagine themselves taking them.

It is easiest to get compliance when the patient is likely to need the opioid for only a short time. In such circumstances, you can reassure the patient that you'll taper him off the drugs as soon as he doesn't need them anymore. For example, to someone receiving radiation therapy to a bone metastasis you might say, *"You are very likely to have less and less pain as the radiation treatment works. I'll follow your progress closely and decrease the medication as you find you need it less. If you don't need the opioids anymore, I'll stop them the way I do any other medication."* It seems easier for patients to preserve their self-esteem if they consider that they are taking opioids to relieve the pain "just until the treatment has time to work." Your assurance that you will wean them gradually and safely usually removes the last obstacle to their accepting your recommendation.

FEAR OF EXHAUSTING EFFECTIVE PAIN MEDICATION

Patients who resist taking opioids may be thinking, "I can stand this pain now. But what if it becomes worse later?" Their pain may be "only" moderate now, and they fear that if they take *any* opioid now they will have "used up" the strongest medication available. Perhaps you, too, have had patients say, "But if I take this now, what will be left if the pain gets worse?" And family members' past experiences may have contributed to such concerns. The mother-in-law of one of my patients had died fifteen years before from cancer, with a course marked by uninterrupted pain. Having seen her mother's suffering, this patient's wife was understandably skeptical about my ability to provide comfort for her husband as the disease progressed.

You can reassure patients and their families that many pain-relieving medications are now available that you'll be able to give them later on (I will discuss these in detail in later chapters). They can go ahead and take the recommended medicine now, knowing that if the pain becomes worse, there will always be a medication strong enough to relieve it.

Unfortunately, as you know, many patients may not be willing or able to articulate this concern to you. To anticipate and allay it for them, you might say something like: *"You cannot use up pain medicine; there's always plenty more where that came from. I've prescribed a low dose of the opioid for*

now and I can always give you more of it, or we can change to a stronger medicine later if you need one."
By thus encouraging patients to take opioids early in the course of their disease, you will be able to restore to them months or years of virtually normal, functional life. Their cancer burden is at its lowest and, because you have eliminated the pain, they will be able to work, perform most normal everyday tasks, and enjoy life. During this time they can be virtually pain-free and reassured that they have in no way diminished their chance for effective pain relief in the future.

MISCONCEPTIONS ABOUT SIDE EFFECTS

Patients may also resist taking opioids because of adverse side effects they have experienced in the past when taking a mild opioid, for example after a tooth extraction. I remember well the experience of a colleague of mine with codeine. When she was ending her intern year, her L5–S1 disk herniated—she had fallen on the ice that winter and, over the following months, had apparently lifted too many patients. At any rate, she was unable to stand and, as she was living alone at the time, was admitted to the hospital. After the first shot of morphine, which relieved her pain, she was given one or two shots of meperidine (Demerol). But upon awakening the next morning in severe pain, she was offered only codeine. She found it so profoundly nauseating that she took it as infrequently as possible. What was worse though, she said, was her realization, two weeks into her hospital course, that she hadn't had a bowel movement. She had never thought to ask for a laxative and one had never been offered. The discomfort of the eventual evacuation, exacerbated by her herniated disk, convinced her that opioids were something she'd *never* accept again.

And she is a physician. It is easy to understand why patients with similar experiences may refuse to consider opioids, even though they may be suffering from moderate to severe pain. Even the anticipation of uncontrolled constipation, nausea, or a "doped up" feeling is often unpleasant enough to prompt patients to refuse. Thus we must let patients know that we are aware of these side effects and intend to prevent as many as we can, and that we will offer treatment for those we cannot prevent. (A full discussion of the prevention of constipation and the treatment of nausea and other opioid-induced side effects is given in Chapter 5.)

CONSTIPATION.   I have found that the anticipation of constipation can be an especially serious problem in the elderly, for whom the daily bowel movement seems necessary to a sense of well-being. One of my patients, Mr. Salieri, had pain that was well controlled by 90 mg of oral sustained-release morphine twice a day. But because he could not alleviate the accompanying constipation using only "natural means" (prunes, fiber cereals), he refused to take anything stronger than ibuprofen, despite the intensity of his pain. Eventually, he agreed to take the morphine because his constipation was relieved using Senokot. He considered this an acceptable drug because he found its active ingredient, senna, in a health food store.

OTHER SIDE EFFECTS.   You can also reassure patients about the other common side effects: feeling "doped up" or sedated or having nausea. The "doped up" feeling usually goes away after the first few days of therapy. The other side effects are usually relieved by switching to another opioid, since each opioid has a different side-effect profile. Opioid-induced nightmares and hallucinations, for example, may disappear if the opioid is changed. Urge your patients to let you or your nurse know if problems persist so that you can prescribe a different agent that will relieve the pain just as well without causing the troublesome side effect (see Chapter 5).

MISCONCEPTIONS ABOUT RELIGIOUS TEACHINGS

Finally, patients and their families, and even health care professionals, may be leery about pain medicines because they have misinterpreted or are misinformed about what their religion teaches on the subjects of drugs, pain, suicide, and euthanasia. There are strictures in some religions, such as Roman Catholicism, against suicide, euthanasia, and the use of illicit drugs. Patients and their families may mistakenly think that these prohibitions apply to opioids prescribed for pain relief. They may believe that they cannot take (or give) doses of opioids that would relieve pain but might shorten life, because they would be committing suicide or assisting euthanasia.

The Church's position was stated first by Pius XII in 1957 and reiterated in the 1994 Catechism (*Catechism of the Catholic Church* 1994, Subheading I, Euthanasia, 2279):

> Even if death is thought imminent, the ordinary care owed to a sick person cannot be legitimately interrupted. The use of painkillers to alleviate the

sufferings of the dying, even at the risk of shortening their days, can be morally in conformity with human dignity if death is not willed as either an end or a means, but only foreseen and tolerated as inevitable. Palliative care is a special form of disinterested charity. As such, it should be encouraged.

This teaching is in contrast to the prohibition of the illicit use of drugs (*Catechism of the Catholic Church* 1994, Subheading II, Respect for the Dignity of Persons, 2291):

> The use *of drugs* inflicts very grave damage on human health and life. Their use, except on strictly therapeutic grounds, is a grave offense. Clandestine production of and trafficking in drugs are scandalous practices. They constitute direct co-operation in evil, since they encourage people to practices gravely contrary to the moral law.

Pain medication given or taken to relieve pain is morally acceptable to the Church, even if its use results in a shortening of life. This is the so-called doctrine of double effect. If the intent of giving the medication is to relieve pain, an unintended shortening of life is acceptable. The stricture against "use of drugs" does not apply in these situations. The physician or family member who gives medication to relieve suffering is not considered to have used drugs illicitly or to have participated in any form of euthanasia; the patient taking such medication is not considered to have committed suicide.

Physicians, nurses, and other health care providers may not be familiar with this teaching. One of the hospital nurses who cared for many of my patients attended an in-service class I was giving about pain, and when I discussed this subject she burst into tears. She told me that for more than ten years she had been giving opioid medication to terminally ill patients to relieve their suffering but had assumed each time that she was committing a mortal sin. The relief she felt was palpable. And as I have pointed out the Church's teaching on this to many Catholic patients and their families, their relief was apparent as well.

Most Orthodox Jewish opinion, as well as that of Islamic leaders, also supports this doctrine of double effect. Pain medicine can be given even at the risk of shortening life. Intent is the key in all these cases. And as one of the Islamic opinions clearly stated, "Intention is beyond the verification by the law," but according to Islam, "it cannot escape the ever watchful eye of God Who according to the Qur'an 'knows the treachery of the eyes, and all that hearts conceal'" (Qur'an 40:19). Some Muslims who need pain medication, however, will resist accepting even parenteral doses during the month of Ramadan. They may not be aware that the Qur'an relieves the sick of the burden of fasting during this month.

Eliminating these powerful misconceptions can allow Catholic, Jewish, and Muslim patients to attain the relief they need, along with the spiritual reassurance that what they and their families are doing is right. Observant Buddhists pose a more serious challenge. Their search for awareness may induce them to refuse pain medication if it interferes with the required meditation practices. Here, the suffering may affect the staff more than the patient, who accepts it as a necessary part of being alive.

OTHER TECHNIQUES TO ENHANCE COMPLIANCE

Even after you have dispelled the fears of patients and their families, answered their unasked questions, and corrected their misconceptions about opioids, you are likely to find some patients who continue to resist taking opioid medications. Many patients are discouraged from trying them because they assume the discomfort they suffer is part of their condition and cannot be improved. Others harbor hidden agendas that we must bring to light.

PRACTICE POINTS: ENHANCING COMPLIANCE

- Reassure patients that taking opioids now will not preclude their obtaining relief later, even if they develop more severe pain.
- Reassure patients that opioid-induced side effects can be managed with additional medications or by using a different opioid.
- Explain the doctrine of double effect and correct misconceptions about religious teachings on opioids.
- Help patients identify a meaningful functional goal that can be accomplished only if their pain is relieved.
- Enlist the help of family and friends to obtain a more nearly correct assessment of the patient who does not wish to distress you by admitting he is still in pain.
- Reassure patients that pain and disease severity are not related.
- Use careful questioning to uncover any guilt, denial, or anger.

Develop a Functional Goal

Unrelieved pain can be a major cause of disability for many cancer patients, but some patients incorrectly assume that their *cancer* has caused all the deterioration in their physical abilities. They feel that they have no choice but to accept their new limitations and learn to live with them, since they cannot even remember what life was like without the pain. They thus have no incentive to take pain medicine, because they think this would involve accepting side effects without gaining any meaningful benefits: "What good is it to me to be bedridden and pain-free but doped up?"

For many of these patients, however, the pain, not the cancer, is the problem. If they took opioids and their pain were relieved, they would no longer be bedridden and could function much more effectively in their families and communities. However, they have lost the ability to set goals for themselves outside some narrow limits. I suggest that you help such patients set functional goals. You might ask, *"What would you like to do that you can't now do because of the pain?"* Then, depending on the patient, suggest something like:

> *"Would you like to make breakfast for your husband?"*
> *"Would you like to take the kids to a ball game?"*
> *"Would you like to go fishing?"*
> *"Could you go to church and sit through the service?"*

Patients will often choose one of these or offer another reasonable goal. Using that goal, you can encourage them to take the pain medications by saying, "If *you take the medicines I've prescribed, you'll be able to do that—and other things you haven't been able to do for some time."* I have found this to be a very successful technique to motivate patients who really would be able to function if they were out of pain. Even some people who have felt such despair at their helplessness and inactivity that they have expressed suicidal ideas have responded to these questions by setting realistic goals and, after taking appropriate pain medications, accomplishing them. Patients who had lost the support of their spiritual community were able to regain it and the comfort it provided.

Persuade Patients to Admit They Are Having Pain

GOOD PATIENTS.   Some people simply want to be Good Patients. Despite their considerable pain, they appear brave, cheerful, and grateful during their visits with you and want to make you feel good when you see them. They are usually successful in this deception until you receive a call from the family, desperate because once again they have been up all night with the patient clearly in agony.

I believe that, on some level, these patients fear telling us that the medication we prescribed isn't working, because they are afraid we will become angry and reject them. I don't mean that they think we'll throw them out of the office, but they do feel we will be less glad to see them if they come with complaints instead of praise.

Even when the patient insists on continuing in the Good Patient role, the family can be of great help. I find it useful to include them in my initial pain-management discussions with the patient. I believe this lets family members know that I place a high priority on making the patient comfortable, and they are then more likely to tell me if the treatment regimen is not successful.

I have several patients whose families call before the patient's scheduled appointment to let me know how things are really going at home. They always insist I not tell the patient that they called, and during the patient's visit I usually can find something that "leads" me to the problem the family has identified. Patients will then often admit that a family member has urged them to mention the problem, but say, "I didn't think it was worth bothering you about." I let patients know that after the visit, I plan a follow-up call to the family to inform them of changes in the management plan. I also explain that it's really less bother if they tell me about the problems themselves, and in time some actually do.

PAIN SEVERITY DOESN'T EQUAL DISEASE SEVERITY.   Other patients are unable to admit how much pain they're actually experiencing because they fear that severe pain equals severe disease, and that the worse the pain, the sooner they are going to die. Such patients, understandably, will be afraid to admit to you how much pain they are having.

Just as you need to dispel patients' misconceptions about opioids, you may also need to anticipate this usually unstated misconception about pain. You can remind them that a very small injury in the wrong place (such as a damaged nerve or a broken bone) can cause very severe pain. This analogy may help them to understand that the severity of the pain is not related to the extent of their disease or to their prognosis. They may then be more willing to tell you honestly how much pain they are having.

Unearth Hidden Agendas

Finally, some patients seem inexplicably resistant to accepting pain medications. I have sometimes been successful in discovering their unexpressed agendas, among which I have most commonly found guilt, denial, and anger.

GUILT.   Some patients, despite our best efforts, seem to resist all attempts to relieve their pain. I have been amazed at the range of reasons for this. One Vietnam War veteran finally admitted to me, "I'd rather burn now than burn later." He never told me what it was he thought he needed to atone for, but he clearly felt that the suffering he was now experiencing would save him from an eternity of punishment after he died. A week or so after our discussion, he allowed me to prescribe medication; several weeks later he died pain-free.

The key here was to convince the patient to trust me enough to reveal his feelings. If I initially had had more insight into his distress, I could have enlisted the aid of a psychologist or chaplain to help him uncover, share, and perhaps relieve his spiritual suffering.

DENIAL.   Other patients seem to be using the pain to help them deny the extent of the disability caused by the cancer. The family of a woman who had widely metastatic breast cancer and had been bedridden for months was distraught at my seeming inability to decrease her pain. Whatever treatment we tried, the pain was always a "10" or "excruciating." When I finally asked the patient what she would do if she didn't have the pain, she told me quite seriously that she would be skiing in Vermont. Her answer told me that her complaint of pain would never cease because, if it did, denial, her main defense mechanism, would disappear. She would then have to deal with what the *cancer*, not the pain, had done to her.

Once I understood this and explained it to her family, they were able to use other measures to assess the efficacy of the pain medicines (see Chapter 4). Functional measures (was she eating? sleeping? interacting with others?) revealed that the opioids were, on some level, working. Her family began to feel comfortable using these measures to adjust the drugs and became satisfied that they were providing all the comfort they could.

ANGER.   Some patients are angry at us, or at medicine, but either do not find it acceptable to tell us or have buried their feelings so deeply that they don't realize how hostile they are. They do know they feel bad and they want us to relieve their distress. They are likely, therefore, to continue to complain of "pain" until we are able to eliminate the source of the rage.

I find that asking *"What do you think is causing the pain?"* is a good way of detecting the anger in cancer patients who complain of pain but in whom I cannot find an anatomic source. Once the cause is elucidated, it often can be eliminated.

Anger Masked by a Complaint of Pain

Mrs. Lange reported persistent abdominal pain one month after a complete resection of what was found to be a localized recurrence of colon cancer at the anastomotic site. To my surprise, in answer to my question on what she thought was causing the pain she replied, *"I think that the pain is from cancer that Dr. Shore left in there and that you're all hiding it from me. When I had my first operation, the doctor told me he 'got it all.' Now I find out he lied to me. It came back, and I had to have another operation. Why should I believe you now when you tell me that there's no cancer left?"* A frank, open discussion about her anger toward, disappointment in, and distrust of all doctors followed. At future visits we continued our discussions, and the pain complaints ceased.

Discovering the source and letting her express her hostility was more effective in relieving her distress than any opioids I might have mistakenly offered.

FOR THESE PATIENTS SUFFERING from guilt, denial, or anger, the pain served its purpose so well that, on some level, they did not want it to be relieved. Your efforts need to be directed at understanding their complicated agendas. Once you do, they may allow you to relieve much of their distress.

EDUCATING COLLEAGUES

All these concerns about giving or taking opioids are shared not only by patients and families but also by physicians and the nursing and other staff encountered by patients in the hospital, the emergency room, or other physicians' offices. Even if you are comfortable with prescribing opioids and have explained their importance to your patients and their families, your best efforts can still be undone if any member of the health care team is not "on board."

Physicians and nurse practitioners may still harbor misconceptions about their legal liability when they prescribe effective doses of opioids, even for patients with far-advanced disease. They may feel that the high doses these patients need will cause the prescriber to be investigated, prosecuted, and even disciplined. *Undertreatment* of a patient dying with cancer, however, is more likely to result in legal consequences. The U.S. Supreme Court recognized the right to maximal pain and symptom relief in *Vacco v. Quill*, which supported the use of whatever medication was needed to relieve suffering, even if there was a chance of hastening death. In 1999, Oregon's Board of Medical Examiners disciplined a physician who grossly undertreated the pain of six of his patients. In California, a suit brought by the family of a patient who was undertreated resulted in continuing medical education (CME) requirements in pain management and care at the end of life.

Staff nurses or interns, too, can unwittingly sabotage the pain management plan and the patient's trust in the physician.

How Uninformed Staff Contribute to Patient Distress

One of my saddest memories is of a patient with extensive multiple myeloma who had been admitted for an unrelated condition, biliary obstruction due to gallstones. Mr. Hines had a previous history of alcohol abuse. One of his sons had been a heroin addict, and this had severely affected Mr. Hines's entire family. It had taken me a while, but I had finally convinced Mr. Hines that to achieve his goals, he needed the 90 mg of sustained-release morphine he was taking three times a day. Prior to his hospitalization for biliary obstruction, he had been active, pain-free, and free of any significant side effects from the medication.

But when I visited him after he was settled into his hospital bed, he was a very depressed and angry man. He greeted me with, "I'm not going to take that morphine anymore, ever!" I asked him, "Why? What happened?" He replied,

> I told the intern what my usual medications were, and she said, "Isn't that an awful lot of morphine? I've never seen anyone who took that much morphine. Are you sure you really need it?" And then I heard her repeat the same thing to the nurses outside my door. They all looked in at me like I was the world's worst person. They think I'm an addict!
>
> Are they right? You made the morphine seem like any other medicine. You didn't seem to think that the dose I was taking was unusual, so it never occurred to me that it was a particularly high dose. But I don't want to go through what my son went through or shame my family. So I don't want any more of that morphine; I'd rather deal with the pain.

In one short conversation, the intern had unwittingly undone everything I had worked so hard to achieve with Mr. Hines. He felt terrible about himself and was angry at me for misleading and betraying him. Fortunately, he and I had a relationship of many years' standing. I was able to convince him that the dose he was taking was not at all unusual for someone with his condition, that I had many patients using much higher doses of opioids, and that if the intern had not yet taken care of anyone taking that dose of morphine, it was due to her lack of experience with cancer patients in pain, not to any problems in his character. I promised I would speak to the intern and the nursing staff, and he finally agreed to continue taking the morphine.

Despite the many advances in understanding and treating cancer pain, we still have a long way to go. We should not be surprised if some of our co-workers still harbor fears and misconceptions about opioids and the patients who take them. I try to be attuned to comments that reveal these underlying feelings on the part of the physicians or other staff who care for patients, and use such occurrences as opportunities to teach and to explain my position.

Years ago, I focused my efforts on the nurses who were caring for my patients while they were hospitalized. I used the rather crude device of taping a note to the front of the patient's chart, which said, "If you feel uncomfortable ordering or giving the opioid dose we recommend, please page me." This engendered a number of conversations and prompted several lectures and in-service classes on nursing units. In these sessions I tried to explore all the issues mentioned in this chapter, and asked nursing staff to share their reservations with me so that we could work to resolve them.

Now, we give house staff, attending physicians, and nurses pocket-sized, laminated copies of Table 5.5, Commonly Used Opioids: Equianalgesic Doses (see p. XXX), on the back of which is a visual analog scale and a listing of basic pain management principles. Our palliative care team has developed a pocket-sized booklet about pain management for all hospital staff. The nurses and house staff, in turn, become the teachers. And when new house staff who are uninformed about correct pain management come on service, the nurses and the knowledgeable house staff are in a position to educate them. The palliative care team remains available to back them up, but the well-informed nurses and house staff are now the vanguard of our pain management efforts.

SUMMARY

Even when we wish to relieve our patients' pain, their fears and misconceptions about opioids can prevent them from taking our advice. By addressing these issues when we first prescribe opioids, helping patients set functional goals, getting them to admit they are having pain, unearthing their hidden agendas, and educating our colleagues, we will have done our best to make it possible for patients and their families to accept the help we have to offer. By bringing house staff and nurses onto the pain management team, we increase the efficacy of our pain relief program.

Bibliography

Abrahm JL, Snyder L. 2001. Pain assessment and management. *Primary Care: Clinics in Office Practice* 28:269–297.

Calman K. 2004. Cultural and spiritual aspects of palliative medicine. In *Oxford Textbook of Palliative Medicine,* 3rd ed, Doyle D, Hanks G, Cherny N, Calman K (eds). Oxford: Oxford University Press.

Catechism of the Catholic Church. 1994. Part Three, Life in Christ, Section 2, Chapter 2, Article 5. Pauline, St. Paul Books and Media.

Kanner RM, Foley KM. 1981. Patterns of narcotic use in a cancer pain clinic. *Ann NY Acad Sci* 362:161–172.

Meisel A, Snyder L, Quill TE. 2000. Seven legal barriers to end-of-life care: myths, realities and grains of truth. *JAMA* 284:2495–2501.

Miaskowski C, Cleary J, Burney R, et al. 2005. *Guideline for the Management of Cancer Pain in Adults and Children.* APS Clinical Practice Guidelines Series, No. 3. Glenview, Ill.: American Pain Society. www.ampainsoc.org.

Rhiner M, Coluzzi PH. 1995. Family issues influencing management of cancer pain. In *Cancer Pain Management,* 2nd ed, McGuire DB, Yarbro CH, Ferrell BR (eds). Boston: Jones and Bartlett.

Vacco v. Quill, 177 S. Ct. 2293 (1997).

Von Roenn JH, Cleeland CS, Gonin R, et al. 1993. Physician attitudes and practice in cancer pain management. *Ann Intern Med* 119:121–126.

Weissman DE, Dahl JL. 1990. Attitudes about cancer pain: a survey of Wisconsin. *J Pain Symptom Manage* 5:345–349.

Approaching the End

COMPONENTS OF A "GOOD DEATH"

We cannot change the downhill course of some patients with far-advanced illnesses. We can, however, strive to provide all patients with care and comfort as they die. Marilyn Webb, in the conclusion to her book *The Good Death: The New American Search to Reshape the End of Life*, lists ten components that she has found to be present when someone died a "good death":

- Open, ongoing communication
- Preservation of the patient's decision-making power
- Sophisticated symptom control
- Limits on excessive treatment
- A focus on preserving the patient's quality of life
- Emotional support
- Financial support
- Family support
- Spiritual support
- The medical staff's not abandoning the patient even when curative treatment is no longer required

I too have found that, as in the initial days when the patient was adjusting to the diagnosis of cancer, communication is often at the heart of good patient care as death approaches. Providing family support, helping patients and families who have been abandoned by other physicians to regain a sense of trust, and limiting unnecessary treatment are also crucial. I have included these components of a good death among the issues discussed early in this chapter.

Many of the problems that occur in the terminal phases of illness are due to problems in communication—communication between you and the patient, between you and the family, and between the patient and his or her family and friends. Some of these difficulties may arise because each of us (physician, patient, family member, friend) has a different view of the stage of the patient's illness and the remaining options for care. Others are unintended consequences of family members' efforts to protect one another from depressing information. Sometimes problems occur because the true source of distress is not clearly communicated. At other times we physicians are to blame, because the words we use convey the opposite of what we feel or what we are trying to say, especially when attempting to explain why comfort care is the only remaining reasonable option. I will discuss each of these communication problems.

I also review in this chapter what for me has been a very distressing matter—a patient's request that I help him kill himself or, worse, that I end his life. I examine why patients ask this of us and suggest how we can respond—whether or not we accede to their wishes.

DEALING WITH THE CONFLICTING VIEWS OF PHYSICIAN, PATIENT, FAMILY, AND FRIENDS

Consequences of Emotional Asynchrony

My uncle John visited his neurologist because he was having difficulty speaking and right-side weakness, and he was found to have numerous brain metastases. Despite an extensive search, no primary cancer was found. He received palliative cranial irradiation, which gave some improvement. As an oncologist, I was called upon to coordinate communication from his physicians to the family.

I had explained to family and friends that Uncle John was getting appropriate care but that his chances for prolonged survival, or even survival beyond six months, were small. His general internist, medical oncologist, radiation oncologist, neurologist, and I all agreed that there was no indication for further antineoplastic treatments, that symptom management should be our goal, and that his internist was in the best position to manage this. My husband and I, visiting my uncle, had found him to be comfortable but mildly confused, and exhausted by minor exertions such as going out to eat. His main source of distress, however, was the feeling that he ought to be doing something to fight the cancer—the implication of the advice he had been getting from friends and other members of the family.

Some had suggested he go immediately to a nearby university-affiliated Cancer Center and sign up for experimental therapy. Others insisted that the N.I.H. in Bethesda, Maryland, was the only place to be. Still others sent Uncle John alternative-medicine pamphlets and catalogues, extolling "natural products" and diet regimens that were sure to be effective. Uncle John expressed to me his dismay at all this: *"I am so confused. The family and my friends keep telling me what I ought to be doing, and each one has a different idea. What do you think I should be doing?"* Although I explained to him that we could not cure his cancer or delay its recurrence, he continued to ask me repeatedly, *"But shouldn't I be doing something?"*

THE SPECTRUM OF RESPONSES TO A TERMINAL CANCER DIAGNOSIS

At first I could not understand why Uncle John was dismissing the unanimous advice of all his physicians, and I was furious at our family and his friends for supporting his "delusions." What was causing this breakdown in communication?

The answer, I later realized, could be found by analyzing our family's behavior using the framework of the emotional stages cancer patients often experience after they are told they have a terminal illness. Dr. Elizabeth Kübler-Ross first described these stages in her seminal book *On Death and Dying:* they include *denial, anger, bargaining, depression,* and *acceptance.* In this first book, Dr. Kübler-Ross cautioned that some patients do not experience all stages and that some experience them in a different order, or even simultaneously (e.g., anger and bargaining). She later expanded her conception of the emotional processes that occur as a person faces death, but this first formulation still provides a useful framework for understanding the spectrum of patients' feelings.

I began to notice that our family members and friends were going through these same emotional stages, but we were going through them at different rates. Our problems of communication arose because we almost never were in the same stage of the process at the same time. (I suspect that some physicians who care for patients with far-advanced disease also go through these stages to some degree, and a similar mismatch in stages may compromise their ability to understand patient and family goals.)

DENIAL. *(What do you mean I have cancer? I just came here for a checkup and now you tell me I'm going to die!)* My uncle was not denying that he had cancer, but he was denying the grimness of the prognosis. Despite his symptoms and debility, he simply could not accept that he might not get entirely better after radiation therapy, could not be "cured," and was likely to die.

ANGER. *(Why me?)* Anger can be directed at God, at the doctor, at the patient himself *(Why didn't I get that colonoscopy?)*, or at whoever is unlucky enough to be the one who tells the patient something he very much wants not to hear. This is what happened to my husband, Fred (not his real name). During a phone call, Uncle John repeatedly asked Fred to tell him his prognosis. So Fred finally did. *"Fred,"* Uncle John bellowed, *"What are you telling me? That I'm not going to make it to Christmas?! That's only six months away! Who died and made you king? You're not even a doctor! How dare you tell me such a thing!"* And he slammed the phone down.

We are all familiar with what is likely to happen to the "bearer of bad news," and thus I might have expected this response from my uncle. But I did not expect it from the family, too. As we soon discovered, they were also in denial—less than he was, perhaps, but more so than we were—

about Uncle John's prognosis. They were furious that we had presumed to tell him that he might die of his illness in a relatively short time. There were several suggestions that my husband was an unfeeling brute who had recklessly removed whatever hope my uncle might have had left.

Unlike the other relatives, my husband and I had already passed through the first two stages of reaction to a terminal prognosis—*denial* and *anger*—and were even past *bargaining (if he goes through all his treatments and is a good patient, the cancer will miraculously disappear)*. We were now experiencing a little *depression* and *acceptance*. Because we had accepted Uncle John's grim prognosis and had begun grieving, my husband and I were focused on making his remaining days as comfortable and rewarding as possible. The rest of the family was still in a bit of denial and were not ready to talk about such matters. They were still focused on fighting his disease and were urging him to seek treatments that might at least delay the disease's progression.

My uncle, though still not sure about his ultimate prognosis, had accepted that his tumor was unlikely to respond to any antineoplastic chemotherapy. By insisting otherwise, family members were denying him an important avenue of support. Instead of letting him share with them his daily progress in overcoming the side effects of radiation and dexamethasone, they were making him feel worse by implying that he wasn't doing everything possible to obtain a cure (or to cure himself).

THE IMPACT OF DISTANCE IN SPACE AND TIME

An additional principle was operating here, one that is probably very familiar to those of you who have taken care of patients whose immediate relatives live at some distance: the intensity of the therapy family members demand varies directly with their distance from the patient and with the length of time since their last visit.

My uncle lived in Massachusetts. His relatives in Florida, who had not seen him for several years, wanted everything done and no expense spared in prolonging his life; those who lived in Washington, D.C., demanded somewhat less intensity of diagnostic and therapeutic interventions; we, who had seen him most recently, knew hospice care was most appropriate.

Once I understood what was underlying our various positions, I was able to explain to other family members why their efforts were counterproductive and to convince them to stop hounding my uncle to seek out

a miracle cure. His anxiety decreased when they stopped raising questions that he thought had already been answered satisfactorily. He
sought psychological counseling to help him deal with his overwhelming situation and focused on the remaining goals he wished to achieve
before he died.

ISOLATION: AN UNINTENDED CONSEQUENCE OF PROTECTION
    As it becomes clearer that the final months are approaching, patients
and their families often seek to protect each other from the impending
loss.

The Case of the Disappearing Walls

One morning I had to tell John Babar, a patient with colon cancer and extensive
metastases to his liver, that the chemotherapy no longer appeared to be working—
the metastases in his liver had become larger. I added that there were no other therapies that were likely to stop the tumor from growing and I felt he was likely to die
within the next few months. John said that he was not really surprised, because he
had been feeling weaker and had almost no appetite. He said he was OK with the
news, but asked me not to share this information with his family.

Similarly, when I have had to inform a family of bad news before I've
been able to talk with the patient, some have asked me not to share the
information with the patient, going so far as threatening to sue me if I
did. Whether or not it is understood as such, in both types of situations
the underlying motivation is to protect the loved one(s). Patients and
families are often unaware of this protective instinct; they are worried
that if the truth were known, either the family would decompensate
from grief or the patient would "give up" and die precipitously.

Rather than betray John's trust, I tried to help him understand that he would be
hurting his wife and children more by keeping the grim prognosis from them than
by telling them. I probably said something along the following lines:

> I realize that you want your wife and children to be spared the pain that
> you're now feeling. And I can certainly understand that impulse. But your
> family is pretty smart and must have a sense of what has been going on. Your
> weight loss, your increased pain, and your profound weakness are hard to ig-
> nore. But by pretending they're not happening, you make it impossible for your

family to talk with you about what they're feeling. They are unlikely to initiate the conversation because they want to protect your feelings as much as you want to protect theirs.

By shielding them, you are isolating them from you, leaving them to face their fears and grief alone. They want to comfort you, to help you set and reach goals for the time you have left. There may be things they want to say to you, and you to them, that have been hard to say before but would be easier to say now.

When you don't talk to them about something as important as the fact that you're dying, it's as though you are building a room around them without doors or windows. But when you tell them how serious things are, you are letting them know that it's OK to talk with you about it. You create a door in one of the walls through which they can come out and join you. Then, instead of being isolated from your family, you can share your love and concern and can comfort each other.

John thought over what I'd said, then asked me to be present when he shared the information with his family, who were waiting outside my office. He said that he hadn't wanted me to tell them because, somehow, if he didn't talk about it, nothing would change. He didn't want his family feeling sorry for him, treating him differently, or being sad because he was dying. But he now realized that they probably did know that his illness had gotten much worse, and he welcomed the chance to get everything out into the open. Before I let in his wife and children, he joked, *"Go ahead and open the door, doc. I'm ready to blow down all four of those lousy walls!"*

AVOIDING PATIENT ABANDONMENT

Sometimes a physician can be the source of unnecessary distress to a patient with far-advanced cancer. I heard a very sad example of this from a colleague of mine who is a general internist.

Abandonment

Several years earlier, the internist had detected a prostate nodule during a routine examination of one of his patients, Mr. Smith, and had referred him to a urologist for evaluation. The urologist had confirmed the diagnosis of prostate cancer, performed appropriate surgery, and administered monthly hormonal therapy. My friend did not see Mr. Smith during this time, but several days before our conversation Mr. Smith and his wife had reappeared in my friend's office.

Mr. Smith was not in pain, but both he and his wife appeared very depressed. On further questioning, it became clear that the circumstances of the referral were partially responsible. *"Mr. Smith, your last bone scan showed progressive disease,"* the urologist had told them. *"I'm sorry, but there's nothing more I can do for you. I think it would be better if, in the future, you went to your internist for care."*

Unfortunately, this is not an uncommon story. A patient participates in numerous therapeutic trials at a university center, for example, but is "sent back" to his community physician when he is no longer eligible for any new protocols. Patients sometimes came to me at the Veterans Administration hospital when their insurance would not pay for more therapy—sometimes in the middle of a series of chemotherapy treatments.

Even if a subspecialist would like to continue to care for a patient, this may not be possible in today's managed care environment. If Mr. Smith had been enrolled in a managed care plan, when his disease reached the stage at which no specific anticancer therapies were indicated he might have been forced to leave the care of his urologist. And, unless his internist were one of the plan's approved physicians, Mr. Smith might not have been able to return to his care but instead might have been assigned to a new primary care physician.

The Smiths had been crushed by their last visit to the urologist: not only was the cancer progressing but there was "nothing more to be done." The physician they had trusted no longer even wanted to see them. By the time they saw my friend, they were virtually in despair.

My friend reassured them that he was delighted to resume Mr. Smith's care and that there was a great deal he could do for them. He suggested that while the urologist was an expert in the aggressive treatment of the cancer, he, their internist, could offer therapy that was just as aggressive to control any cancer-related symptoms that arose at this stage of the disease.

He also encouraged them to tell him more about how they felt when they were asked to change physicians. The Smiths admitted that they felt abandoned, worthless, and hopeless. Under the same circumstances, other patients might reveal similar signs or symptoms of anxiety or depression. If these are severe, a referral to a psychologist, psychiatrist, pastoral counselor, or social worker with psychological training may be needed.

It may take several months, but you will most likely be able to reestablish the hope and trust of patients like the Smiths. By continuing to show sensitivity to their feelings and by meticulous attention to their medical as well as psychosocial and spiritual concerns, you can help them regain feelings of worth and hope and can demonstrate the array of effective therapies remaining for them.

PRIORITIZED SYMPTOM LISTS

"I know what the therapeutic goals are for my patients with diabetes or heart failure, but how do I get a handle on managing the symptoms of patients who have widespread cancer?"

When you assume the care of patients with advanced cancer, you may find yourself wondering where to concentrate your efforts. Patients and their families may come with a seemingly insurmountable symptom list, including physical, social, spiritual, and emotional problems. Dr. Russell Portenoy (currently professor of neurology at Albert Einstein College of Medicine and chairman of the Department of Pain Medicine and Palliative Care at Beth Israel Medical Center in New York) and other members of the Pain and Palliative Care Service at Memorial Sloan-Kettering Cancer Center taught me how to prioritize these complaints.

Physicians, families, and patients first determine which symptoms are most troublesome and which are likely to respond to therapy, and which, if any, aggressive diagnostic evaluations and therapies the patient is still willing to accept. They use this information to rank the problems in order of both import to the patient and ease of reversal (Portenoy 1993). Using this "prioritized symptom list" as a guide, your efforts can be focused on controlling the most distressing and the most reversible problems.

THE PATIENT'S LIST

As Mr. Smith's prostate cancer progressed, his symptom list included:

- Pain
- Dry mouth
- Constipation
- Weakness

My friend (his internist) reassured Mr. Smith that his pain could be relieved to a degree that would be satisfactory to him. As later chapters will show, with appropriate therapies you can expect to relieve the pain of 90 percent of your patients with cancer. Constipation, whether due to hypercalcemia, inactivity, or opioids, is even more likely to be entirely relieved. The mouth dryness will lessen if the patient discontinues medications with anticholinergic properties (such as Benadryl) or adds agents that stimulate saliva production—pilocarpine or sour candies, for instance. (Later chapters provide more details on the therapies that are effective for these complaints.) Unless it is caused by anemia, however, the weakness is likely to be more difficult to reverse.

In that case, what can be done? I'd tell Mr. Smith that I was confident we could treat the first three symptoms successfully, but I'd admit that his weakness was less likely to be reversible. My patients usually appreciate such frankness and are often willing to redirect their energy toward ameliorating symptoms that are likely to respond to therapy.

THE FAMILY'S LIST

The family's list is rarely as straightforward as the patient's. Underlying the problems they report are the hidden concerns and unasked questions that are usually equally troubling and even harder to address. One family with such concerns was the Hermans.

Unspoken Family Expectations

Mr. Herman was a 65-year-old man whose metastatic lung cancer had progressed despite therapy. He had the same complaints as Mr. Smith (pain, dry mouth, constipation, weakness), but he seemed very satisfied with the treatment regimen I had instituted. I looked forward to his weekly visits. But at one visit, his wife and daughters accompanied him and they were by no means pleased with his progress. The daughters detailed their concerns:

> Dad is not eating enough and is spending most of his day in bed because he's so weak. We don't understand why you haven't given him something to increase his appetite, or maybe put a feeding tube in his stomach. If he got more food, we're sure he'd get stronger and feel much better. Also, Mom tells us that he keeps her up half the night, helping him to the bathroom or worrying that he needs something as he tosses and turns. She thinks this means he's still in pain, though he's taking the medicine you gave him.
>
> We know there's nothing that will stop the cancer, but he lies around in bed all day. We bring him his favorite foods, but he only picks at them. Can't you do something?

As I listened, I mentally created what you might call "the family's priority list."

THE PATIENT'S LIST	THE FAMILY'S LIST
• Pain	• Weakness
• Dry mouth	• Lack of appetite
• Constipation	• Sleeplessness
• Weakness	• Pain

As you can see, the family's priority list differs significantly from Mr. Herman's. Pain and weakness make it onto the list, but their order of importance is reversed. Mr. Herman's lack of activity was not troublesome to him, but it was severely distressing to his family, as was his sleeplessness. He had *no* complaints of hunger or thirst, and yet his family was asking me to put a feeding tube in him. How was I to meet his family's needs without subjecting Mr. Herman to unnecessary procedures or medications?

The key was to understand the hidden concerns that led to such disparate priority lists. What were the underlying causes of the family's distress? Dr. J. Andrew Billings's *Outpatient Management of Advanced Cancer* offers useful answers in its discussion of the concept of *attribution*—what meaning the family attributes to the patient's actions, rather than what the patient's actions actually mean. Mr. Herman did not eat because he wasn't hungry, but his family was attributing his failure to eat to a rejection of the food they prepared and, by extension, a rejection of the people preparing it. This same reaction manifests in families in which children have made food choices that differ from those of their parents. Meat-eating parents of vegetarian children are often outraged at their offsprings' choice of diet. Why? Not because the diet they have chosen is unhealthy but because, in rejecting their parents' food choices, the children are rejecting their parents and their values.

Mr. Herman is simply not hungry—but his family feels rejected and left out. They also attribute his failure to eat to his "giving up." It feels to them like the first step toward the eventual abandonment his death will bring. They want me to prevent or at least delay this. His staying in bed only serves to reinforce their conviction that he is giving up or, in other words, that he is leaving them before they're ready for him to go. And they can't bear that.

Once I understood these hidden concerns I could address them, rather than just deal with the requests themselves:

I know it must hurt when Mr. Herman doesn't eat much of the foods you prepare especially for him. But as he's told you, he's really not hungry or thirsty. It's very common for people who have as much cancer as your dad does not to feel hungry or thirsty, and to get enjoyment from much less food than we need. But rejecting your food doesn't mean he's rejecting you—he loves you and wants to be with you as long as he can. He is getting weaker, but that is because his cancer is getting worse. Putting a feeding tube in him won't make him live any longer, and it's likely to make him less comfortable in the time he has left. He can already eat anything he wants, and even though he doesn't eat a lot of what you bring him, knowing you make or bring anything he asks for really makes him feel loved and special.

To families for whom "giving up" seems to be an important issue, I might also say:

I know it must seem as if he's giving up—as if he's leaving you—and that hurts, too. But he's fought this cancer a long time and he's tired of fighting now. He loves all of you very much, and that hasn't changed just because he can't fight anymore. Let's all concentrate on helping him have everything he wants and on helping him be as comfortable as possible for as long as he has left.

In my experience, this difference between patient and family priority lists is the rule rather than the exception. Thus it is common for me to have discussions similar to those described above. Almost always during such a talk, family members begin to acknowledge their feelings and to overcome their denial of the seriousness of the patient's condition. Requests for medications to increase appetite or for placement of a feeding tube disappear, as does the need to call in the hospital Ethics Committee.

It would have been simpler for me to accede to the Herman family's requests, but to do so would have been a disservice to Mr. Herman—and to his family as well. I would not have discovered or helped them deal with their feelings of rejection and abandonment. Whether or not they realized they had these feelings, their final days with Mr. Herman might have been marred by their unspoken anger, and their grieving after his death would have been unnecessarily complicated by this anger as well. Uncovering and thereby eliminating these feelings optimized family members' interactions with him in his final days and improved their ability to deal with his eventual death.

THE PHYSICIAN'S LIST

ERRORS OF COMMISSION.   As physicians we are not immune to creating priority lists that differ from both the patient's and the family's. We have had experiences that make us feel we must offer certain treatments to patients, whether or not they express a need for them. This became clear to me when I was working with a surgical chief resident who had admitted one of my patients.

Misdirected Efforts

Mr. Jackson had colon cancer that was metastatic to his peritoneum and liver. He had been admitted for a possible small-bowel obstruction. The obstruction responded to conservative measures, but Mr. Jackson had to remain in the hospital while awaiting placement in a nursing home.

The surgeon complained to me about Mr. Jackson's poor oral intake. I explained to him that the patient told me he was comfortable since the obstruction had resolved and that he was eating all he wanted. To my surprise, however, when I returned three days later from a conference, Mr. Jackson had a feeding tube in place.

I sought out the surgical resident and asked why, despite my express wishes to the contrary, he had placed a feeding tube in Mr. Jackson. At first he reiterated his concerns about Mr. Jackson's poor oral intake, but finally he explained his real reason. It seems that his own grandfather was dying of esophageal cancer and was unable to swallow anything. The surgeon's father was therefore delivering medications via suppository, which the surgeon found extremely degrading. He told me vehemently, *"No other family is going to have to go through what my father is going through!"*

I gently reminded him that my patient had a totally patent esophagus and could swallow perfectly well—he just had no appetite. The surgeon rather sheepishly admitted that Mr. Jackson hadn't needed the tube and that he didn't realize how much his own family situation had clouded his judgment. He promised to try harder in the future to treat the patient's needs rather than his own.

ERRORS OF OMISSION. In addition to errors of commission (such as inserting an unnecessary feeding tube), our own needs can also lead us to equally serious errors of omission. In Chapter 1, for example, I reviewed the barriers that prevent us from discussing advance directives with patients with far-advanced disease. It is even harder for many of us to participate in the emotionally intense and often draining care of patients who are in their final months.

Rachel Naomi Remen, M.D., associate clinical professor of family and community medicine at the University of California, San Francisco, teaches undergraduates, graduates, and practicing physicians about the emotional, psychological, and spiritual aspects of care of the dying. She notes that our problems in this area may arise from our lack of experience in recovering from our own losses. We are not often shown how to process feelings associated with loss and are encouraged to develop defenses designed to deflect them. Rarely are such shields effective; more often, we succeed only in repressing painful feelings. These feelings then become even more powerful, evading our consciousness, resisting cognitive understanding, and yet directing our behavior. We risk becoming blind to the needs of our patients because we cannot risk opening a wound of our own that we do not know how to heal.

Dr. Remen's writings, workshops, and courses help physicians experience the consequences of losses in their own lives and teach them how to heal themselves. They learn to let go of what is past, to feel the pain it caused, and then to emerge safely, healed, on the other side. Physicians who have gone through such experiences are more likely to be sensitive to the needs of their dying patients. They understand that they need not have guilt or shame at death's approach, and they truly understand that while they can't always cure, they can always help.

Eric Cassell, in *The Nature of Suffering and the Goals of Medicine*, offers additional insights into the factors that prevent physicians from appreciating the needs of dying patients. The initial obstacles appear during medical school, where we learn what he calls "The promise of science: to know the disease is to know the illness and its treatment" (p. 20). He notes that "many doctors—perhaps most people—still believe that different persons with the same disease will have the same sickness" (p. x). But a disease such as pneumonia, he explains, can cause very different illnesses in different people. Moreover, science is value-free and objective, but doctors are in the business of treating *people*, who are value-laden and, by their very nature, subjective. A sick person, he says, is the subject not the object of care. There is no population for whom this is more true than the dying.

But how are we to know our patients' values? We no longer have the luxury of longitudinal relationships with them. In the past, we came to know their values through the choices they made as we treated their various acute medical problems or guided them through a chronic illness. Are they risk-takers? Is quality of life of paramount importance, or quantity? How were treatment-related side effects tolerated? Did incapacity affect their sense of self-worth? And so on.

This knowledge is invaluable if we seek to understand how best to serve our dying patients and their families. We must elicit the information doctors formerly obtained by experience through careful questioning of patients about the goals they wish to achieve, and we must take care not simply to substitute our values for theirs.

MOVING FORWARD TO "COMFORT CARE"

MAKING THE TRANSITION

There comes a time when the burdens of antineoplastic treatment begin to outweigh the benefits. Even when the treatment itself has few side effects, the frequent trips for therapy, and the constant monitoring of blood counts and renal and hepatic function, become a drain on precious energy reserves. How can patients and their physicians make the transition to care without chemotherapy and avoid risking their relationship? Sara Bloom's story is illustrative of the dilemma.

Sara was a 53-year-old widow with a Ph.D. in psychology. She had been diagnosed with colon cancer five years before, received adjuvant chemotherapy, and for the last three years had received treatment for metastatic colon cancer. Her tumor had slowly progressed despite a series of chemotherapy agents, and she was now on a regimen that required weekly infusions and was complicated by intermittent diarrhea and mouth sores. She needed monthly taps of her ascites, and her fatigue was increasing despite erythropoietin and red blood cell transfusions about every six weeks. Sara was quite sensitive to the cognitive effects of the opioids she needed for pain control. Dr. Olinsky, her oncologist, asked us to work with Sara to identify a regimen that would be less sedating. Sara had three adult children, one of whom always accompanied her to her office visits.

During a follow-up visit with all of us, Dr. Olinsky told Sara that her recent CT scan showed slight progression and added that, as Sara knew, her ascites now needed to be tapped every two weeks to control the discomfort it caused. Dr. Olinsky added that he thought Sara should stop her current therapy and take a break for a while to "regain her strength," after which they could consider adding something new. Sara was very upset. She angrily accused Dr. Olinsky of abandoning her now that she was no longer eligible for experimental therapy trials. She directed her daughter to wheel her "out of here," and, glaring at Dr. Olinsky and me, said, *"What do you all expect me to do now . . . just sit by the window waiting to die?"*

The work of Schou and Hewison (1999) can help us understand Sara's outburst. These sociologists have studied patients receiving radiation therapy, and their families. The families were negotiating the care systems for the first time, and Schou and Hewison tried to determine which elements of the experience contributed to or detracted from the patients' quality of life. Their insights are equally applicable to patients like Sara who are undergoing chemotherapy regimens.

The demands of chemotherapy tend to isolate patients and their families, and to focus all their hopes on disease remission. They may have forgotten how to hope for anything else. Before they began treatment, of course, patients usually had a variety of plans for the future that filled their lives. Schou and Hewison suggest we think in terms of calendars by which patients and families run their lives: the *sociocultural calendar*, which includes holidays like Thanksgiving, Christmas, and Passover; the *personal and private calendar*, which includes birthdays, anniversaries, weddings, and graduations; and the *life calendar*, with church, soccer practice, and play dates. In addition to these events of daily living the life calendar also includes plans for achieving goals in the realms of work and relationships.

Once chemotherapy treatment starts, they argue, all these calendars are superseded by the *illness calendar* and the *treatment calendar*. The illness calendar begins during diagnosis and continues as long as the patient requires medical check-ups. Of more immediate concern to patients and families, however, are the treatment calendars which they create each time they begin a new therapy. Patients and their families vest the current treatment calendar with the magical power to bring about a cure. Any disruption in that calendar is therefore very distressing: they strive to complete the treatments "on time" so that all will be well. When white blood cell or platelet counts are too low, patients see the nutritionist and ask what they can do to "get back on schedule." Oncologists may know that the dates are not so important for most treatment regimens, but patients do not know this, and they rarely ask to delay a treatment in order to feel better for an important event. For example, offers to delay chemotherapy until after Thanksgiving are often met by patients with a puzzled refusal. It is as though the doctor were thoughtlessly jeopardizing the patient's future.

Dr. Olinsky and his team needed a plan for when they resumed Sara's chemotherapy. To prevent a recurrence of her feeling of abandonment, they needed to encourage her to reintegrate into her daily life the activities that were meaningful before treatment began. Sara and her family could work with his team to schedule treatment sessions to accommodate important family celebrations or holidays. When he reinitiates treatment, Dr. Olinsky should reassure Sara and her children that minor alterations in the schedule will not affect the efficacy of the treatment. In this way, Dr. Olinsky will be able to help Sara rebuild her personal calendar, and as that calendar fills up, the importance of the treatment calendar is likely to fade.

In the meantime, we encouraged Sara to use the energy she has during this break to think about which important events she would like to be a part of, and how to create her legacy. Some patients hope they can participate in a child's graduation, or be present for the birth of a grandchild. For Sara, the event was her daughter's wedding, planned for four months hence, although the odds were that she would not survive that long. We therefore urged Sara to make use of her time before the next treatment started to ensure she would have some presence at the wedding, in case it could not be the presence she wanted. We helped her children make videotapes with her, including one in which she narrated the family scrapbook as part of her wedding gift.

We suggest that our patients with young children or grandchildren consider writing letters to them for events far into the future, or create or purchase gifts that will embody their love and ensure that they will be there in spirit. For patients who assure us they will be there in person, we reply that if all goes as they hope, the children will simply have extra gifts to enjoy, knowing they were in the patient's thoughts even when things looked darkest.

As disease progresses despite ongoing treatment, patients who, like Sara, have begun to reengage in non-treatment-related activities and have developed a broader relationship with their oncology team are more likely to understand that, later, the oncologist is not abandoning them when he says that the burden of another therapy is much greater than the potential benefit. When Dr. Olinsky next proposed that chemotherapy be discontinued, Sara would be less likely to complain that stopping treatment was "waiting around to die," because she had found other activities to fill her days.

This shift from chemotherapy or other antineoplastic treatment to comfort care is the last important hurdle as you and your patient approach her death. Discussions about this shift often take place when the patient is hospitalized, when it is clear that further therapy directed at the cancer, an underlying infection, or anything other than comfort is no longer appropriate. House officers usually are unsure of how to approach the family with their concerns about the appropriate level of care, and they can benefit from the guidance of a more experienced physician.

Physicians do best when they express themselves by using words that convey concern rather than words that imply a lack of concern. Physicians want to provide *comfort* and *care,* yet they may speak only in terms of *withdrawing* care. Their conversations with patients and their families seem to focus on what they don't want to do rather than on what they do want to do.

Phrases such as *"We want to stop the antibiotics and blood transfusions"* and *"We won't be doing any more tests"* may lead the family to conclude erroneously that *all* care is going to be stopped. Families can easily focus on the *stop* part of the message and respond, *"But we want everything done. How can you deny our father the care that he's entitled to?"*

Substituting phrases such as the following conveys a more accurate idea of caring and support and enhances the likelihood that the family will agree that "comfort care" is best for the patient: *"We want to care for your father as you would at home if you had all the help we do here. We'll do all we can to make sure he is comfortable, and we'll only do things that will make him feel better."*

It is also important, before proceeding, to evaluate the burdens and benefits of each diagnostic test and of each treatment. The burden/benefit ratio will vary depending on the patient's goals and values, her mental and physical condition, whether the problem is likely to be reversible, and how far the underlying disease has advanced.

As you would expect, these burden/benefit dilemmas become more frequent as the disease progresses. For some patients with shortness of breath from a pleural effusion, a chest tube is the answer. For others,

---

PRACTICE POINTS: MOVING TO COMFORT CARE

- Convey concern.
- Reassure the patient and family that you will do everything possible to keep the patient comfortable.
- Consult with the patient and family to determine the burden/benefit ratio of each test and treatment.
- Work with them to tailor the diagnostic and treatment plan toward achieving and maintaining an acceptable quality of life.
- Explore the patient's and family's religious beliefs about the significance of accepting comfort care.
- Reassure the patient and family that you will not abandon them.
- Be open to discussions of psychological, financial, spiritual, and existential concerns.
- Readily refer patients and their families to hospice or to individual professionals who can address these concerns.

---

oxygen and morphine given at home provide more appropriate palliation. Two patients, one with newly diagnosed lung cancer and one bedridden with widely metastatic, refractory breast cancer, might have the same cancerous invasion and pathologic fracture of the T10 vertebra, without spinal cord compression. Neither has been irradiated in that area and thus both are candidates for radiation therapy. For the patient who has no other complications from lung cancer and has an active life and no other sources of pain or disability, the choice is clear—the spinal metastasis should be irradiated to prevent the spinal cord compression that is otherwise likely to follow. But for the patient riddled with multiple painful bone metastases from refractory breast cancer, pain medication alone may be preferable.

How do we know which therapy is appropriate? We must review the overall condition of the patient as dispassionately as we can and, whenever possible, make the patient an active participant in the discussion. We will then be most likely to tailor all evaluations and treatments to achieve a quality of life that is acceptable to the patient.

IMPACT OF RELIGIOUS VIEWS

An exploration into the patient's religious beliefs is an important prelude to suggesting that the goals be shifted to those of comfort care.

Sometimes you will discover a deep faith in a loving God who is expected to "take me home." These patients are often happy to accept symptomatic care. Others, however, hold tenets that make the transition almost impossible. Some patients, for example, feel that their religion prohibits them from accepting any course of treatment that might shorten their life. As I reviewed in Chapters 1 and 2, most Christian, Jewish, and Islamic teachings support the right of the patient to refuse futile and excessively burdensome treatments and to accept pain relief even if they risk an earlier death. But some Orthodox Jewish rabbis and some Evangelical or Pentecostal Christian sects regard all God-given life as sacred, and nothing that would diminish it by even a moment is acceptable. Patients of those faiths might feel that accepting comfort care is tantamount to admitting they no longer have faith in God. Should this be the case, it may be helpful to confer with the patient, the family, and their spiritual leader to clarify the acceptable goals of care. In the worst case, if you do not feel you can abide by a patient's wishes, you may have to identify another physician who can.

A patient's beliefs about the nature of an afterlife and the effects of one's past activities on it can also enhance or inhibit the acceptance of death, and consequently can affect the patient's ability to accept comfort measures. Religious Christians or Muslims who expect to be judged and sent to heaven or hell based on their actions, or Buddhists, who believe that the sum of the worth of their deeds (karma) will determine the nature of their reincarnation, may fear death if they judge themselves to have led a life that will be found morally wanting. They will seek any treatment to defer a death that is terrifying to them. In Chapter 4 you will find questions that can help in determining whether patients have unresolved, distressing, existential or spiritual concerns that prevent them from accepting the reality of their medical situation.

READDRESSING RESUSCITATION

I work with many patients who have far-advanced disease but choose to be resuscitated when they die, despite even their oncologist's explanations, in advance, that they will end their days in an ICU. As you might expect, the concerns that lead younger patients (especially young parents) to refuse to name a health proxy or consider DNR status usually differ significantly from those of older patients. For some patients, the struggle that prevents their consideration of an advance care plan manifests as daytime anxiety or insomnia. For others, the barrier lies in gaining an understanding of the true nature of the miracle they are waiting for.

YOUNG PARENTS.   Young adult patients (35 years old or younger) are often just beginning to have their hard work pay off in successful careers or growing families. They seem to be trying to make sense of their short lives, or wondering how they can possibly leave their children. Some have no religious tradition that can help them make sense of what is happening to them. For patients with existential distress, we can offer to help them tell their stories, to bring meaning to the short lives they have had, as I discuss in Chapter 7.

Young parents, especially single parents, present a heartrending challenge. We always explore whether we can help them with concerns about their children. We try to ensure that the children are offered counseling, at least from their school counselors, who should be aware of the parent's serious illness. Dr. Paula Rauch, director of the Cancer Center Parenting Program and chief of Child Psychiatry Consultation Service at Massachusetts General Hospital, developed and directs the PACT program at the hospital. PACT is for children with a dying parent or for parents with cancer who need help learning how to talk with their children about their illness and even their impending death. Rauch's guidelines for clinicians who work with these parents and their children include six steps.

PRACTICE POINTS: PARENTS WITH YOUNG CHILDREN

- Learn about the children.
- Maximize the child's support system.
- Facilitate honest communication about the illness.
- Address common questions.
- Prepare for hospital visits.
- Saying good-bye.

(From Rauch et al. 2002)

"*(1) Learn about the children.*" Start with something simple like asking the parent to tell you about their children, including their ages and how they coped with previous personal or family challenges.

"*(2) Maximize the child's support system.*" A mainstay of a support system for children is maintaining their normal routine. Help the parents identify who among their family and friends can help keep the children's schedules as close to normal as possible, including sleeping, eating, school, friends, and out-of-school activities. If the ill parent encourages the children to form relationships with these nonparental friends, they won't feel disloyal in doing so.

"*(3) Facilitate honest communication about the illness.*" Parents need to spend as much time as is needed to ensure that their children have all their questions answered in a way that is appropriate for their ages. Children from 3 to 7 years old may mistakenly feel that they are the cause of their parent's illness. These children may be expressing their guilt by "anxious, inhibited behavior or outbursts of angry, oppositional behavior." Their parents need to ask the children what they think caused the cancer, so they can correct their misunderstandings. Young children do not understand that death is permanent, so death need not be part of the discussions while the ill parent is alive. Older children (7 to 12) may also fear that their behavior contributed to the cancer, and they also need to be reassured that "the cancer is not contagious and that not all cancers are caused by cigarette smoking." They do know that death is permanent, and so may need to discuss their fears and concerns about their parent leaving them. Children should be encouraged to share any stories they have heard but don't understand, to ask any questions they want to. Parents, however, have to be careful to understand what the real question is, and should feel free not to answer every question right away. Saying, "That is an important question. Let me think about it," is fine, so long as you remember to give an answer at a later time.

"*(4) Address common questions.*" Parents often ask Dr. Rauch, "What do we call the illness?" She encourages them not to use euphemisms, but rather to name the cancer specifically. Calling it a "boo-boo" or bump may scare and confuse children who themselves have had many a boo-boo or bump. Parents also ask, "How much should we share with the children?" Dr. Rauch says, "Assume that whatever the adults are discussing will be heard by the children." They are likely to feel more frightened by being left to interpret the information alone than if they are present, informed, and can be comforted should they show distress. Another question from parents is, "Should I make my child talk about the illness?" While it is very important to let children know a parent is available to talk if they want to, Rauch advises parents to let their children initiate the discussions. "Are you going to die?" is, Rauch says, "the question most commonly feared by parents." She advises parents to ask about "specific worries about what would happen if the parent died" (such as whom the children would live with), and to share that although the illness might be fatal, they're doing all they can to live as long as possible and as well as possible.

"(5) Prepare for hospital visits." Children should be allowed to visit the hospital if they want to, except when a parent is confused or agitated, which a young child is unlikely to understand. But they need special preparation for what they are about to see, including a discussion of their fears and expectations, and they should be taken there by someone who can leave when the child is ready to leave. After the visit, the child should be asked to discuss any parts that were difficult or enjoyable, or were different from what he or she expected. For children who do not want to visit, a family member or other trusted adult can help them communicate with the ill parent by preparing letters, drawings, or other gifts, making tapes or videotapes, or talking on the phone or videophone.

"(6) Saying goodbye." Rauch says, "If one's children know they are loved, and why they are loved, there is usually no need to say the word 'goodbye.'" But she encourages parents and their children to say a last "I love you" in person whenever possible. If necessary, a child can say it to a parent in a coma, or after the parent has died. Children should also be given "a road map for the grief process ahead," and the surviving parent can help the children feel comfortable about going on with school and other activities after the death by encouraging them to talk about what they have been doing, just as that parent did before the death.

Using these guidelines, clinicians can often help parents make the plans needed for care of their children when they are gone. Although they face their deaths with undiminished sadness, parents are able to say what their children need to hear. Sometimes, when appropriate plans have been made, these patients will see the benefit of appointing a health care proxy and, when appropriate, of asking not to be resuscitated.

OLDER PATIENTS.   Family concerns can also cause older patients to demand resuscitation. Some are the center of their family constellation, the matriarch or patriarch to whom everyone has turned for advice, validation, and love. They have directed careers, patched up marriages, managed divorces, run the family business, comforted angry teenagers, and made peace between generations. When disease overwhelms such a person and there has been insufficient time to delegate that role and its responsibilities, dying is not an option. Despite being told repeatedly by their trusted oncologist that resuscitation is futile, such patients cannot accept DNR orders. For them, communication even while intubated is preferable to death. Sometimes, through intensive work by the social worker with the family and the patient, the burden of leadership can be transferred to one or more family members. Encouraging family members to let the patient know that they will take care of each other, and that the patient's spirit will continue to guide them, can sometimes release the patient from the strongly felt obligation. When these older patients remain unconvinced, you may have to resuscitate them against your better judgment.

For other patients, it is a religious belief that is tormenting them. Molly was a 77-year-old woman with end-stage breast cancer that had infiltrated her lungs to the degree that she required maximum respiratory support and was nearing the point of needing noninvasive positive pressure ventilation (BiPAP) or even intubation. We were unable to relieve any of her anxiety or insomnia with medications and relaxation techniques. Her concerns became clear only when we visited Molly with our chaplain. In response to questioning, Molly said that she did believe in God, but immediately burst into tears; she told us how she could not sleep because she saw the fires of hell that were going to consume her when she died. She declined to share with us what it was that she had done, but when the chaplain asked whether the God she believed in was a vengeful or a forgiving God, Molly said it was a forgiving God. The chaplain then told her the story of the prodigal son, reminding Molly that God waits for even the worst sinners to come back to him so that he can glory in their return. She asked Molly whether she would like to pray together, which they did. Molly did not sleep soundly that night, or come any closer to making an advance care plan, but she did begin a dialogue with the chaplain that led to a marked decrease in her anxiety, and eventually to an improvement in her terror and her visions. And she was no longer afraid to ask her own pastor to visit.

For another family, the promise of a miracle was their source of torment.

Recognizing the Miracle

Jonathan was a 20-year-old man with recurrent, refractory lymphoma that was progressing rapidly and causing increasing respiratory distress from pleural effusions and interstitial disease. The attending physician who preceded me had tried repeatedly to obtain consent for a DNR/DNI (do not resuscitate or intubate) order from Jon's health proxy, his mother. She and his aunts and uncles were always at his side, and when I met them for the first time, they were clear that they had a very strong belief that Jon would be saved by a miracle. They were also clear that they did not want to discuss the DNR question further, intimating that we were trying to deny Jon the care he deserved. Jon was so ill that he was not able to communicate verbally with us, though his family felt he could communicate discomfort to them.

Our team decided it might help our relationship with the family if we were careful to demonstrate how much we did care for them and for Jon. We began twice daily meetings with family members to assess their understanding of Jon's condition and to tell them about the measures we were taking and any plans for studies or changes in his regimen. We demonstrated that we had widened the focus of our care, asking how they were doing, what their hopes and fears for Jon were, and whether they thought Jon had any spiritual needs that were being unmet. One of their hopes was that Jon would come home, so we introduced them to hospice, reassuring them that they need not opt for DNR to enroll. That was news to them, and they were very interested in the support hospice programs could offer.

As we expected, Jon's condition suddenly worsened, and he was unable to communicate in any fashion. I received a 1 a.m. phone call from the covering resident, saying that unless Jon were intubated very soon, he would die. I told Jon's mother, who was staying in the hospital with him, of the impending crisis, and for the first time asked her whether we should intubate him. She calmly and sadly refused, adding that the family had noticed the change in Jon that day. *"The miracle we asked for has come,"* she said tearfully. *"He is peaceful at last."*

We can sometimes gain the trust of families who are waiting for a miracle by providing meticulous patient care, respecting their views, and attempting to fulfill their needs. When we let go of the "DNR agenda," our compassion can shine through. Families who are not spending their time fighting us can, with assistance from their pastor or social worker, reflect on what is best for their loved one and reconcile their loss and their beliefs. When the end nears, they and the health care team can arrive at the same place, albeit by very different roads.

ANTICIPATING FAMILY CONCERNS

Once family members have accepted comfort care as a goal, they want to be sure that they are doing everything possible to help the dying patient. Billings (1985) suggests that when a family experiences insecurity, it generally arises from a combination of factors: (1) anticipation of problems (i.e., anything they can imagine happening might indeed happen); (2) a sense of isolation combined with an overwhelming sense of responsibility; and (3) vulnerability and helplessness, which can lead to outrage and even anger.

BENEFITS OF HOSPICE CARE

- The hospice philosophy is to ensure the best quality of life for patients with terminal illnesses. Patients are eligible for the Medicare hospice benefit if they are expected to live for six months or less.
- Multidisciplinary team care usually takes place in the patient's home. The team includes nurses, social workers, nursing aides, chaplains, volunteers, and physicians (including the referring M.D.).
- Care is centered on the goals and values of patients and their families.
- Attention is paid to the physical, psychological, social, financial, spiritual, and existential causes of distress.
- All medications, equipment, and supplies needed to maintain patient comfort are provided.
- If needed, 24-hour home nursing or hospitalization of the patient for uncontrollable symptoms is available.
- Respite care is available, if needed by the family.
- The patient does not always have to request DNR to enroll.
- Support for the bereaved is routinely provided.

To help a family avoid feeling insecure, Billings suggests that the medical team must (1) be available, (2) be consistent and dependable, (3) anticipate problems and rehearse responses, (4) elicit and address attributions (misinterpretations of what the patient's actions mean), and (5) offer reassurance, encouragement, and hopefulness. Hospice teams incorporate all these components in their plans of care. Their goals, as stated by the National Hospice Organization (1997), include self-determined life closure, safe and comfortable dying, and effective grieving.

Rather than waiting until death is imminent, I encourage patients to accept hospice care as soon as I determine that they are likely to live for six months or less if the disease takes its expected course. Families and hospice workers report that having this time to get to know one another enhances the hospice team's understanding of the patient's and family's

- **Heart Disease**
  - Optimal diuretic and vasodilator Rx
  - Class 4 congestive heart failure
  - Ejection fraction <20% (if available)
  - Refractory angina
  - Not a revascularization candidate
  - Not a transplant candidate

- **Pulmonary Disease**
  - Not a lung transplant candidate
  - Disabling dyspnea at rest
  - Poor response to bronchodilators
  - Hypoxemia at rest while on oxygen (pO_2 ≤55; O_2 sat. ≤88 on O_2)
  - Hypercapnia (pCO_2 ≥50)
  - FEV1 after bronchodilator ≤30% predicted
  - Serial decrease of FEV1 >40 ml/yr
  - Cor pulmonale/right heart failure
  - Hospitalizations for lung problems

- **Renal Disease**
  - Not a renal transplant candidate
  - Dialysis refused/NR
  - CrCl <10 ml/min (<15 ml/min diabetics)
  - With CHF: CrCl <15 ml/min in (20 ml/min in diabetics)
  - Cr >8 mg/dl (>6 mg/dl in diabetics)

- **Liver Disease**
  - May be awaiting liver transplant
  - PT >5 sec over control, or INR >1.5
  - Serum albumin <2.5 mg/dl
  - One of the following:
    Ascites despite diuretics
    Bacterial peritonitis
    Hepatorenal syndrome
    Hepatic encephalopathy
    Recurrent variceal bleeding

- **HIV**
  - CD4 <25 cells/μl
  - Viral load >100,000 copies/ml
    And one of the following:
  - Wasting (>33% loss of lean body mass) despite medications
  - Cryptosporidium
  - CNS or systemic lymphoma
  - Unresponsive MAC bacteremia or toxoplasmosis
  - PML
  - Visceral KS, unresponsive
  - Karnovsky perf status ≤50

- **Dementia**
  - Unable to walk, dress, or bathe without assistance
  - Urinary and fecal incontinence
  - Unable to speak or communicate meaningfully, or using ≤6 meaningful words
  - Medical complications within the past year:
    Aspiration pneumonia
    Pyelonephritis
    Septicemia
    Multiple stage 3–4 decubitus ulcers
    Recurrent fevers
    Difficulty swallowing food or refusal to eat
    Refusing tube feeds
    Weight loss >10% despite tube feeds
    Albumin <2.5 mg/dl

- **Stroke, Acute Phase**
  - Coma or persistent vegetative state for ≥3 days
  - In post-anoxic stroke, coma or severe obtundation with severe myoclonus for ≥3 days post anoxic event
  - Dysphagia preventing adequate intake without artificial feeding or hydration

- **Stroke, Chronic Phase**
  - Poor functional status (KPS ≤40)
  - Dementia, with FAST score >7
  - Unable to ambulate, dress, bathe without assistance
  - Urinary and fecal incontinence
  - Speech limited to ≤6 intelligible words
  - Poor nutritional status/weight loss >10% in past 6 months or serum albumin <2.5 mg/dl

- **Coma**
  - Coma or persistent vegetative state for >3 days, *with any three of the following:*
    Abnormal brainstem response
    Absent verbal response
    Absent withdrawal response to pain
    Cr >1.5 mg/dl

3.1 Medicare Hospice Eligibility Criteria, 1998. Adapted from Wellmark, Inc., Federal Medicare Intermediary and Carrier.

Table 3.1   Levels of Clinical Care Provided by Hospice Programs

	Routine	Continuous	Inpatient	Respite
24-hr "on call"	✓	✓	✓	✓
Home health aide	≤2 hr/day			
R.N. visits	≤3/wk + p.r.n.			
Social worker visits	q2wk			
Chaplain visits	q2–4 wk			
Volunteer	2–4 hr/wk			
M.D.	p.r.n.			
Occupational/physical/ respiratory therapy	p.r.n.			
Continuous nursing		≥8 hr R.N./day		
Inpatient care			p.r.n.	
Respite care				5 days/month

Note: *Continuous home care* is for patients with, for example, refractory cough, dyspnea, pain, or delirium; they can receive 24-hour nursing and home health aide services.

Inpatient care, rarely utilized, is for refractory symptoms that cannot be controlled at home, even with continuous care. The referring physician admits the patient and may bill for services under Medicare Part B.

The goal of *respite care* (in a community skilled or intermediate nursing facility) is either to provide a rest for the caregiver or to remove the patient to an adequate facility when the home is temporarily inadequate to meet the patient's care needs.

needs and its efficacy in providing help during the last days. It is usually not difficult to determine when cancer patients are eligible for hospice, but for patients with nonmalignant terminal illnesses this can be difficult. In 1995 and 1996, the National Hospice Organization published guidelines designed to help clinicians with this decision; in 1997 these were codified by Medicare into eligibility criteria (Figure 3.1). The levels of clinical care that hospice programs provide are indicated in Table 3.1.

Despite my best efforts, some patients are simply not willing to agree to hospice care. Our palliative care team, therefore, has incorporated hospice principles into our practice. We remind the patient and family that they can reach one of us at any time, 24 hours a day (including weekends), and encourage them to call us. We do this even for families who are receiving home nursing services. One member of the team makes the phone calls to patients with difficult symptom-management problems, to families when they need extra support, or to patients who are in their last few weeks of life. We establish a mutually convenient time and overcome any resistance by assuring the family that this is not a bother for us, that we feel better if they allow us to "check in" every day to be sure things are going well. If a nurse is going to be in the home, we schedule the call so that we can also speak with the nurse. We try to be sure that social, financial, and spiritual issues are being addressed along with the physical and psychological. If the call reveals problems in these areas, we encourage the patient or a family member to meet with a social worker or chaplain or to confer with his or her own rabbi, pastor, or priest.

During these calls we try to anticipate problems and rehearse solutions, which is what a hospice team does when it visits each patient at home. If, for example, the patient is likely to become delirious, the family is told how to identify delirium and whom to call, and is reassured that, if necessary, we will tell them how to administer the psychotropic medications that are in the home. We also use the calls to reassure family members that they are doing a wonderful job, that they are special people for assuming this responsibility and, by doing so, they are enabling their loved one to remain at home. We remind them that they are not expected to be experts and that we and the visiting nursing personnel will be there to help with the technical details. It is more than enough that they are managing all the other problems.

To help prevent family burnout, we urge family members to leave the house for at least an hour or two during the day. We remind them that they must stay mentally and physically healthy and that full-time care of a patient with advanced cancer is exhausting. They are often reluctant to leave the patient alone, and so we urge them to allow a friend, relative, or, if the patient is enrolled in a hospice program, a trained hospice volunteer to stay with the patient for a while each day to enable them to get the break they need. Hospice can also arrange for respite care for the family. The patient is cared for in a nursing home for several days (usually five), and caregivers can then go to a family reunion, graduation, or wedding or just catch up on some much-needed sleep.

We also try to counter families' fears about our ability to manage the patient's symptoms and try to help the family cope with the responsibility of providing so much of the patient's care. We reiterate the commitment of the hospice program and of our team to symptom control, and assure them that both teams have a great deal of competence in responding to such needs as they arise. We let them know that we consider symptom control to be as important as the choice of a chemotherapy regimen, and that we will work closely with the home care nurses or the hospice team to ensure that the patient receives the best symptom control we can deliver.

Finally, our team or the hospice team tries to ensure that families are comfortable with the choices they have made about the patient's care so that they will have no guilt about these choices when the patient dies. In *Dying Well*, Dr. Ira Byock shares an important technique he uses for helping families explore these issues. For example, when asking a family to consider discontinuation of tube feedings, he says to them, "This is wrenching stuff, so take as much time as you need. None of us, in the months to come, and especially after [the patient] has died, wants to look back and wonder whether we did the right thing."

I have begun using this approach each time I ask for family input in a significant decision, such as *"Should she be hospitalized to treat this problem?"* or *"Should a feeding tube be placed?"* or *"Will you be able to keep him here at home when he is dying?"* I ask the family to imagine that the patient has died and that they are reconsidering the choices they made: *"How do you feel about this decision? Do you still think we did the right thing? Was everything we did in agreement with [the patient's] values and goals, and with yours?"* If they are able to answer yes to these questions, they are much more likely to remain at peace with their decisions after the patient dies.

ANTICIPATING HOUSE STAFF'S CONCERNS
"How do you know when it's time to stop what we normally do?"

Our palliative care team had been consulting on the care of Oma, a young woman dying from a refractory metastatic gynecologic cancer. She was much loved by her house staff and the nurses on the unit, who had known her for several months. She and her family had come from the Dominican Republic to seek help for her condition, but it appeared no help was possible. The tumor had continued to grow despite everyone's best efforts. It swelled her abdomen and afflicted her with abdominal pain and finally with hypercalcemia, which, too, was refractory to medical efforts at correction.

Oma was well supported by her family and friends. Her mother had been with her throughout the months of her stay in the United States. In her last weeks of life, Oma reunited with her estranged husband. Her family was allowed to be in close attendance, and together, we were able to give her the comfort she needed, and she died peacefully under our care in the hospital.

But we did not achieve this easily, even though Oma had accepted comfort care, understanding that there was no further antineoplastic therapy to try. While the house staff and nurses shared the goals of our palliative care team, they were often puzzled by and resisted implementing our recommendations. At the time, I did not understand why. Though our approach was very different from theirs, it provided the comfort they said they were seeking for Oma.

The answer appeared only after her death, while we were meeting with members of the gynecologic oncology team at their request. They could not understand how we and they had observed the same patient and yet found different problems that required totally different solutions. They were saddened by Oma's death and realized they wanted to understand better how to help future patients. This was the first time they had worked with a palliative care team, and so they asked us, *"How do you know when it's time to stop what we normally do?"* How should they think about caring for someone who was on "comfort care"? What criteria did we use as we made our recommendations? For example, why didn't we want them to monitor her calcium and potassium levels? Why did we oppose "fluid challenges" (i.e., rapid infusions of 500-ml bolus doses of IV fluid) when she was tachycardic, up to 150/min? "Why," the nurses had asked, "do they want us to do an enema in someone only days from death?"

It was not the details of day-to-day management that they needed from us, but a new understanding of the different philosophy of caring for their dying hospitalized patients. We suggested that the gynecologic oncology team treat these patients as though they were caring for them at home, perhaps with the help of a hospice team. There, the goals and priorities of the patient and family—not the disease or metabolic abnormalities—are paramount. We suggested that they ask themselves, before each possible intervention, what is the burden versus the benefit of this intervention? How will it help us further the patient's and family's goals? Understandably, this focus was very different from their standard management goals, and yet they seemed to accept its relevance for this situation.

We also emphasized that assessing the burden/benefit ratio was very different from assessing risk/benefit, with which they were more familiar. After all, only minimal risk is entailed in a venipuncture or a fluid challenge. But there is a great deal of potential burden, especially in someone whose ascites, pulmonary secretions, and edema are going to be markedly exacerbated by the fluid.

House staff, it seems, spend much less time visiting the rooms of patients who are receiving comfort care than those of other patients (Mills et al. 1994). That may be because the house staff do not know how they can be of help. The gynecologic oncology team was troubled about its role in providing comfort care for Oma: "If we aren't drawing blood, or monitoring her vital signs, what should we do?" They felt helpless and at sea; they felt they'd had no more to offer, to Oma or her family. We explained that there are many other ways to show concern. Providing excellent comfort care, for example, requires frequent observations of patients and their families and an understanding of what causes distress for dying patients. We explained that we'd asked them to stop the fluids to prevent her having breathing difficulties due to the excess hydration, and asked for the enema because we surmised that obstipation due to the continuous opioid infusion and refractory hypercalcemia was causing her significant discomfort. We also explained how the house staff's frequent visits to Oma and obvious concern for her had provided comfort to her family. By the end of this meeting, the team members felt they had begun to understand the other forms that care could take, and we promised more sessions about caring for dying patients.

PHYSICIAN-ASSISTED SUICIDE

REQUESTS

Anticipating family concerns and enabling the family and the home care and inpatient teams to provide expert symptom management may not be enough to convince some patients that life is still worthwhile.

The Patient Who Asks for Help in Committing Suicide

I was caring for Mr. D'Angelo, a 55-year-old man with Waldenström's macroglobulinemia. Plasmapheresis controlled his blood viscosity, but he had anemia, massive splenomegaly, and an acquired coagulation inhibitor that caused a von Willebrand's–like disease that was refractory to clotting factor replacement. His only symptoms were weakness and shortness of breath when the anemia became too severe. Splenectomy might have helped, but his coagulopathy made the operation impossible.

Mr. D, as he asked us to call him, was an active gardener and had often brought me home-grown vegetables and herbs. Now, however, even with transfusions, he noted he was getting weaker, and one day, even using his walker, he felt too weak to ambulate. He asked whether he would ever get out of his wheelchair again and I told him that I didn't think he would. He replied, *"Fine, doc. Then I guess it's about time for you to help me to 'get out' permanently. Life in a wheelchair is not for me."*

I was taken aback. Other than being in a wheelchair, he did not seem to me to have a life that was not worth living. Except for his weakness, his symptoms were easily controlled, and his mind was working very well. At the time, projecting my standards of an acceptable quality of life onto Mr. D, it seemed inconceivable that someone would want to die just because he had to use a wheelchair to get around. If he had been closer to the other end of the spectrum—bedridden or in severe pain—I could have understood his request. But for Mr. D, the wheelchair created limitations that were simply not acceptable; his quality of life was unsatisfactory and he wanted to die.

I did not act on his request and I was unable to comfort him. He refused psychological help but said he would allow a visit from his parish priest. A week later his wife found him dead in his wheelchair. The autopsy, which she requested, revealed a massive myocardial infarction.

CAUSES OF REQUESTS FOR PHYSICIAN-ASSISTED SUICIDE.   Mr. D'Angelo was the first, but since then, like many other physicians, I have had other patients ask me to kill them or to help them kill themselves. Studies indicate a number of reasons why patients make such requests.

WHY PATIENTS REQUEST PHYSICIAN-ASSISTED SUICIDE

- Patients lack technical expertise.
- The physician is expected to serve as "guide, companion, and caretaker."
- Patients worry about adequate symptom control now and in the future.
- Patients worry that the family will be unable to care for them.
- Patients do not wish to burden the family.
- Patients experience loss of "personhood," sense of worth, and meaning in life.
- The physician's attention to the patient's concerns is felt to be inadequate.

In their 1994 paper on this subject, Block and Billings suggest that patients ask us to kill them because they expect us "to be a guide, companion, and caretaker in their final passage. Patients, in fact, lack the technical knowledge to kill themselves quickly and comfortably." Since we have been managing their care throughout the treatment phase of their illness, they expect us now to provide the expertise to help them die.

Block and Billings also list a number of reasons that patients who seem to have a lot to live for, like Mr. D, want to end their lives. Some may be concerned that as they get sicker, we will not provide effective control of their symptoms. They may have had bad experiences with the health care system in the past, feel that their symptoms were inadequately treated, and fear a prolonged period of unalleviated suffering.

They may also fear that their family will fail them. The diagnosis of cancer and the side effects of the treatments may have stressed the family's emotional and financial resources already. Patients may feel their family is overwhelmed or resentful. Even patients being well cared for may feel that in the future they will become too great a burden. They cannot risk putting it to the test: failure would be too painful.

Since they may also fear that I will abandon them, I let my patients know almost from their first visit that I'll be there "for the duration." I half jokingly say, *"You know, once you're in my care there's nothing you can do to get out. You can take or reject my suggestions for treatment, but you can't get rid of me. You're stuck with me until the end."* Often just my willingness to listen and to give them the security that I will not abandon them offers enough comfort.

I am also convinced that for patients who know they are dying, there are unique opportunities for growth. Patients should be encouraged to search for new meaning in altered life roles, to accept borrowed strength, and to pursue transcendence (Cassell 1991). And they can replace some of their losses by filling a new role in their community and within the family (Byock 1997). In Byock's *Dying Well*, for example, Mayor Burke came to understand that by accepting help from a hospice program, his neighbors, and his family, he was filling an important community role and bringing satisfaction to a number of people. It was his final gift to them. As he said, "I guess it's time to be on the receiving end" (p. 97). The dignity that he sought lay not in his physical condition (he was dying of amyotrophic lateral sclerosis [ALS]) but in something larger, which had, if anything, grown as his health had worsened.

Finally, there are patients who simply want us to pay more attention to their concerns and use the request for physician-assisted suicide to shock us into doing so. While we were concentrating on their physical problems, we may have overlooked their psychological, spiritual, or even financial concerns. Requests for euthanasia or assisted suicide suggest that the patient harbors such concerns and that they are very serious. Asking us to end their lives may be the only way patients feel they can enlist our aid in ending their suffering.

Other contributing factors include physical or psychological disorders and the patient's personal values. Patients suffering from uncontrolled pain, depression, anxiety, organic mental disorders (such as delirium or brain metastases), or personality disorders are more likely to want to die. And unfortunately, both inadequately controlled pain and psychiatric disorders are common in the terminally ill patient population. In addition, patients who are grieving the many losses associated with their illness (loss of "personhood," as described above, and physical, social, financial, and spiritual losses) may feel that death offers the best answer.

When you encounter patients in this kind of despair, you should, in addition to evaluating them for reversible causes, have a low threshold for referring them to professionals skilled in treating psychological, social, and spiritual problems. In most cases you or these other professionals will be able to reduce the suffering of these patients, and they will no longer want to hasten their death.

Patients' personal values also may lead to requests for euthanasia or assisted suicide. People for whom remaining in control is especially important may feel that relinquishing control or their independence is worse than dying. They cannot be dependent on anyone. Patients who have always been self-reliant, who have had trouble accepting help from others, or who have never been comfortable with the disabilities of others may find it intolerable to be in such a position themselves. That is what they are asking you to prevent. In retrospect, I think Mr. D may have been such a person.

There are also narcissistic people whose view of an acceptable life is different from their physicians'. A narcissist has "a pathologic need for control, a dysfunctional sense of entitlement, a basic sense that nothing is good enough, and a profound difficulty in trusting others . . . Clinicians may perceive such patients as cold, ungrateful, demeaning, or help-rejecting . . . [Such patients] also may be relatively assertive and demanding toward health care workers, and unwilling to accept professional opinion" (Block and Billings 1994). Euthanasia requests from such difficult patients may be among the hardest to handle.

HOW TO RESPOND TO SUCH REQUESTS.   Physicians' personal responses to requests to assist in a suicide vary widely (Block and Billings 1994). Some of us avoid the subject and deny to ourselves that it was even raised. Others feel guilty or depressed about forcing the patient to continue an unwanted, suffering-filled existence. From time to time, a few of us, especially those of us who know the patient well, comply.

There are several ways to deal with such a request other than acceding to it (Block and Billings 1994). First, acknowledge it and encourage the patient to talk about what has prompted it. Then offer a compassionate, consistent presence to the patient and his family. Next, be clear about what you will and won't do. While you might be willing, for example, to provide pain medicine, the patient should not expect that you will actually administer a bolus of drug intended to kill him.

Finally, address the change in your relationship with the patient that results from a request for euthanasia or assisted suicide. Ask how he will feel about you if you reject his request—how it will affect future requests of other kinds, and whether it diminishes his trust. Reiterate your offer of help, short of killing him, and let him know that if he now feels he needs to see another physician, you will understand.

LEGALIZING PHYSICIAN-ASSISTED SUICIDE AND EUTHANASIA

As I prepare the second edition of this book, physicians, ethicists, lawyers, politicians, and the public are still engaged in a heated debate about legalizing physician-assisted suicide and euthanasia. Issues of patient autonomy have come to the forefront, with increasing expressions of concern among our patients that we will force them to stay alive despite their wishes to the contrary. To protect themselves, many people are completing living wills and assigning powers of attorney for health care.

Disturbingly, there is evidence from several studies that these concerns are not unfounded: we physicians do not always make it our business to know our patients' wishes about resuscitation or life support measures. Even if patients have a living will, many doctors fail to honor their requests to withdraw or withhold life support measures.

This withholding or withdrawing of treatment (sometimes called "passive euthanasia") is *legal*, even if it means that the patient will die as a result. Religious leaders as well as legal experts and ethicists agree that withholding or withdrawing such therapy should be distinguished from euthanasia and from physician-assisted suicide. Euthanasia is currently *illegal* in all fifty states, and in thirty-one there are statutes that expressly forbid physician-assisted suicide. Oregon is the only state that permits physician-assisted suicide for mentally competent adults suffering from a terminal illness—defined as likely to result in death within six months. Patients must consult with two physicians and wait fifteen days.

The American Cancer Society, the American College of Physicians, and many individual palliative care and pain experts, such as Dr. Kathleen Foley, professor of neurology and neurosciences and professor of clinical pharmacology at Cornell University Medical College and former chief of the Pain and Palliative Care Service at Memorial Sloan-Kettering Cancer Center, all oppose legalizing physician-assisted suicide and euthanasia. As the American Cancer Society stated in its 1995 position paper, "We believe these acts are contrary to the ethical traditions and threaten the moral integrity of health care professionals. We assert that it is the responsibility of all organizations concerned with cancer care to work to improve care at the end of life, and to undertake broad educational programs for patients, families, and health care professionals concerning care at the end of life."

Dr. Foley is also concerned that with legalization, euthanasia would replace other, more appropriate treatment of a patient's symptoms. She argues that the state of education of most health professionals in palliative care is woefully inadequate, as is their ability to recognize chronic pain, depression, or "existential" suffering in many of their patients (Foley 1991, 1995, 1997). Most patients do not understand that, with expert palliative care, their suffering can be relieved, no matter what its cause. Even proponents of legalization of physician-assisted suicide, such as Dr. Timothy Quill (1993), agree that up to 95 percent of patients should be able to die with their symptoms controlled to their satisfaction.

Several surveys of both generalists and specialists reveal that many physicians would be willing to participate in physician-assisted suicide or euthanasia if it were legal. It may be that since most physicians don't know other ways to relieve suffering, they feel that death is the only humane option. According to these surveys, hospice physicians, in contrast to physicians who knew or felt they knew little about symptom control, understood that death was not the more humane option, and they were less likely to agree to participate in assisted suicide or euthanasia.

That is why Dr. Foley and others assert that physician education in how to recognize and relieve suffering, and public education about the efficacy of currently available symptomatic treatments, must precede any legislation that makes assisted suicide or euthanasia more readily available. We need to understand, and to help our patients understand, that we can already achieve symptom control for 95 percent of them.

What to do about the other 5 percent? Palliative sedation is a technique that can provide comfort for all patients. It can be given in the home or in a health care facility by skilled clinicians employing appropriate medications. I will review the details of the technique in Chapter 8. For some, however, this technique is tantamount to physician-assisted suicide. This remains a matter of individual conscience. Many respected physicians believe that they should have the legal option to help someone who asks for help ending his life and for whom all available expert palliative care has not led to a satisfactory quality of life. They do not disagree with Dr. Foley or the American Cancer Society about the need for better education in the provision of care. But when that care has not produced a satisfactory outcome, they do not think it morally wrong to help patients end their life, or to end it for them.

This debate, regardless of its outcome, has raised the level of public discussion about the importance of providing an acceptable quality of life for patients with advanced cancer. I am hopeful that as the availability of comprehensive palliative care for patients improves, requests for euthanasia and physician-assisted suicide will decrease.

SELF-CARE

Caring for even one patient who is dying with advanced cancer can be intellectually and emotionally exhausting. Like the families you work with, you may need to develop some "self-care" techniques. In the course of trying to help house officers maintain their emotional equilibrium as they work with increasingly large numbers of extremely sick patients, I needed to analyze how I managed not to "burn out." As I thought back, I realized that my initial self-care strategy was a disaster.

The first time I recall needing a strategy for self-care was in 1971, when I was a second-year medical student taking my first clinical rotation: pediatrics. But this pediatrics was not in an outpatient office or even community hospital setting. The children I saw had been admitted to a tertiary care hospital to be treated for leukemia, which at that time was almost invariably fatal, or illnesses of similar severity and complexity. The "general pediatrics" ward was filled with children with cystic fibrosis. Women were scarce in medicine back then, so I instinctively knew that crying in response to what I was dealing with "was not an option." But a great deal of what I saw called for tears. I eventually found a place to shed them in private, when I was relaxed, and I could take my time to review the emotionally charged events. Sometimes I found myself crying silently during a concert, and feeling better when the concert ended. That safety valve seemed to work so well that I used it throughout pediatrics.

But many years later, when I was in the midst of my first year of clinical training in oncology, an odd thing started to happen. I found myself dreading attending concerts. Both my husband and I had looked forward to summer evenings spent at an outdoor orchestral performance, but I began to find reasons not to go. Finally, one evening, I said, "I'm just not up to that tonight!" My husband, quite puzzled, replied, "Up to what? Why would anyone not be 'up to' hearing Mozart?" It was only then that I realized what had happened. To deal with the troubling feelings aroused by the tragic stories of the cancer patients I was caring for, I had automatically reactivated my earlier mechanism: grieve them in private, usually during the slow moments of symphonies. What I wasn't "up to" was a mental review of the patients I'd seen recently or the full experience of the grief I had suppressed so that I could get through the work.

Once I understood what I'd been doing, I was able to devise other strategies for dealing with my grief much closer to when it occurred. After someone died, I cried if I needed to, and even found a few minutes to give full vent to my sadness. I found private places around the hospital, or confided in colleagues who then felt free to share their stories with me.

Grief Rounds

Given these experiences, you can imagine how delighted I was when the chief medical residents at Brigham and Women's Hospital, where I currently work, asked my colleague Dr. Susan Block and me whether we could offer any source of support for the house staff on the oncology and bone marrow transplant teams. Dr. Block had completed an intensive study of the reactions of house staff to the deaths of their patients, and had found that they often had unresolved feelings of grief or guilt or anger about these deaths. The attending rounds in ICUs and in oncology rarely made room for a discussion of the events surrounding a death, for airing of house staff's concerns, and for education about the grief and bereavement not only of families but of professional caregivers such as nurses and physicians.

We therefore began to conduct grief rounds every other week, to which the interns were invited. The discussions were confidential and, of course, food and drink were provided. The chief residents, who arranged for the food, also reminded the busy interns to come to the rounds, instructing them to sign out their beepers to their residents for the hour. These rounds have been very well attended, and are continuing. Interns are able to share their concerns, learn that many of their colleagues have the same concerns, and work out ways to interact more comfortably with patients who are dying and their families. My hope is that this forum will prevent them from developing the kind of dysfunctional mechanism I had used to protect myself from the grief I was feeling.

OTHER TECHNIQUES

My colleagues in palliative care stress that each of us needs to identify a way to process the intense emotions the work entails. Some meditate, others exercise, but all recognize that unless we grieve our losses, we will no longer be able to remain present in the face of suffering, or to offer compassion. We need to be attentive to our own emotional and spiritual needs, as, I imagine, do my oncology colleagues. Part of the training we offer our oncology fellows teaches a respect for self-care and the importance of recognizing the stresses that their choice of profession will entail. My advice to the fellows is summarized here:

Clues for Self-Preservation
- Recognize how stressful caring for dying patients can be.
- Give yourself credit for the work you are doing.
- Learn how to work with a team; delegate and thereby diffuse responsibilities; let other team members help you.
- Monitor your emotional reactions and take time for yourself when you need it.
- Set appropriate goals; acknowledge medicine's and your own limitations.

SUMMARY

Communication among patients, families, and clinicians is crucial as patients approach the end of life. By avoiding misunderstandings about the goals of therapy, by clarifying patients', families', and clinicians' priorities, and by reinstating patients' personal calendars, clinicians can help patients and their families make the transition to comfort care. Readdressing the issues of resuscitation, and reviewing the concerns of dying parents who have young children, of family elders, and of families and patients who are waiting for a miracle, can help them make truly informed choices. Once the patient and family have accepted comfort care, hospice programs can help alleviate family insecurities. House staff are equally in need of our support and education. We can provide these by answering their question, "How do we know when it's time to stop what we normally do?"; we can offer a forum such as grief rounds, where they can share difficult experiences and gain skills in difficult communication tasks. With the help of the hospice team (for patients at home or in a long-term care facility) and the palliative care team (for those in the hospital), clinicians can provide comprehensive assessment and sophisticated management of patients' concerns; patients and families can be helped to reach their final goals; and requests for physician-assisted suicide can be minimized. Using self-care techniques to renew and reenergize themselves clinicians can continue to accompany their patients during their last journey.

Bibliography

American Cancer Society Advisory Group on Cancer Pain Relief. 1995. *American Cancer Society Position Statement on Assisted Suicide and Euthanasia.* Atlanta: American Cancer Society.

Angell M. 1997. The Supreme Court and physician-assisted suicide—the ultimate right. *N Engl J Med* 336:50–53.

Asch DA. 1996. The role of critical care nurses in euthanasia and assisted suicide. *N Engl J Med* 334:1374–1379.

Billings JA. 1985. *Outpatient Management of Advanced Cancer: Symptom Control, Support, and Hospice-in-the-Home.* Philadelphia: JB Lippincott.

Blank LL (ed). 1996. *Caring for the Dying: Identification and Promotion of Physician Competency,* (1) Educational Resource Document [250 references and listings of other information resources] and (2) Personal Narratives of Physicians Caring for Dying Patients. Philadelphia: American Board of Internal Medicine.

Block SD. 2001. Psychological considerations, growth, and transcendance at the end of life: the art of the possible. *JAMA* 285:2898–2905.

Block SD, Billings JA. 1994. Patient requests to hasten death: evaluation and management in terminal care. *Arch Intern Med* 154:2039–2047.

Byock I. 1997. *Dying Well: Peace and Possibilities at the End of Life.* New York: Riverhead Books.

Cassell E. 1991. *The Nature of Suffering and the Goals of Medicine*. New York: Oxford University Press.

Cherny NI, Coyle N, Foley KM. 1994. Suffering in the advanced cancer patient: a definition and taxonomy. *J Palliat Care* 10:57–70.

Cherny NI, Coyle N, Foley KM. 1996. Guidelines in the care of the dying cancer patient. *Hematol Oncol Clin North Am* 10:261–286.

Covinsky KE, Landefeld CS, Teno J, et al., SUPPORT Investigators. 1996. Is economic hardship on the families of the seriously ill associated with patient and surrogate care preferences? *Arch Intern Med* 156:1737–1741.

Emanuel EJ, Battin MP. 1998. What are the potential cost savings from legalizing physician-assisted suicide? *N Engl J Med* 339:167–172.

Foley KM. 1991. The relationship of pain and symptom management to patient requests for physician-assisted suicide. *J Pain Symptom Manage* 6:289–297.

Foley KM. 1995. Pain, physician-assisted suicide, and euthanasia. *Pain Forum* 4:163–178.

Foley KM. 1997. Competent care for the dying instead of physician-assisted suicide. *N Engl J Med* 336:54–58.

Hamel RP, Lysaught MT. 1994. Choosing palliative care: do religious beliefs make a difference? *J Palliat Care* 10(3):61–66.

Health Care Financing Administration, Department of Health and Human Services. 1993. *Title 42 of the Code of Federal Regulations, Part 418 (Medicare Hospice Certification)*. Baltimore: Health Care Financing Administration.

Hiller RJ. 1991. Ethics and hospice physicians. *Am J Hospice Palliat Care* Jan/Feb:17–26.

Kübler-Ross E. 1969. *On Death and Dying*. New York: Collier Books, Macmillan.

Lynn J. 2001. Serving patients who may die soon and their families: the role of hospice and other services. *JAMA* 85:925–932.

Mills M, Davies HTO, Macrae WA. 1994. Care of dying patients in the hospital. *BMJ* 309:583–586.

National Hospice Organization. 1997. *A Pathway for Patients and Families Facing Terminal Illness*. Arlington, Va.: National Hospice Organization.

Portenoy RK. 1993. Chronic pain management. In *Medical Psychiatric Practice*, vol 2, Stoudemire GA, Fogel BS (eds). Washington, D.C.: American Psychiatric Press.

Quill TE. 1993. *Death and Dignity*. New York: WW Norton.

Quill TE, Brody H. 1996. Physician recommendations and patient autonomy: finding a balance between physician power and patient choice. *Ann Intern Med* 125:763–769.

Rauch PK, Muriel AC, Cassem NH. 2002. Parents with cancer: who's looking after the children? *J Clin Oncol* 20:4399–4402.

Remen RN. 1996. *Kitchen Table Wisdom: Stories That Heal*. New York: Riverhead Books.

Rinpoche S. 1993. *The Tibetan Book of Living and Dying*, Gaffney P, Harvey A (eds). New York: Harper San Francisco.

Schou KC, Hewison J. 1999. *Experiencing Cancer: Quality of Life in Cancer Treatment*. Buckingham, England: Open University Press.

Stuart B, Connor S, Kinzbrunner BM, et al. 1996. *Medical Guidelines for Determining Prognosis in Selected Non-cancer Diseases*, 2nd ed. Arlington, Va.: National Hospice Organization.

Suarez-Almazor ME, Belzile M, Bruera E. 1997. Euthanasia and physician-assisted suicide: a comparative survey of physicians, terminally ill cancer patients, and the general population. *J Clin Oncol* 15:418–427.

The SUPPORT Principal Investigators. 1995. A controlled trial to improve care for seriously ill hospitalized patients. *JAMA* 274:1591–1598.

Teno JM, Clarridge BR, Casey V, et al. 2004. Family perspectives on end-of-life care at the last place of care. *JAMA* 291:88–93.

US Department of Health and Human Services. 1992. *Medicare Hospice Manual*, Section 230.3 (revised). Springfield, Ill.: US Department of Commerce.

Webb M. 1997. *The Good Death: The New American Search to Reshape the End of Life*. New York: Bantam.

Weir RF (ed). 1997. *Physician-Assisted Suicide*. Medical Ethics Series. Bloomington: Indiana University Press.

PART II

Pain Control and
Symptom Management

4

ASSESSING THE PATIENT IN PAIN

Why an entire chapter devoted to assessing pain in cancer patients? Pain, after all, is something physicians already know a lot about. It is one of the most common complaints for which patients seek their help, and physicians routinely elicit comprehensive descriptions of the pain to aid them in diagnosis.

But the causes of pain are different in oncology patients. Only about 5 to 10 percent of pain in these patients is caused by diseases common in patients who don't have cancer. Ninety to 95 percent of cancer pain is due to the cancer, resulting either directly from tumor involvement (about 75 percent) or from treatments for the disease (about 15 to 20 percent), such as mucositis caused by chemotherapy or radiation therapy. The procedures needed to stage the cancer also cause significant distress. Pain was reported by almost 70 percent of patients undergoing bone marrow aspirate or biopsy, 14 percent undergoing lumbar puncture, and 10 percent having catheters placed (Portnow et al. 2003). In 25 percent the pain was moderate and in 25 percent it was severe. Oncology patients' pain is frequently exacerbated by the psychological, social, and spiritual stresses of their disease.

In addition, a number of pain syndromes are typically seen in cancer patients. Mr. Young, for example, a patient of mine with lung cancer, had a referred pain syndrome peculiar to patients with cancer. About three months after completing radiation therapy to his lung lesion, he developed severe right hip pain. Findings from x-rays of his hip and pelvis were entirely normal, and the bone scan confirmed the absence of metastases in this region. But the scan did reveal a metastasis in his thoracic spine, at T12. After radiation therapy to this lesion, the referred hip pain entirely resolved.

For all these reasons, the complex pain problems of many cancer patients are difficult to evaluate. Inasmuch as an accurate pain assessment is the key to effective therapy, this chapter delineates the elements of a comprehensive pain assessment in cancer patients.

TYPES OF CANCER PATIENTS WITH PAIN

Cancer patients who develop pain vary in their personalities and past experiences, as well as in the nature of their disease, its stage, and where they are in their course of treatment. Pain assessments should take into account not only the stage of the disease but also the current pain syndrome and any past history of pain or substance abuse (Foley 2004). Patients with acute cancer-related pain, for example, usually tolerate their pain well psychologically. They know that the pain is likely to respond to antineoplastic therapy or, for those with treatment-related complications, likely to resolve entirely with time.

Patients with chronic cancer-associated pain (lasting more than three months) have "meaningless" pain: the pain does not alert the patient to something that can be fixed. Therefore, the assessment of the psychological, social, and spiritual responses of the patient to this "meaningless pain" must be very extensive. I discuss these evaluations in more detail later in the chapter. Since the source of the pain in these patients can rarely be eliminated, treatment is usually focused on maximizing function and minimizing symptoms.

Two groups of patients—those with a history of nonmalignant chronic pain who now have, in addition, chronic cancer pain, and those with a history of drug dependence—require special management techniques, discussed in Chapter 5. Finally, for dying patients, for whom the sole goal is to maintain comfort, we must address all causes of suffering related to dying, including the psychological and the spiritual.

GUIDELINES FOR ASSESSMENT OF CANCER PAIN

CLINICAL GUIDELINES

Experts with years of experience in pain research and in consultation and treatment of patients with pain emphasize the importance of a thorough pain assessment. Most mistakes in diagnosing the cause of a pain syndrome and failure to manage the problem effectively stem from neglecting one or more components of the following assessments:

Clinical Guidelines for Assessment of Pain
1. Believe the patient's complaint of pain.
2. Take a careful history of the pain complaint to place it temporally in the patient's cancer history.
3. Assess the characteristics of each pain, including its site, its pattern of referral, its aggravating and relieving factors.
4. Clarify the temporal aspects of the pain: acute, subacute, chronic, episodic, intermittent, breakthrough, or incident.
5. List and prioritize each pain complaint.
6. Evaluate the response to previous and current analgesic therapies.
7. Evaluate the psychological state of the patient.
8. Ask if the patient has a past history of alcohol or drug dependence.
9. Perform a careful medical and neurological examination.
10. Order and personally review the appropriate diagnostic procedures.
11. Treat the patient's pain to facilitate the necessary work-up.
12. Design the diagnostic and therapeutic approach to suit the individual.
13. Provide continuity of care from evaluation to treatment, to ensure patient compliance and to reduce patient anxiety.

14. Reassess the patient's response to pain therapy.
15. Discuss advance directives with the patient and the family.*

AHCPR Guidelines

The pain assessment recommendations in the Agency for Health Care Policy and Research (AHCPR) guidelines, *Management of Cancer Pain*, incorporate those listed above, but they are stated slightly differently. The six AHCPR recommendations for pain assessment are:

1. Health professionals should ask about pain, and the patient's self-report should be the primary source of assessment.
2. Clinicians should assess pain with easily administered rating scales and should document the efficacy of pain relief at regular intervals after starting or changing treatment. Documentation forms should be readily accessible to all clinicians involved in the patient's care.
3. Clinicians should teach patients and their families to use assessment tools in their homes in order to promote continuity of effective pain management across all settings.
4. The initial evaluation of the pain should include:
   - A detailed history, including an assessment of pain intensity and characteristics
   - A physical examination
   - A psychosocial assessment
   - A diagnostic evaluation of signs and symptoms associated with the common cancer pain syndromes
5. Clinicians should be aware of common pain syndromes: this prompt recognition may hasten therapy and minimize the morbidity of unrelieved pain.
6. Changes in pain patterns or the development of new pain should trigger a diagnostic evaluation and modification of the treatment plan.†

---

*From K. M. Foley, Acute and chronic cancer pain syndromes, in *Oxford Textbook of Palliative Medicine*, 3rd ed., D. Doyle, G. W. C. Hanks, N. I. Cherny, K. Calman (eds). Oxford: Oxford University Press, 2004.

†From A. Jacox, D. B. Carr, R. Payne, et al., *Management of Cancer Pain: Clinical Practice Guideline No. 9*, p. 23, Rockville, Md.: Agency for Health Care and Policy Research, U.S. Department of Health and Human Services, Public Health Service, 1994. AHCPR publication 94-0592.

The remainder of this chapter considers each of these recommendations in more detail.

ASK ABOUT THE PAIN

Strangely enough, cancer patients, especially those with chronic pain, seldom complain about their pain during routine office visits. Often, they assume that pain is an inevitable, irreversible part of having cancer, and they see no reason to waste their few minutes with us talking about something they don't think we can change. Instead, they ask about the progress of their disease, their prognosis, their increasing debility, or problems with their medications. Some may fear that we will think less of them if they are unable to deal with their pain, so do not reveal it even if asked how they are feeling.

It is up to us, then, to ask our patients directly whether they are having pain, especially if we know they have lesions that are likely to cause discomfort. We need to teach them that we don't consider it shameful to have pain, any more than it is shameful to have a cough or a broken arm. By carefully questioning them and being attentive to their responses, we can demonstrate that we consider pain to be a legitimate complaint. And by successfully managing their complaints, we can correct their misconception that pain is a necessary part of the cancer process.

BELIEVE THE PATIENT

Cancer patients may also be reluctant to report their pain to us because they suspect that we won't believe them. They may be reluctant to admit they need a stronger opioid to relieve their pain, because they fear we will treat them as though they are drug addicts. We must believe the patient's complaint of pain, however, because doing so is crucial to an accurate pain assessment.

But this is not as easy as it may seem. Some people, albeit unconsciously, use cultural stereotypes that affect how they interpret someone else's pain complaint. They may think, for example, that patients from Jewish or Italian backgrounds are more likely to exaggerate the pain they are feeling than are the more stoic Scots or Swedes. One study showed that adequate pain medication was more often prescribed to nonminority than to minority patients, but the authors stated that their study did not take into account reluctance of patients or their families to report pain, take the opioid prescribed, or pay for it (Cleeland et al. 1997). Numerous other studies were similarly not controlled for important variables that affect patients' pain complaints. The few studies that have had proper controls have not shown cultural differences in pain threshold, pain expression, or coping ability. (Other ways in which culture influences pain assessment are discussed later in the chapter.)

In addition, whether or not a patient "looks" as if he is in pain may affect whether you believe his complaint. For example, you are very likely to believe complaints of pain from a patient with a broken arm, because people with *acute* pain look as if they're in pain: they appear uncomfortable and anxious and are often sweating. People with acute pain look this way because their activated sympathetic nervous system causes sweating and an increase in pulse and blood pressure. When we observe these findings, we usually believe complaints of pain.

But what about patients with *chronic* pain who do not "look" as if they are in pain? Their complaints often seem out of proportion to the amount of disease that can be documented by physical exam or x-rays. Consider the patient with severe arthritis or advanced osteoporosis with compression fractures. Her pulse and blood pressure are normal; she's not particularly anxious and she's not sweating. Don't you find it a little harder to believe that she is in severe pain?

And don't you find it harder to treat her with opioids? After all, as I discussed in Chapter 2, many of us find it difficult to prescribe opioids when we are not sure someone is having pain, because we suspect she is using our prescriptions to "get high." Given this suspicion, we want to be confident that someone is really experiencing pain before we prescribe an opioid.

We don't have resistance like this to prescribing most other drugs, and so we don't have to be quite as sure of the diagnosis before prescribing them. If, for example, you see someone who has orthopnea and paroxysmal nocturnal dyspnea but whose physical and x-ray findings don't fully substantiate a diagnosis of congestive heart failure, you have no problem prescribing appropriate medications and monitoring the patient's response. If his symptoms improve, great! If not, you simply pursue other diagnostic possibilities.

But even if the osteoporotic patient has equally compelling pain symptoms, if you think the objective findings don't substantiate her complaint you might well be reluctant to treat her empirically with opioids. But what are the objective findings for someone with chronic pain? What should you be looking for to substantiate her pain complaint, or the complaint of an oncology patient with chronic, severe pain? Being familiar with the presentation of patients in severe *chronic* pain makes it easier for us to decide how to treat the patient.

The Problem of Neuropathic Pain

It was hard for Mr. Cirelli's physicians to believe he was in pain, though that was what led him to see his doctor. Mr. Cirelli was thought to have a Pancoast tumor, a lung cancer that, because of its location in the lung apex, often infiltrates the chest wall and the nerves of the brachial plexus. When the admitting resident called to ask me to see him, she apologized that no pathologic diagnosis had yet been made: *"His chest film shows a mass in the right lung apex, but I really haven't been able to do a thorough exam or obtain any tissue because Mr. Cirelli won't cooperate."* When I went to his ward, his nurses confirmed the physician's impression, adding that Mr. Cirelli was short-tempered and demanding, and that I was unlikely to get much conversation from him.

On entering his room, what I saw was a man lying very quietly in bed staring at the TV mounted on the wall. In answer to my greeting, he slowly turned his head toward me, but the rest of his body stayed very still. He looked exhausted, but he was not grimacing or wincing. He kept his right elbow bent with his right forearm across his chest, supported by his left hand.

In response to my questions, he said that he had been well until four months earlier when he had noticed a mild aching pain in his right shoulder area. The discomfort had progressed, and when he developed weakness in his right hand grip he saw an orthopedist, who treated him for an injured rotator cuff. When the pain worsened and a shoulder film suggested a mass in the apex of the lung, he was referred for further evaluation. He now described the pain as excruciating (the choices I gave him were mild, moderate, severe, or excruciating). It was constant, deep, and aching, and it occasionally "shot down" his arm like electricity.

He could not move his right arm without pain and could no longer sleep except for catnaps. He had lost his appetite and ability to concentrate. The pain was his central concern. He told me all this calmly but with a very depressed affect. His pulse and blood pressure were normal and he was not sweating. I tried to examine his right shoulder area, but he could not tolerate any evaluation of his neck, right supraclavicular area, right shoulder, or right axilla, and he would not sit up for a lung examination. His right hand showed muscle atrophy typical of the C7–T1 distribution.

Mr. Cirelli's symptoms and signs were typical of someone with chronic severe neuropathic pain arising from tumor infiltration into the nerves of his right brachial plexus. His physicians and nurses were not familiar with the presentation of neuropathic pain and so could not have known how agonizing for him was any examination of the shoulder area. Since he didn't resemble patients with acute pain, they mistook his distress for obstreperousness.

Patients like Mr. Cirelli who have severe chronic pain do not sweat or have tachycardia or hypertension but they usually guard the part that hurts and often have a generalized lack of spontaneous movement. They may appear anxious or depressed, withdrawn or angry, and may have difficulty relating to others, sleeping, concentrating, or eating.

Since I frequently work with patients who have chronic neuropathic pain, I was able to believe Mr. Cirelli. I pointed out my findings to his physicians and nurses, and suggested that his personality might be very different if he had less severe pain. They were still skeptical but concurred that we would not be able to make a diagnosis unless we relieved his pain. At my recommendation they agreed to initiate opioids and high-dose corticosteroids, which are often effective for neuropathic pain.

Within 48 hours Mr. Cirelli was a different person. His pain was now only mild, which was acceptable to him. He showed me how he could now put his right arm above his head with little discomfort. He readily agreed to a physical examination and to the CT scan and biopsy necessary to make a diagnosis. The nurses remarked on how affable and talkative he was and how helpful he had been to other patients on the ward. He was able to sleep through the night, eat, and interact with others. The relief of his chronic pain had been dramatic and, according to his family, he had become himself again.

Mr. Cirelli's neuropathic pain was a clue to his underlying pathology. Had it been recognized sooner, he would have suffered less, his lung cancer may have been discovered sooner, and his hand strength might have been preserved. When sought for, the signs of chronic pain are often apparent in a variety of cancer patients whose complaints might otherwise seem unfounded. They may also be recognized in patients with intense pain of nonmalignant origin, such as chronic arthritis, diabetic neuropathy, or post-herpetic neuralgia.

MEASURE THE PAIN AND THE DISTRESS IT CAUSES

The AHCPR guidelines stress that "the patient's self-report should be the primary source of assessment." In this respect, pain is unique. While we do ask a diabetic patient about his symptoms, physicians usually rely on the blood glucose and ketone levels to adjust insulin doses. But to determine the effectiveness of a pain-relief regimen, we must rely on the patient to *tell us* how his pain has changed after therapy. No one but the patient can accurately report his pain—not the nurses caring for him, not his family, not his friends. No matter how well trained we are or how well we know our patients, numerous studies have shown that all of us significantly underestimate the intensity of patients' pain.

Of course, people differ in how they experience pain. If you ask five people with broken arms to rate how much pain they are having, you are likely to get five different answers. But if you give them nothing to relieve their pain and ask them to rate it again sometime later, each patient is extremely likely to give you exactly the same rating as the first time. Numerous studies have shown, in fact, that a patient's reports of pain are consistent, reproducible, and reliable. Pain ratings after treatment are just as accurate and are used to indicate the effectiveness of a specific treatment for that patient.

Pain rating scales are subjective, not objective. But they are still *accurate* and they provide a *number* that represents the intensity of a patient's pain. Just as they use blood glucose levels to gauge a patient's response to insulin, doctors and nurses can judge a patient's response to pain therapy by noting how the pain-intensity number changes. (I describe several types of rating scales below.)

Equally importantly, physicians and nurses can ask patients whether the degree of pain relief *is satisfactory to them.* For some patients, a pain rating of 6 on a scale from 0 (no pain) to 10 (the worst pain you can imagine) is fine. These patients can tolerate the pain better than they can the side effects caused by higher doses of analgesic. For others, a level of 2 or 3 must be achieved. Mr. Cirelli, for example, told me he had "no pain" after he began taking the corticosteroids and opioids. When I pressed him for a number, he said it was a 2 or a 3. In my experience, he is typical of patients with well-controlled chronic pain, for whom "no pain" is a level 2 or 3.

I often find it necessary to explain these concepts to those I work with so that they can help me relieve a patient's pain as quickly as possible. If nurses and house staff in your hospital are similarly unfamiliar with the importance of measuring pain, you might find the diabetes analogy useful. You might say something like,

> *If you were taking care of someone with diabetes, you wouldn't call his doctor and say, "The patient's blood glucose was bad, so I gave him some insulin and it got a little better." The doctor would have no idea how effective the insulin was or what the next dose of insulin should be. Well, it also makes no sense to say, "The patient's pain was bad, so I gave him a Percocet and now it's better."*
>
> *The tools we have to measure a patient's pain are just as reliable as those we use to measure his blood glucose. We just have to ask the patient to tell us how severe his pain is. Wouldn't it be better to be able to say to his doctor, "The patient said his pain was a 9 out of 10. I gave him two Percocet, and an hour later he said his pain level was a 7 and that he was not satisfied with that degree of pain relief"? This gives the doctor much more information: the two Percocet were inadequate and stronger medication will be required.*

I also encourage house staff to include a quantitative pain assessment in the daily progress notes of all patients with a significant complaint of pain, just as they would include the blood glucose level in the progress notes of a patient with diabetes. Since the Joint Commission on Accreditation of Healthcare Organizations (JCAHO) has mandated the documentation of the level of pain and pain relief, many hospitals have modified their TPR (temperature, pulse, and respiration) sheets to include a continuous record of patients' pain level and whether or not the degree of pain relief is satisfactory to them (Figure 4.1). Studies have shown that as a result, pain control and patient satisfaction significantly increased.

The word scales and numerical scales used in the examples above are only two of a number of tools that patients can use to measure their pain. These tools have been extensively tested in research settings and found to be valid and reliable; they are easy to administer and to understand. They are designed to be used by patients, their families, their physicians, and other health professionals. If you offer a variety of types of scales and tools, patients and their families can choose one that makes the most sense to them and then learn from someone in your office exactly how to use it.

TEMPERATURE

		Month-Day-Year
		Post Adm/Post-Op

Hours of Day: 4 8 12 4 8 12 4 8 12 4 8 12 4 8 12 4 8 12 4 8 12 4 8 12 4 8 12 4 8 12 4 8 12 4 8 12 4 8 12 4 8 12 4 8 12 4 8 12

PULSE (RED) 160 ... 150 ... 140 ... 130 ... 120 ... 110 ... 100 ... 90 ... 80 ... 70 ... 60 ... 50 ... 40

TEMP C: 41 40 39 38 37 36 35

RECTAL ○ - RECTAL X - TYMPANIC ○ - ORAL

Respiration: 10

Pain Intensity: 10 5 0

Relief Acceptable (Y/N)

Weight

N D E N D E N D E N D E N D E N D E N D E

Blood Pressure

INTAKE
- Oral
- Tube Feeding
- Supplements
- Intravenous
- Blood Products
- TPN/PPN/Lipids
- 8 Hour Total
- 24 Hour Total

OUTPUT
- Urine
- Emesis/NG
- Stool
- 8 Hour Total
- 24 Hour Total

FORM 56-09805 TEMP A

4.1 Memorial Sloan-Kettering Vital Sign Sheet Incorporating a Pain Documentation Form. From M. Bookbinder, M. Kiss, N. Coyle, et al., Improving pain management practices, in *Cancer Pain Management,* 2nd ed., D. B. McGuire, C. H. Yarbo, and B. R. Ferrell (eds), Sudbury, Mass.: Jones and Bartlett, 1995; reprinted with permission.

INTENSITY SCALES

VISUAL ANALOG SCALE.   A Visual Analog Scale (VAS) is a 10-cm hor-
izontal or vertical unruled line anchored at its ends by numbers or
words describing the two extremes of a symptom. In the case of pain, for
example, one end is labeled "0" or "No pain" and the other end "10" or
"Worst possible pain" (Figure 4.2a).

But patients with cancer often have more than one pain. While the
pains might be equally intense, one may be more *distressing* than another. For example, neuropathic pain, such as Mr. Cirelli's, is usually
more distressing than visceral pain, such as that caused by an enlarged
liver. To unravel complex pain syndromes, it is useful to determine not
only the intensity of various pains but the associated distress. A VAS can
also be used here; the ends would be labeled "No distress" and "Un-
bearable distress" (Figure 4.2b).

Patients usually need instruction in using a VAS for the first time.
After explaining the meaning of the two ends of the scale, the clinician
asks the patient to make a mark on the line that reflects his present pain
intensity, then to use a ruler to measure how far this mark is from the
"No pain" end of the scale. This distance is the *pain intensity rating*. The
process can be repeated to determine the average, worst, and mildest
pain intensity over the preceding few weeks and to measure the effectiveness of drugs and of nonpharmacologic therapies.

For example, a patient with breast cancer metastatic to her bones who
is taking only acetaminophen might have largely uncontrolled pain. She
would indicate this on a VAS by making a mark close to the "Worst possible pain" end of the scale. If the mark were 8.5 cm from the "No pain"
end, her pain intensity would be 8.5. An hour or so after taking two pills
of acetaminophen with oxycodone, the patient would make a new mark
to represent how much pain she was having, then remeasure. The distance might now be 4 cm, and her pain intensity would be 4. The drop
from 8.5 to 4 indicates that the pills have been quite effective.

If you feel that a patient will not be able to do these measurements
easily, choose a scale that is already ruled in 1-cm increments, with each
mark numbered (0, 1, 2, etc., as shown in Figure 4.2a and b). This ruled
scale is not quite as accurate as the unruled one, because patients tend
to choose a whole number rather than a fraction of one, but it is adequate
for clinical purposes and is very reliable.

Most patients have no difficulty using a VAS. The scales are nonin-
trusive, and patients understand the concepts of assigning a number to

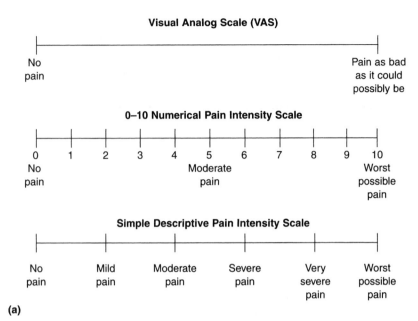

Visual Analog Scale (VAS)

No	Pain as bad
pain	as it could
	possibly be

0–10 Numerical Pain Intensity Scale

0	1	2	3	4	5	6	7	8	9	10
No					Moderate					Worst
pain					pain					possible
										pain

Simple Descriptive Pain Intensity Scale

No	Mild	Moderate	Severe	Very	Worst
pain	pain	pain	pain	severe	possible
				pain	pain

(a)

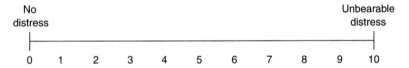

Visual Analog Scale (VAS)

No	Unbearable
distress	distress

0	1	2	3	4	5	6	7	8	9	10

0–10 Numerical Pain Distress Scale

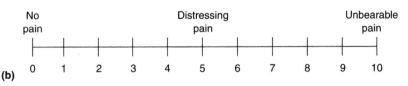

No	Distressing	Unbearable
pain	pain	pain

0	1	2	3	4	5	6	7	8	9	10

(b)

4.2 (a) Pain Intensity Scales and (b) Pain Distress Scales. A 10-cm baseline is recommended for VAS scales and for numerical and descriptive scales used as graphic rating scales. From the Acute Pain Management Guideline Panel, Agency for Health Care Policy and Research, Rockville, Md., 1992 and 1994.

reflect the intensity of their pain and using the scales to help them communicate how effective the pain therapy has been. A disadvantage sometimes noted for these scales is that they rate only the intensity of the pain, not its quality or the degree of functional or psychological and social disability it induces. And some people cannot understand the abstract concept that a larger or smaller number reflects increasing or decreasing pain. These patients always assign the same number even though they clearly are experiencing varying pain intensities.

WORD SCALES.   For some people, it is simpler and more intuitive to rate their pain or distress on a scale that uses words instead of numbers. Word scales (descriptive scales) have been found to be particularly useful for patients over 70. Instead of asking them to make a mark on a line or assign a number to quantitate the pain, ask them whether they have *No pain* or pain that is *Mild, Moderate, Severe, Very severe,* or *Worst possible.* This scale is called a Simple Descriptive Pain Intensity Scale (Figure 4.2a). Another word scale gives the patient the choice of *None, Mild, Moderate, Severe,* or *Excruciating* to describe his pain.

There is also a word scale for the distress caused by the pain. The patient chooses a word to indicate whether his distress level is *None, Annoying, Uncomfortable, Dreadful, Horrible,* or *Agonizing.* These words have been extensively tested for their ability to discriminate among different degrees of pain intensity; to maintain the reliability of the scale, these specific words must be used.

Just as with the number scales, physicians can use any of these word scales to get an idea of the range of pain and its associated distress that a patient has experienced throughout the day. Patients simply select which word best describes the most severe and which describes the mildest pain they have had that day.

PAIN ASSESSMENT FORMS

A minority of patients cannot use numbers or words to quantify their pain, the distress it is causing, or the efficacy of therapy. For them, I rely on comprehensive assessment forms (or tools) that include a measure not only of pain intensity but also of other functional dimensions that reflect the impact of the pain on the patient's day-to-day life. These tools are also easy to use and take no more than five to ten minutes to complete.

MEMORIAL PAIN ASSESSMENT CARD.   The Memorial Pain Assessment Card (MPAC) (Figure 4.3) was originally developed by the Analgesic

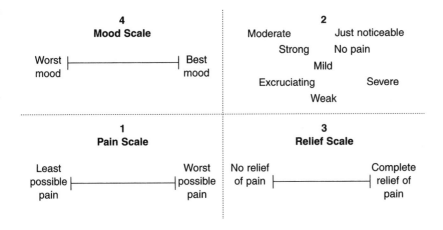

4.3 Memorial Sloan-Kettering Pain Assessment Card. The card is folded along the dotted line so that each measure is presented to the patient separately in the numbered order. From B. Fishman, S. Pasternak, S. L. Wallenstein, R. W. Houde, F. C. Holland, and K. M. Foley, The Memorial Pain Assessment Card: a valid instrument for the evaluation of cancer pain, *Cancer*, 60:1151–1158, 1987; copyright © 1987 American Cancer Society; with permission of Wiley-Liss, Inc., a subsidiary of John Wiley & Sons, Inc.

Studies Section of Memorial Sloan-Kettering Cancer Center to evaluate the relative potencies of new drugs. It was found, however, to correlate well with other validated measures of pain and psychological distress that take much longer to complete. It's portable—it fits in a coat or jacket pocket—and, when folded to allow each scale to be shown to the patient separately, allows measurement not only of pain *intensity* but also of pain *quality*, pain *relief*, and patient *mood*.

WISCONSIN BRIEF PAIN INVENTORY. One of the most widely used forms, which is extremely useful in unraveling and managing complicated pain problems, is the tool developed by the Pain Research Group at the University of Wisconsin–Madison Medical School (Figure 4.4). This Brief Pain Inventory, which can be reproduced for inclusion in the patient's chart, records the location of each pain (on a diagram); the worst, least, and average pain intensity and the level "right now"; the degree of relief that pain treatments have provided; and the functional consequences of the pain.

The functional consequences, such as disturbances in physical activity, mood, walking ability, relationships with others, sleep, and enjoy-

Brief Pain Inventory (Short Form)

Date:_____/_____/_____   Time:_____

Name:_____ _____ _____

Last   First   Middle Initial

1. Throughout our lives, most of us have had pain from time to time (such as minor headaches, sprains, and toothaches). Have you had pain other than these everyday kinds of pain today?

    1.   Yes   2.   No

2. On the diagram, shade in the areas where you feel pain. Put an X on the area that hurts the most.

3. Please rate your pain by circling the one number that best describes your pain at its **worst** in the last 24 hours.

0	1	2	3	4	5	6	7	8	9	10
No Pain										Pain as bad as you can imagine

4. Please rate your pain by circling the one number that best describes your pain at its **least** in the last 24 hours.

0	1	2	3	4	5	6	7	8	9	10
No Pain										Pain as bad as you can imagine

5. Please rate your pain by circling the one number that best describes your pain on the **average.**

0	1	2	3	4	5	6	7	8	9	10
No Pain										Pain as bad as you can imagine

6. Please rate your pain by circling the one number that tells how much pain you have **right now.**

0	1	2	3	4	5	6	7	8	9	10
No Pain										Pain as bad as you can imagine

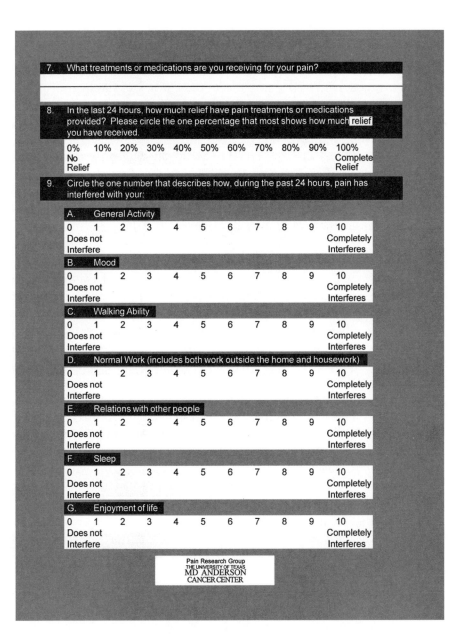

7. What treatments or medications are you receiving for your pain?

8. In the last 24 hours, how much relief have pain treatments or medications provided? Please circle the one percentage that most shows how much relief you have received.

0%	10%	20%	30%	40%	50%	60%	70%	80%	90%	100%
No Relief										Complete Relief

9. Circle the one number that describes how, during the past 24 hours, pain has interfered with your:

A. General Activity

0	1	2	3	4	5	6	7	8	9	10
Does not Interfere										Completely Interferes

B. Mood

0	1	2	3	4	5	6	7	8	9	10
Does not Interfere										Completely Interferes

C. Walking Ability

0	1	2	3	4	5	6	7	8	9	10
Does not Interfere										Completely Interferes

D. Normal Work (includes both work outside the home and housework)

0	1	2	3	4	5	6	7	8	9	10
Does not Interfere										Completely Interferes

E. Relations with other people

0	1	2	3	4	5	6	7	8	9	10
Does not Interfere										Completely Interferes

F. Sleep

0	1	2	3	4	5	6	7	8	9	10
Does not Interfere										Completely Interferes

G. Enjoyment of life

0	1	2	3	4	5	6	7	8	9	10
Does not Interfere										Completely Interferes

Pain Research Group
THE UNIVERSITY OF TEXAS
MD ANDERSON
CANCER CENTER

4.4 Wisconsin Brief Pain Inventory. From the University of Texas M. D. Anderson Cancer Center; reprinted with permission.

ment of life, can be very sensitive indicators that a patient's pain is unrelieved. Even patients who cannot tell you whether their pain "number" has changed, or cannot give you a word to describe it, report changes in their functional levels that indicate the efficacy of the treatment. Patients' families can help as well, completing the assessments at home after changes in the patient's pain-relief regimen and reporting the results to you by phone.

The functional changes noted in Mr. Cirelli's behavior, for example, heralded the relief of his pain. From a bedridden, depressed, withdrawn person with a very short temper and attention span he became someone who was voluble, helpful, interactive, and cooperative. When his pain was relieved, the disturbances disappeared.

PAIN DIARIES

The VAS, word scales, MPAC, and Wisconsin Brief Pain Inventory provide sufficient information for designing pain-relief regimens for most patients. But there can be cases in which the regimen seems to be working only part of the time. Pain diaries are useful here. In the diary, patients record the time of day they took their pain medicine, the pain intensity rating before and after they took it, the type of pain medicine, and any other comments they feel are relevant (e.g., what they were doing when the pain occurred). A sample diary page is shown in Figure 4.5.

For patients who complain of being too sedated, diaries can help determine whether they're taking too much medicine, or taking the correct dose but too often. And diaries are useful for patients who have so-called *breakthrough pains*, moderate to excruciating acute pains that occur intermittently, often on a background of well-controlled chronic pain. There are three types of breakthrough pain: *end-of-dose pain*, which is pain that recurs before the next regularly scheduled dose of medication is due; *incident pain*, which is directly related to an activity (such as turning over in bed); and *spontaneous pain*, which occurs unpredictably.

Diaries are helpful in determining which kind(s) of breakthrough pain(s) patients are experiencing. For many, the pattern that emerges will reveal end-of-dose pain or incident pain. You can then devise a plan to prevent the anticipated pains. For example, if the pain recurs four hours before the next sustained-release morphine pill is due (i.e., is end-of-dose pain), you can decrease the dosing interval to eight hours. Or if a patient's pain reliably exacerbates with movement (i.e., is incident pain), a short-acting medication can be given thirty minutes to an hour

You can use a chart like this to rate your pain and to keep a record of how well the medicine is working. Write the information in the chart. Use the pain intensity scale to rate your pain before and after you take the medicine.

Pain Intensity Scale

0   1   2   3   4   5   6   7   8   9   10

No pain   Medium pain   Worst pain

Date	Time	Pain intensity scale rating.	Medicine I took.	Pain intensity scale rating 1 hour after taking the medicine.	What I was doing when I felt the pain.
1/3/94	2:35	6	two aspirin tablets	3	Sitting at my desk and reading.

4.5 Pain Diary. From the Agency for Health Care Policy and Research, Rockville, Md.

before the patient gets out of bed, or an immediate-acting agent can be given five or ten minutes before.

Finally, diaries are essential to solve the mysteries of those few patients who have a pain recurrence pattern that seems to make no pharmacologic sense. Miss Alexander was such a patient.

The Problem of the Pain Pattern That Makes No Sense

Miss Alexander was a 32-year-old woman receiving chemotherapy for metastatic ovarian cancer. She had worked in her father's business since her high school graduation, and had lived in her own apartment until the side effects of the chemotherapy forced her to move back to her parents' home.

Miss Alexander had abdominal pain that, despite my efforts at changing her medication dose and schedule, seemed never to come under satisfactory control. I asked her to keep a pain diary. In the diary she recorded that she took sustained-release morphine at 6 a.m., 2 p.m., and 10 p.m. At 7 a.m., before setting out for work, she usually took a dose of immediate-acting morphine. Using a scale of 0 to 10, she recorded her pain intensity before each dose of morphine and its intensity an hour or so later.

She had been taking the same morphine doses for about a week when she came to the office. I reviewed the diary and graphed the pain intensity (0 to 10) on the y axis and the time of day on the x axis (Figure 4.6). I noted that her pain intensity was highest on weekends and between 7 p.m. and 10 p.m. on weekdays. Her pain relief was satisfactory at all other times.

There is nothing I know about morphine's pharmacology that could explain why sustained-release morphine would be effective for eight hours in the daytime on weekdays and overnight, but not on weekends or weekday evenings. As I wondered what other factors might be involved, I considered that it might be difficult for Miss Alexander, a formerly independent, lively young woman, to have to return from work to her conservative family home every night and weekend. So I questioned her about this. She replied,

> When I'm at Dad's office, there's plenty to keep me occupied. I do some work, though not as much as before, and I can visit with my friends. But there's not much to do at home. And Mom keeps asking me all the time, "How are you doing? Are you having any pain? Is there anything I can get you?" or "What did the doctor say today, honey?" Oh, sometimes there's a TV program I like, or I can get caught up in a book I'm reading. The pain's not so bad, then—kind of like it is at the office. But most of the time, it's much worse.

At home, it seemed, there wasn't much to take her mind off her cancer or her loss of independence, and her pain was more intense and caused her more distress. Since she had found a few things that helped, I suggested she try to continue to fill her evenings and weekends watching rented movies or listening to books on tape, and to ask her friends from the office to visit or take her with them on weekend outings. Happily, this strategy was effective and her pain came under satisfactory con-

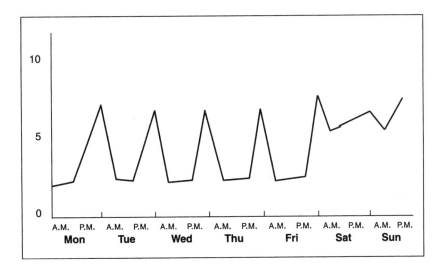

4.6   Miss Alexander's Pain Pattern

trol without any further changes in dose or timing of medication. The diary was the key—once I knew *when* it hurt, I could figure out *why*.

COMPREHENSIVELY EVALUATE THE PATIENT

Further questioning includes exploring (1) the temporal aspects of the pain (is it acute, chronic, or breakthrough pain?), (2) its quality (is it somatic, visceral, or neuropathic?), and (3) its similarity to pain syndromes typically seen in cancer patients. Depending on the causes you think likely, other diagnostic tests should follow. Finally, to uncover sources of anxiety and distress not caused by pain (but potentially making the pain worse), patients are evaluated for psychological, social, financial, and spiritual problems.

TEMPORAL ASPECTS OF PAIN: ACUTE, CHRONIC, OR BREAKTHROUGH

Cancer patients usually have a mixture of chronic and breakthrough pains. To maximize pain relief while minimizing side effects, it is useful to determine both the intensity of the chronic pain and the characteristics of the breakthrough pains and to treat each with agents appropriate for them.

Long-acting agents (e.g., methadone) or sustained-release formulations of short-acting agents (e.g., transdermal fentanyl, sustained-release oxycodone or morphine) are used to keep the chronic pain at an acceptably low level (e.g., level 2 or 3). The peak blood level of opioids delivered in these preparations is lower than with the other formulations and they are therefore less sedating.

End-of-dose breakthrough pains, once recognized, are easy to prevent by increasing the frequency of dosing of long-acting or sustained-release agents. Spontaneous pains and incident pains, which can be precipitated by movement, the Valsalva maneuver, or even flatulence, are more difficult to manage. A patient with bony metastases, for example, may have reasonable control of chronic pain without excessive sedation but develop severe pain when rising from a bed or chair. Agents with a quick onset of action (hydromorphone, morphine, oxycodone) and immediate-acting agents (the transmucosal formulation of fentanyl citrate) can be added either prophylactically for activities expected to cause incident pain or episodically when spontaneous pains occur. But the higher peak opioid levels associated with these agents often cause sedation. Patients often must endure this increased sedation to achieve acceptable pain relief.

Pain Quality: Somatic, Visceral, or Neuropathic

Determining the quality of cancer pain is often helpful in identifying the site of tissue injury, because somatic, visceral, and neuropathic pains each have a characteristic presentation. Somatic and visceral pains are common in people who do not have cancer. Other than in patients with disk disease, diabetic neuropathy, or herpes zoster, however, lesions that cause neuropathic pain rarely occur in people who do not have cancer or AIDS.

SOMATIC PAIN.   Somatic pain arises from skin and subcutaneous tissues, bone, muscle, blood vessels, and connective tissues. It is usually described as *constant, dull,* and *aching, increased by movement,* and *localized to the area of the lesion.* Patients with arthritis or bony metastases will describe their chronic pain in words similar to these. Incident pain (described above), however, is not dull but rather a sharp, intense somatic pain caused by movement of a bone containing a metastasis.

VISCERAL PAIN.   Visceral pain arises from organs and the lining of body cavities. The pain caused by a myocardial infarction is a typical example of a visceral pain. It is often a *poorly localized, deep, aching* discom-

---

PRACTICE POINTS: DISTINGUISHING AMONG SOMATIC, VISCERAL, AND NEUROPATHIC PAINS

- Somatic pain (e.g., arthritis, bone metastases) is constant, dull, and aching, increased by movement, and localized to the area of the lesion.
- Visceral pain (e.g., myocardial ischemia, liver metastases) is poorly localized, deep, aching, cramping, twisting, or tearing.
- Neuropathic pain (e.g., sciatica, brachial plexus metastases) is burning, sharp, shooting, tingling, electrical, or shock-like.

---

fort, but it can feel like *cramping, squeezing, twisting,* or *tearing.* Patients with kidney invasion by tumor or a distended liver filled with metastases will have this type of pain. Visceral pain can localize to more superficial structures and, if it is intense, often radiates to larger areas, usually the muscle or skin innervated by the same spinal nerves that innervate the viscus. Pain in the left shoulder and arm of a patient with myocardial ischemia is an example of this phenomenon. Abdominal pains due to bowel obstruction by tumor also are visceral, but they have the intermittent, cycling quality that characterizes an obstruction from any cause.

NEUROPATHIC PAIN.   Neuropathic pain, the kind from which Mr. Cirelli was suffering, arises from peripheral nerves, the spinal cord, and the central nervous system. It is the most distressing type of pain. Neuropathic pain is usually poorly localized; it is often *burning* (as typically seen in diabetic neuropathy or herpes zoster) but can be described as *sharp, shooting, tingling, electrical,* or *shock-like.* With sufficient nerve damage, there may be associated *paresthesias, painful numbness, hyperesthesia,* or *sensory loss,* and, as in Mr. Cirelli, *weakness* and *muscle wasting. Allodynia,* pain caused by normal touch or by clothing, can also occur. Neuropathic pain can be limited to the site of the lesion, but it often radiates or is completely referred to distant sites.

RECOGNIZING CANCER-RELATED PAIN SYNDROMES

Cancer-related pain syndromes are most often caused by nerve damage. The cancer usually has spread to the bone or tissue adjacent to the nerve, and as it grows it compresses the nerve or its blood supply, causing neuropathic pain and eventual nerve death. Recognizing neuropathic pain, therefore, is crucial to identifying patients with lesions of (1) cranial nerves as they exit the skull, (2) nerve plexi (cervical, brachial, and lumbosacral), (3) peripheral nerves, and, most dangerously, (4) the spinal cord (from tumors in vertebral bodies and the epidural space) (Foley 1987).

CRANIAL NERVES.　Metastases to the *jugular foramen* cause occipital and ipsilateral shoulder pain along with dysfunction of cranial nerves 9 to 12 that exit through the foramen. Disease of the *sphenoid sinus* mimics sinusitis, but patients with tumor infiltration usually have a more severe headache and they may have diplopia due to infiltration or edema of the sixth cranial nerve. Patients with tumor infiltration of the cranial nerves have pain in the head and face in the distribution of the nerve involved, often the ninth or the trigeminal.

NERVE PLEXI.　Brachial or lumbosacral plexus infiltration can be particularly difficult to diagnose, but it can herald primary or recurrent tumors. In the brachial plexus, the nerves lower in the plexus (C7 and T1) are most likely to be directly invaded by tumor, as were Mr. Cirelli's. Patients with either brachial or lumbosacral plexus infiltrations present, as did Mr. Cirelli, with deep, aching, often shooting pains and, later, muscle atrophy in the groups innervated. MRI (magnetic resonance imaging) may reveal tumor infiltration, and treatment can be planned.

The pain of radiation fibrosis may mimic that of recurrent cancer in the brachial plexus, but it has a different distribution. Because the clavicle protects the nerves lower in the plexus, nerves located in the upper part of the plexus (C5 and C6) are most commonly affected by radiation damage. The pain and weakness will be in the C5,6 distribution; an EMG (electromyogram) will document the abnormality.

PERIPHERAL NERVES.　The *post-mastectomy* and *post-thoracotomy* pain syndromes are caused by diseases of peripheral nerves. Prompt recognition of these syndromes is particularly important because treatment within six months of their onset is usually very effective.

The term *post-mastectomy* syndrome is something of a misnomer because it can occur in women who undergo any type of breast surgery, from lumpectomy to radical mastectomy. It is a common problem: 4 to 10 percent of women who undergo breast surgery develop this syndrome. The pain can appear immediately or as late as six months after the surgery. A patient with post-mastectomy syndrome feels a burning, constricting sensation in her posterior arm, axilla, and anterior chest wall in the area where she has lost sensation due to the surgery. Her chest wall may be hyperesthetic or dysesthetic. The patient finds it most comfortable to keep her arm flexed, and she may therefore develop a frozen shoulder. Post-mastectomy pain is caused by a neuroma of the intercostobrachial nerve (a branch of T1,2), which was cut during surgery. There is often an associated trigger point (a place where the pain can be reproduced by touching that part of the skin) in the axilla or anterior chest wall.

Similarly, patients who have had thoracotomies can develop post-thoracotomy syndrome. These patients describe an aching and burning sensation in the distribution of the incision and numbness of the skin in that area. There is exquisite point tenderness at both ends of the scar. The post-thoracotomy syndrome is caused by pulling or cutting of the intercostal nerve.

As you can imagine, suffering caused by either of these syndromes can be extreme, especially for those whose cancer has been cured. For these patients, the pain serves as a reminder both of the experience and of the potential for cancer recurrence. Early diagnosis and prompt treatment can eliminate this pain.

VERTEBRAL LESIONS.   Patients with *odontoid* and *atlas* fractures present with severe neck pain radiating over the posterior part of the skull to the vertex, and neck stiffness. The symptoms may mimic meningitis and are particularly dangerous because the patient is at risk for developing paraplegia or quadriplegia from the subluxation and spinal cord or brainstem compression.

Metastases to C7 often do not cause neck pain, but patients experience pain between the scapulae. Early detection will prevent cervical cord compression, but these lesions are often missed because films are taken only of the thoracic spine and, if the findings are normal, no bone scan is done. Similarly, *lesions of T12* can present as isolated hip pain, as occurred in Mr. Young (described at the beginning of this chapter). Here also, if hip, pelvis, and thoracic spine films reveal no abnormalities, a bone scan is indicated. For either lesion, CT or MRI will be required to plan therapy. The C7 and T12 referred pain syndromes are important to recognize, but are rare.

Epidural disease in cancer patients usually does not cause a unique pain syndrome. It presents most commonly as *back pain* in the area of the vertebral metastasis, with or without radiation in the distribution of the spinal nerves exiting the spinal cord at that level. Its similarity to the pain of benign disk disease is a source of dangerous diagnostic confusion.

PRACTICE POINTS: RECOGNIZING SPINAL CORD COMPRESSION

- Back pain may be the only finding.
- In a patient with back pain and findings consistent with metastases on a plain film of the spine in the area of the pain, the probability of invasion of the epidural space is approximately 70 percent. A radiculopathy raises this probability to 90 percent.
- Emergency MRI is indicated in these patients even when the neurologic exam is completely normal.
- Prompt recognition and therapy is the key to preserving ambulation; only 10 percent of patients with spinal cord compression who lose their ability to ambulate will ever regain it.

If a patient without cancer complains of back pain and there are no abnormal neurologic findings, most physicians would not order a plain film of the spine, let alone an MRI. They would treat him symptomatically. But in a cancer patient, back pain may be the only clue that he has a malignant epidural process and an impending cord compression. Thus evaluation of the back pain of a cancer patient must be much more aggressive than that of the patient without cancer.

Even with completely normal neurologic findings, there is about a 70 percent chance that a cancer patient with back pain and abnormal plain films of the spine has epidural metastases. This very important fact is not widely known, and many physicians wait for abnormal physical findings before pursuing further diagnostic tests. Some let the decision rest on the results of the bone scan, but as many as 5 percent of cancer patients with normal findings will have metastatic bony disease demonstrated on MRI. Bone scans are of very little value as a screening test for patients with multiple myeloma, because the results are usually normal even in the presence of extensive bony disease.

MRI of the entire spine should be obtained immediately (Janjan 1997). MRI is as sensitive and specific as CT myelography, which is a more uncomfortable procedure and potentially associated with more complications. Further, in patients whose cancer involves more than one epidural site, MRI can reveal additional lesions above and below the area of pain that will need to be included in the radiation field.

Epidural metastatic disease must be diagnosed and treated before any neurologic abnormalities develop, because, once they appear, they are often irreversible. If patients are treated while they are still ambulatory, they have about a 90 percent chance of remaining so. If they become paraparetic the odds drop to 40 to 50 percent, and only 10 percent of patients who lose their ability to walk because cancer is compressing their spinal cord will ever walk again.

PSYCHOLOGICAL, SOCIAL, FINANCIAL, AND SPIRITUAL SOURCES OF ANXIETY OR DISTRESS

Asking "How are you within yourself?" (Byock 1997) is a wonderful way to start a conversation designed to detect the psychological, social, financial, or spiritual problems that often occur in cancer patients with pain and that by themselves can cause distress even in those without pain. An evaluation in each of these areas completes the initial pain assessment. And, because patients' reactions to pain are modified by their families' reactions and abilities to cope with someone in pain, a determination must be made of how the family is functioning. For patients cared for by hospice teams, the nurse, social worker, and chaplain will routinely do these assessments and communicate the results to you.

The model developed by Betty Rolling Ferrell, Ph.D., R.N., F.A.A.N., associate research scientist at City of Hope National Medical Center, provides a framework for the assessment (Figure 4.7). This model explores the extensive impact of pain on all dimensions of the quality of a patient's life: physical, psychological, social, and spiritual (Ferrell and Rhiner 1991). We have already reviewed how to assess the physical impairments induced by pain; I discuss here how to assess the psychological, social, and spiritual causes.

PSYCHOLOGICAL CAUSES. Psychological effects of cancer pain include both the emotional response to the pain (the affective dimension) and how the patient thinks about the pain (the cognitive dimension). Delirium, an organic mental disorder that particularly affects cancer patients, is not caused by the pain itself but is a source of great distress.

Affective Dimension. People who have uncontrolled pain are usually unable to feel much pleasure. Happiness, even of a momentary kind, is very hard for them to imagine. In addition, patients in pain are often

<table>
<tr><td>
**Physical Well-Being
and Associated Symptoms**
Functional Ability
Strength/Fatigue
Sleep and Rest
Nausea
Appetite
Constipation
</td><td>
Psychological Well-Being
Anxiety
Depression
Enjoyment/Leisure
Pain Distress
Happiness
Fear
Cognition/Attention
</td></tr>
</table>

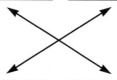

<table>
<tr><td>
Social Concerns
Caregiver Burden
Roles and Relationships
Affection/Sexual Function
Appearance
</td><td>
Spiritual Well-Being
Suffering
Meaning of Pain
Religiosity
</td></tr>
</table>

4.7   Effects of Pain on Dimensions of the Quality of Life.   From B. R. Ferrell and M. Rhiner, High-tech comfort: ethical issues in cancer pain management for the 1990s, *Journal of Clinical Ethics,* 2:108–112, 1991; copyright 1991 by *The Journal of Clinical Ethics;* all rights reserved.

anxious or depressed and are unable to focus their attention on anything other than the pain. Pain also exacerbates depression, which is the strongest contributing factor to suicidal ideation in cancer patients.

Anxiety and depression are, of course, not limited to cancer patients with pain—they are the most common psychological problems of all patients with cancer. Assessment and management of patients with depression and anxiety will be discussed in Chapter 7.

Cognitive Dimension.   The cognitive dimension, which includes families' and patients' attitudes, beliefs, and knowledge about pain and its treatment, affects their interpretation of new pains and their acceptance of proposed changes in treatment regimens. For example, it may be psychologically easier for the family to ignore worsening pain than to face the implications of the patient's worsening condition. In their denial of the patient's impending death, they may not adequately treat his escalating pain. Families are no better than physicians at guessing the intensity of the patient's pain, and the more different their perception is from what the patient is actually feeling, the more stress they experience (Miaskowki et al. 1997).

PRACTICE POINTS: ASSESSING THE COGNITIVE DIMENSIONS OF PAIN

- Assess the family's desire for information, willingness to acquire new skills, and psychological needs.
- Assess the family caregiver's personal characteristics (e.g., age, sex) and how those characteristics affect caregiving efforts.
- Take the opportunity to reassure the patient and family that the patient's pain will be controlled and that the family will be supported in its caregiving efforts.
- Discover what the pain means to the patient; it will affect both emotional response to pain and ability to cope with it.
- Determine the patient's expectations about the extent of pain relief, and work to align these expectations with what you know to be clinical reality.

Gaining a family's cooperation begins with assessing its desire for information, willingness to acquire new skills, and psychological needs. Physicians can begin this process by addressing unasked family questions such as:

"How bad is his pain likely to get in the future?"
"Will we have help managing Mom's pain at home?"
"Who will answer our questions as they arise?"

Family members can be reassured that we will be able to relieve the pain, no matter how intense it becomes, and that we will not abandon them. They will know that we'll work with them and help them cope with the stresses they are likely to experience as they care for the patient at home.

A number of personal characteristics can help us anticipate how caregivers are likely to help manage the patient's pain. Younger couples, for example, are more likely to be frustrated and angry, but they are less likely than older couples to be overwhelmed and feel depressed. Women tend to experience and express more distress and depression but are more understanding of the patient's physical and emotional needs, while men focus on financial matters and household chores.

In addition to the family assessment, we also need to know what patients are thinking and feeling. We have to determine what the pain means to them, because this will affect their emotional response to and ability to cope with the pain. Does the patient, for example, believe his pain to be a manifestation of progressive disease? People who have this belief are more likely to be depressed or anxious or to report more pain than those who do not. Alternatively, the patient may regard his pain as a challenge. If so, he will probably cope better and be less depressed than someone who views pain as a punishment.

We must also ascertain patients' therapeutic expectations. A patient with extensive bony metastases is unlikely to achieve complete pain relief without side effects if the only medication she takes is a sustained-release morphine preparation. She may have such an expectation, however, and question the polypharmacy that is prescribed. Once the source of confusion is elicited, the patient's expectations can be better aligned with the physician's.

Presentations of Delirium. Delirium is the most common organic mental disorder affecting cancer patients. While not caused by pain, delirium can be caused by the medicines used to treat it, and it can present as uncontrolled pain. Metabolic disruptions and the dying process itself also cause delirium. Miss Monroe was a patient of mine who experienced delirium from a number of causes.

The Problem of Delirium

Miss Monroe was a 62-year-old elementary school teacher who developed multiple myeloma. She was sent to me from her general internist, who had made the diagnosis during his evaluation of her complaints of back pain and anemia. MRI revealed that her pain was due to an epidural spinal cord compression, and she was just finishing radiation therapy for this when she had her first episode of delirium.

Miss Monroe was accompanied on her visit by her niece, Sara, who lived with her while going to college. Sara had noted that her aunt was not always herself these days. Miss Monroe had previously been a very steady, matter-of-fact kind of person, friendly, generous, and caring. Her students loved her and her colleagues respected her. Lately, however, her behavior had become erratic. While much of the time she seemed her old self, at other times she appeared euphoric, at others depressed and tearful, and at still others angry for no apparent reason. She forgot things she never would have forgotten before and, increasingly, seemed distant. Sara missed the nightly talks they used to have about school and the strategy sessions for getting through the next day or week.

What Sara had noticed were the early signs of delirium. Miss Monroe's memory was impaired; she wasn't thinking clearly; she had poor judgment; and her mental status varied from normal to abnormal throughout the course of the day. Because her calcium, sodium, and blood glucose levels were normal, we believed her delirium was caused by the high-dose corticosteroids she had begun taking when her spinal cord compression was diagnosed. Steroid-induced delirium is by no means rare: in one study, as many as one-quarter of the cancer patients treated with high-dose prednisone or dexamethasone developed delirium.

Because her radiation therapy treatments were completed, her corticosteroids were tapered rapidly—and her mental status quickly returned to normal. But later in the course of her illness she had progressive bony disease that was refractory to therapy and began taking sustained-release morphine preparations for the pain. When the dose was escalated to improve pain control, Miss Monroe herself noticed a problem.

"I think I must be going crazy," she told me at one clinic visit. "A few months ago I was having nightmares, but that sort of made sense to me. After all, I'm under a lot of strain here; my cancer seems to be getting worse and not better, and a few bad dreams were not something I even considered mentioning to you. But lately, I'm seeing things that Sara doesn't see and talking with people I know can't be real because they died years ago! What is happening to me?"

Once again, Miss Monroe was suffering from delirium, manifested this time by hallucinations. The morphine was responsible. Her earlier nightmares had been caused by the morphine, and raising her dose had made the problem even worse. Her symptoms disappeared when she was switched to a different opioid.

Her final bout with delirium occurred as she was dying at home. Sara called me in tears one night at 3 a.m. to report a sudden major change in her aunt. Earlier that day Miss Monroe had been resting comfortably. Now, when Sara had tried to give her some pain medication, she refused and accused Sara of trying to poison her. Sara wasn't even sure that her aunt recognized her. Miss Monroe was restless, throwing off the bedcovers or "picking" at them, and was shouting at her, swearing, and refusing to be touched. Sara said she was about to call the police, but thought maybe I had some idea of what was going on.

I told her that the symptoms and signs indicated that her aunt had another, more severe form of delirium: Miss Monroe was confused and disoriented; her speech was not always coherent; she got worse at night; and she had no insight into her problem. I reassured Sara that none of this was her fault, that over three-quarters of dying patients experience delirium. I advised her to call the hospice nurse, and told her which medication to administer while she waited. Miss Monroe responded promptly. Three days later, she died peacefully at home.

During her illness, Miss Monroe displayed many of the symptoms of delirium: agitation, hallucinations, paranoid ideation, disordered thinking and perception, delusions, labile mood, and what is termed "psychomotor behavior"—picking at bedcovers, for example. Some delirious patients, however, experience a quiet delirium that can go undetected unless sought. Such patients are not agitated—they may be curled in bed in the fetal position. But delirium in any of its presentations is distressing and requires therapy. Untreated, both patients and their families suffer.

The causes of Miss Monroe's delirium included corticosteroids, opioids, and the terminal illness itself. She did not receive lorazepam (Ativan), which, paradoxically, can cause an agitated delirium. She also was not receiving anticholinergic agents, which, when combined with drugs with anticholinergic side effects, can cause a "cholinergic crisis," a life-threatening syndrome that includes high fevers and delirium. H_2 blockers (e.g., cimetidine), tricyclic antidepressants, and anticholinergic agents (e.g., diphenhydramine [Benadryl] or hydroxyzine [Atarax, Vistaril]) all have significant anticholinergic side effects and can contribute to a cholinergic crisis.

Other causes of delirium include structural brain lesions, encephalitis, hypoxia, hypercalcemia, renal or hepatic failure, electrolyte imbalance, nutritional deficiency (especially of B vitamins), and infection. As I discuss in Chapters 5 and 7, delirium from a number of these causes can often be treated effectively, even when the underlying problem cannot be reversed.

Role of the Mental Health Professional.   Immediate referral is needed to assess and treat the patient who is suicidal or who is delirious but not actively dying. But for the more routine patient with anxiety or depression, a formal psychological evaluation is not always needed. If pain is controlled but the patient is still anxious or depressed, a trial of one of the psychoactive medications discussed in Chapter 5 is often successful. If this is ineffective, patients often benefit from seeing a psychologist or psychiatrist. As is reviewed in Chapter 7 their anxiety and depression often respond to the therapy and ongoing support these professionals provide.

PRACTICE POINTS: ASSESSING DELIRIUM

- Delirium is characterized by:
  —a change in cognition that cannot be explained by dementia.
  —a disturbance of consciousness with reduced ability to focus, sustain, or shift attention.
  —a disturbance that develops within a short time and fluctuates throughout the day.
- Symptoms include: insomnia and daytime somnolence, nightmares, irritability, distractability, hypersensitivity to light and sound, anxiety, difficulty in concentrating or marshaling thoughts, hallucinations, delusions, emotional lability, attention deficits, and memory disturbances.
- Patients may appear hypoactive or extremely agitated.
- Precipitating factors include: metabolic derangements (hypercalcemia, hypo- or hyperglycemia, hypo- or hypernatremia, hypoxia, renal or hepatic failure), drugs (especially opioids, corticosteroids, and anticholinergic agents), nutritional deficiency (especially of B vitamins), infection, structural brain lesions, and encephalitis.

SOCIAL AND FINANCIAL CAUSES.   Some patients are suffering from what Cassell, in *The Nature of Suffering and the Goals of Medicine,* describes as a loss of "personhood." Cassell has developed a "topology of person" that explores the many dimensions of how illness can affect an individual's "personhood" and cause suffering. Personality and character will affect the response to illness, as will "the lived past . . . a story that has taken place over time, in many places, and involving countless others" (p. 43) and the family's lived past. The patient's cultural background, the many roles he has played (son, father, Little League coach, board chairman), and his associations and relationships are also determinants of suffering in response to illness. Grief over having to relinquish these activities and the accompanying loss of social standing can be a source of significant pain. Other sources include injuries to the body or unconscious mind, diminished possibilities of the self as a political being, loss of a secret life, dashed hopes for the perceived future, or loss of the transcendent dimension—the spirit. When disease progresses, these "aspects of personhood" may become "damaged" or lost. Knowledge that these roles may never be regained becomes an ongoing source of suffering.

Patients and their families also need an evaluation of the social and financial barriers to optimal pain relief. A basic assessment should include the family's living conditions and financial and insurance status. This information helps to determine, for example, whether financial help will be required for patients who need the more expensive pain medicines or a high-tech pain therapy such as intravenous or epidural opioid infusions. It will also reveal whether financial worries are causing insomnia, which exacerbates pain.

Cultural Context. Physicians will benefit from understanding cultural and religious aspects that affect patients' and families' attitudes toward cancer and pain and their ability to communicate their distress. Japanese and Italians, for example, have been found to associate cancer with death. If an Italian patient has pain caused by the cancer, it might serve as a trigger for thoughts of impending death, which would in turn exacerbate the pain experience. In other cultures, the social expectation is that pain should be tolerated; patients in such environments face disapproval from their families if they complain of pain. If you were unaware of the social pressures that led a patient to minimize his pain, you might easily underestimate his true pain intensity.

Similarly, religious teachings may affect a patient's preferences for pain therapy—a Buddhist, for example, may resist strong pain medication because she thinks it will weaken her spirit or cloud her consciousness sufficiently to impair her preparations for dying. An Orthodox Jew may refuse opioids fearing they will hasten his death, and he does not wish to do anything to shorten the life that God has given him.

There are a number of questions that can help us assess the cultural and religious attitudes, beliefs, and coping styles of patients and their families (Fong 1985). Answers to these questions should give us a better idea of how the patient and family communicate about pain and how they wish us to treat it.

Family Disruption. Other social sources of distress arise from disruptions in a person's normal family structure and her place in the community when she becomes a cancer patient. The entire family organization may be turned topsy-turvy when the person who was the breadwinner (or the homemaker) can no longer serve in that capacity.

Others must take over her tasks, which puts both social and financial stress on everyone in the family, including the person who has had to relinquish her accustomed role.

Role of the Social Worker.   Hospital social workers, or the social workers employed by home health agencies or hospice agencies, very effectively perform comprehensive assessments of patients' cultural and psychosocial needs and obtain help for families dealing with these issues. Even if families do not directly express these types of concerns, I encourage them to have at least one consultation with the social worker. This consultation often allows the social worker and the patient's family to develop a relationship that can be renewed as needed throughout the course of the patient's illness.

PRACTICE POINTS: QUESTIONS FOR ASSESSING CULTURAL ATTITUDES OF PATIENTS AND THEIR FAMILIES

- Is touching acceptable to you?
- What word do you use for pain?
- How will we know you are in pain?
- How does your family usually react to pain?
- How do you normally treat or cope with pain?
- Which foods are comforting or healing to you?
- Do you want your family near you when you are hurting?
- How does your family react to your pain?
- Do you see a folk healer when you are sick?
- How do you explain your illness or pain?
- What does the pain mean to you?
- Does the pain mean you are getting better or worse?
- Is it OK to take medication to relieve pain? If not, why?
- Do you want immediate pain relief or do you believe that you must wait until the pain is severe?
- What type of treatment do you want to control your pain?
- Do you read? Which languages?
- How best do you learn (reading, videos, etc.)?

(From Fink and Gates 1995, 34)

At the time of diagnosis and during the early phases of treatment, in addition to performing the psychological and social assessment, social workers may assist in treatment planning, solve insurance and other financial problems, and connect the patient and family with community social service agencies. Social workers can also advise physicians as to which families or patients need more intensive psychological support. They may themselves be able to provide the needed counseling and education in coping skills. If the disease later progresses, the social worker can continue to provide the patient and family members with psychological and social assessments and, for those who need it, intensive counseling or assistance in coping with impending death. I discuss these therapeutic roles of the social worker in more detail in Chapter 6.

SPIRITUAL CAUSES.   Spiritual well-being can modify the experience of pain. Studies have shown that while religious patients reported pain as often as those who were not religious, their pain levels were lower. Moreover, their anxiety, pain frequency, and pain intensity declined as their level of spiritual well-being increased.

Suffering and the Meaning of Pain.   Religious beliefs can have a profound effect on a patient's interpretation of his pain and suffering. Physical pain can exacerbate spiritual concerns, increasing the need for comfort and forgiveness or creating anger at what is perceived as abandonment in a time of need. *Suffering* and the *meaning of the pain* are two areas that are of particular importance to patients who have been referred to me with uncontrolled pain. They seek meaning for their suffering in the context of their religious teachings, and they need to understand the meaning of their pain.

Spiritual assessment is not the sole province of the hospital chaplain. Nurses, social workers, and physicians can assess patients and their families using one of a number of assessment tools, including several designed specifically to determine the interaction of pain and spiritual suffering (Taylor and Ersek 1995) or to identify the presence of spiritual suffering even in the absence of pain (Fitchett and Handzo 1998). As Dr. George Fitchett states, "The aim of spiritual assessment is not to exhaust the complexity or mystery of the spiritual dimension of life. The aim is to organize observations about people's spiritual beliefs, behaviors, and relationships in ways that enhance caregiving" (p. 791). His "7 × 7 model" incorporates spiritual assessment as part of a "holistic" patient assessment, which includes the biological (medical); psychological; family systems; psychosocial; ethnic, racial, and cultural; social issues; and spiritual dimensions. His spiritual assessment tool includes a variety of components that taken together describe the spiritual life of the patient. These include:

- *Belief and Meaning,* and affiliation with a formal religion.
- *Vocation and Obligation,* as these relate to beliefs and sense of meaning.
- *Experience and Emotions,* which identify reactions to direct contact with the sacred, divine, or demonic.
- *Courage and Growth,* which determine the rigidity of the current belief system and willingness to adapt it to new challenges.
- *Ritual and Practice,* which the patient feels should be performed.
- *Community,* the patient's affiliations and the nature of his participation.
- *Authority and Guidance,* which identify the source of authority for the patient's beliefs and his resources (including himself) in times of stress.

PRACTICE POINTS: QUESTIONS FOR REVEALING INTERACTIONS OF PAIN AND SPIRITUAL SUFFERING

- What do your religious teachings say about pain?
- Have your beliefs or values changed since you began having pain?
- Where do you get the strength to live with your pain?
- Do you find any value to living with suffering—has it ennobled you in any way?
- Does the pain affect your ability to practice your religion—does it, for example, interfere with prayer or attending church?
- Does the pain affect your relationship with God?

(From Fink and Gates 1995, 52)

I have heard a variety of answers to the questions developed by Fink and Gates (1995) to determine the interaction of pain and spiritual suffering. Many patients have told me that they had searched their consciences for reasons that God was allowing them to suffer. They felt they were being punished, as they had been as children when they had done something wrong, but they could not think what they had done to deserve such punishment. Some veterans have concluded that it was something they did in the war, saying that they wanted to "burn here" so they wouldn't have to "burn there" (see Chapter 2). They supposed the pain had to be a "just punishment" for their sins. Others have found deficiencies in their former relationships with other people or with God. In many who could find no cause for their suffering, a previously deep faith was profoundly shaken and its comforts were suddenly gone. They told me they felt alone and abandoned.

Role of the Spiritual Counselor.   These people need spiritual counseling and forgiveness if their suffering is to be ameliorated. Chaplains are key members of the hospice team, and our hospital, like many others, has on its staff specially trained pastoral counselors who can discuss with patients their feelings of abandonment by God and of punishment for unknown offenses, their fears of death or the afterlife, or their need for prayer or sacraments. Many patients want to know what they need to do to resolve outstanding spiritual issues before they die; for some this includes a confession or the resolution of outstanding arguments with friends or family members; for others, a marriage in the hospital room. For some, Dr. Ira Byock's "Five things of relationship completion: 'I forgive you'; 'Forgive me'; 'Thank you'; 'I love you'; and 'Good-bye'" are sufficient (Byock 1997, p. 140). For everyone, the chaplain has stressed the forgiving nature of God.

Chaplains can also enhance hope, help families understand how medicine can be a part of what they believe is ultimately God's healing role, and sustain them and their faith when physical healing is no longer possible. Many can provide comforting religious rituals such as meditation, prayer, sacraments, or the reading of sacred texts when the patient cannot participate in public religious services. They can also ascertain which rituals are important to those patients nearing the end of life and communicate these to the other staff working with the patient and family.

I encourage you to urge those of your patients who have good relationships with the clergy to seek increased support from them. Even patients and families who do not consider themselves religious and who have no formal religious affiliation may find relief for existential suffering through expert pastoral counseling. They may receive guidance in their search for the meaning of their suffering. In this way, patients can often receive all the comfort and forgiveness they need and die at peace; in reply to the question "If you died tomorrow, would anything be left undone?" they could answer, "No" (Byock 1997).

REEVALUATE WHEN THE PAIN PATTERN CHANGES

The final recommendation of the AHCPR guidelines is to assess each new pain. Pain assessment is an ongoing process, directed not only at determining the efficacy of the pain-relief regimen but also at detecting new pains so as to identify their causes. When the character, quality, or timing of the patient's pain changes, a new lesion is usually responsible. Disease may be advancing, a bone may have fractured, or a problem unrelated to the cancer may have developed. Frequent reassessment will detect these and enable us to institute effective therapy promptly.

SUMMARY

A comprehensive pain assessment is the foundation of effective pain therapy and is not hard to accomplish. The guidelines from the AHCPR are straightforward, and validated measurement tools are available. In essence, the key to pain assessment is simple: *believe the patient.* If we do that, we can't go far wrong.

Bibliography

Abrahm JL. 2004. Assessment and treatment of patients with malignant spinal cord compression. *J Support Oncol* 2:377–391.

American Pain Society Quality of Care Committee. 1995. Quality improvement guidelines for the treatment of acute pain and cancer pain. *JAMA* 274:1874–1880.

Barkwell DP. 1991. Ascribed meaning: a critical factor in coping and pain attenuation in patients with cancer-related pain. *J Palliat Care* 7:5–14.

Breitbart W, Bruera E, Chochinov H, Lynch M. 1995. Neuropsychiatric syndromes and psychological symptoms in patients with advanced cancer. *J Pain Symptom Manage* 10:131–141.

Breitbart W, Chochinov HM, Passik SD. 2004. Psychiatric symptoms in palliative medicine. In *Oxford Textbook of Palliative Medicine,* 3rd ed, Doyle D, Hanks G, Cherny N, Calman K (eds). Oxford: Oxford University Press.

Breitbart W, Passik SD. 2004. Psychological and psychiatric interventions in pain control. In *Oxford Textbook of Palliative Medicine,* 3rd ed, Doyle D, Hanks G, Cherny N, Calman K (eds). Oxford: Oxford University Press.

Byock I. 1997. *Dying Well: Peace and Possibilities at the End of Life.* New York: Riverhead Books.

Caracini A, Martini C, Simonetti F. 2004. Neurological problems in palliative medicine. In *Oxford Textbook of Palliative Medicine,* 3rd ed, Doyle D, Hanks G, Cherny N, Calman K (eds). Oxford: Oxford University Press.

Cassell E. 1991. *The Nature of Suffering and the Goals of Medicine*. New York: Oxford University Press.

Cleeland CS, Gonin R, Baez L, Loehrer P, Pandya KJ. 1997. Pain and treatment of pain in minority patients with cancer: the Eastern Oncology Group minority outpatient pain study. *Ann Intern Med* 127:813–816.

Daut RL, Cleeland CS, Flanery RC. 1983. The development of the Wisconsin Brief Pain Questionnaire to assess pain in cancer and other diseases. *Pain* 17:197–210.

Derogatis LR, Morrow GR, Feting J, et al. 1983. The prevalence of psychiatric disorders among cancer patients. *JAMA* 249:751–757.

Ferrell BR, Johnston-Taylor EJ, Sattler GR, Fowler M, Cheyney BL. 1993. Searching for the meaning of pain: cancer patients', caregivers' and nurses' perspectives. *Cancer Practice* 1:185–194.

Ferrell BR, Rhiner M. 1991. High-tech comfort: ethical issues in cancer pain management for the 1990s. *J Clin Ethics* 2:108–112.

Ferrell BR, Rhiner M, Zichi-Cohen M, Grant M. 1991. Pain as a metaphor for illness, Part I: impact of cancer pain on family caregivers. *Oncol Nurs Forum* 8:1303–1309.

Fink RS, Gates R. 1995. Cultural diversity and cancer pain. In *Cancer Pain Management*, 2nd ed, McGuire DB, Yarbro CH, Ferrell BR (eds). Boston: Jones and Bartlett.

Fishman B, Pasternak S, Wallenstein SL, Houde RW, Holland JC, Foley KM. 1987. The Memorial Pain Assessment Card: a valid instrument for the evaluation of cancer pain. *Cancer* 60:1151–1158.

Fitchett G, Handzo G. 1998. Spiritual assessment, screening, and intervention. In *Psycho-Oncology*, Holland JC (ed). New York: Oxford University Press.

Foley KM. 1987. Pain syndromes in patients with cancer. *Med Clin North Am* 71:169–184.

Foley KM. 2004. Acute and chronic cancer pain syndromes. In *Oxford Textbook of Palliative Medicine*, 3rd ed, Doyle D, Hanks G, Cherny N, Calman K (eds). Oxford: Oxford University Press.

Fong CM. 1985. Ethnicity and nursing practice. *Top Clin Nurs* 7:1–10.

Galer BS, Jensen MP. 1997. Development and preliminary validation of a pain measure specific to neuropathic pain: the neuropathic pain scale. *Neurology* 48:332–338.

Holland J (ed). 1998. *Psycho-Oncology*. New York: Oxford University Press.

Hoskin PJ. 2004. Radiotherapy in symptom management. In *Oxford Textbook of Palliative Medicine*, 3rd ed, Doyle D, Hanks G, Cherny N, Calman K (eds). Oxford: Oxford University Press.

Ingham JM, Portenoy RK. 2004. The measurement of pain and other symptoms. In *Oxford Textbook of Palliative Medicine*, 3rd ed, Doyle D, Hanks G, Cherny N, Calman K (eds). Oxford: Oxford University Press.

Jacox A, Carr DB, Payne R, et al. 1994. *Management of Cancer Pain: Clinical Practice Guideline No. 9*. Rockville, Md.: Agency for Health Care Policy and Research, US Department of Health and Human Services, Public Health Service. AHCPR publication 94-0592.

Janjan NA. 1997. Radiation for bone metastases: conventional techniques and the role of systemic radiopharmaceuticals. *Cancer* 80:1628–1645.

Lo B, Ruston D, Kates LW, et al. 2002. Discussing religious and spiritual issues at the end of life: a practical guide for physicians. *JAMA* 287:749–754.

Loblaw DA, Laperriere N, Perry J, Chambus A, and Members of the Neuro-Oncology Disease Site Group. 2004. Malignant Extradural Spinal Cord Compression: Diagnosis and Management. Evidence Summary Report #9-9. Cancer Care Ontario. www.cancercare.on.ca/pdf/pebc9-9esf.pdf.

Loblaw DA, Laperriere NJ. 1998. Emergency treatment of malignant extradural spinal cord compression: an evidence-based guideline. *J Clin Oncol* 16:1613–1624.

Loscalzo M, Amendola J. 1990. Psychosocial and behavioral management of cancer pain. *Adv Pain Res Ther* 16:429–442.

McCaffery M, Ferrell BR. 1991. How would you respond to these patients in pain? *Nursing* 21:34–37.

Miaskowski C, Zimmer EF, Barrett KM, Dibble SL, Wallhagen M. 1997. Differences in patients' and family caregivers' perceptions of the pain experience influence patient and caregiver outcomes. *Pain* 72:217–226.

Musick MA, Koenig HG, Larson DB, Matthews D. 1998. Religion and spiritual beliefs. In *Psycho-Oncology*, Holland JC (ed). New York: Oxford University Press.

Peteet J, Tay V, Cohen G, MacIntyre J. 1986. Pain characteristics and treatment in an outpatient cancer population. *Cancer* 57:1259–1265.

Portenoy RK, Hagen NA. 1990. Breakthrough pain: definition, prevalence and characteristics. *Pain* 41:273–282.

Portnow J, Lim C, Grossman SA. 2003. Assessment of pain caused by invasive procedures in cancer patients. *JNCCN* 3:435–439.

Puchalski C, Romer AL. 2000. Taking a spiritual history allows clinicians to understand patients more fully. *J Palliat Med* 3:129–137.

Rhiner M, Coluzzi PH. 1995. Family issues influencing management of cancer pain. In *Cancer Pain Management*, 2nd ed, McGuire DB, Yarbro CH, Ferrell BR (eds). Boston: Jones and Bartlett.

Schiff D. 2003. Spinal cord compression. *Neurol Clin* 21:67–86.

Taylor EJ, Ersek M. 1995. Ethical and spiritual dimensions of cancer pain management. In *Cancer Pain Management*, 2nd ed, McGuire DB, Yarbro CH, Ferrell BR (eds). Boston: Jones and Bartlett.

Pharmacologic Management of Cancer Pain

Pharmacologic therapy is the mainstay of cancer pain relief. Satisfactory pain control for 90 percent of cancer patients can be achieved with a minimum of adverse side effects. A combination of oral or transdermal opioid and adjuvant analgesics is required, along with other agents that prevent or treat opioid-induced constipation, nausea, sedation, and delirium. Only rare patients will need transmucosal, rectal, intravenous, subcutaneous, or spinal routes of opioid administration to achieve pain relief.

In this chapter I discuss the available nonopioid, opioid, and adjuvant analgesic medications, as well as other treatments and the agents that relieve opioid-induced side effects. I also review anesthetic methods that can relieve pain. The special needs of older patients and substance abusers are included. I discuss some common clinical situations: how to start a patient on opioids; how to change opioid doses, routes, or agents; and how to relieve excruciating pain rapidly.

NONSTEROIDAL ANTI-INFLAMMATORY DRUGS (NSAIDs)

Nonsteroidal anti-inflammatory drugs, taken by people with mild to moderate nonmalignant pain, are also very useful alone or combined with an opioid for cancer patients with pain from a variety of sources. They are especially useful for patients with bone pain or tissue inflammation.

The NSAIDs include the *p*-aminophenols (e.g., acetaminophen), the salicylates (e.g., aspirin and the nonacetylated salicylates such as salsalate), the propionic acid derivatives (e.g., ibuprofen), and the acetic acid derivatives (indomethacin, ketorolac) (see Table 5.1; tables begin on p. 254).

Most NSAIDs indirectly inhibit synthesis of prostaglandins. Prostaglandins synthesized as a consequence of injury to bones or joints help mediate the inflammatory response and the transmission of the pain signal. The majority of NSAIDs inhibit the synthesis or the function of both forms of cyclooxygenase (COX) enzymes required for the production of prostaglandins. COX-1 is present in the stomach, kidney, and blood vessels whereas COX-2 is produced only in inflamed tissues. NSAIDs that inhibit COX-2 therefore minimize the inflammation associated with bone or tissue injury, whether from a sports injury, arthritis, or a metastasis. NSAIDs that also inhibit COX-1, however, impair synthesis of the beneficial prostaglandins produced in the stomach and kidney and can therefore cause gastrointestinal distress and renal dysfunction.

USING NSAIDs FOR CANCER PAIN

NSAIDs used alone usually do not provide sufficient relief for patients with cancer pain, though I have had some success with these drugs for patients receiving hormonal therapy for metastatic prostate cancer. When first prescribing an NSAID, generally start with the lowest effective dose and escalate to the maximum 24-hour dose (indicated in Table 5.1). Since both acetaminophen and aspirin have a ceiling effect (1000 mg is the ceiling dose for both agents), a patient gets no more pain relief from a 1500-mg dose of aspirin or acetaminophen than from a 1000-mg dose; he just gets increased toxicity. If the initial agent chosen is ineffective at the maximal recommended dose or the patient develops an intolerable side effect, switch to one of the NSAIDs in a different chemical class (see Table 5.1).

SELECTING AN NSAID

To decide which NSAID to prescribe first, I consider the cause and intensity of the pain, any underlying illnesses that would contraindicate use of an NSAID, and the expected side effects. I also consider whether the patient can take oral medications or will need a rectal preparation.

PRACTICE POINTS: SELECTING AN NSAID FOR CANCER PAIN
- Give NSAIDs alone for mild pain.
- Give indomethacin for gout and pleuritic or pericardial pain.
- Review patients' underlying medical illnesses.
- "Ceiling" effect: the maximum pain relief obtainable from acetaminophen or aspirin is from a 1000-mg dose.
- When pain is refractory to NSAIDs alone, give combination products (NSAID + opioid) for mild to moderate pain.
- Ketorolac is effective for acute severe pain; it should generally not be used for longer than 2 weeks at a time.

Knowing the cause of the pain and its intensity can sometimes help you choose the appropriate NSAID. Indomethacin, for example, is the drug of choice for patients with pleuritic or pericardial pain or gout. It often relieves the pain of these disorders rapidly and completely. Therefore, despite the risk of gastrointestinal side effects and bleeding complications from indomethacin, I recommend it for these patients unless they have a coagulation problem or known ulcer disease.

Underlying illnesses help direct the choice of NSAID. All NSAIDs should be avoided in patients with a known allergy to aspirin or with asthma, as they can produce bronchospasm in up to 20 percent of these patients. Patients at high risk for complications include those over age 60 (those over 70 are at an even higher risk) and those with a history of previous ulcer disease, NSAID-induced bleeding, or cardiovascular disease. These risks are additive. Other risk factors include concomitant use of corticosteroids or anticoagulants and use of multiple NSAIDs. To minimize gastrointestinal ulcers and bleeding frequency, high-risk patients should be started on COX-2 selective agents rather than nonselective NSAIDs (Chan et al. 2002; Laine 2003). The risk is so high for patients taking anticoagulants that they should never take an NSAID that inhibits prostaglandin synthesis.

Patients with moderately reduced platelet counts (<100,000/mm^3) or with inherited coagulation disorders (such as hemophilia) can take COX-2 selective agents (e.g., valdecoxib [Bextra]) or NSAIDs that do not affect cyclooxygenase or prostaglandin synthesis, such as choline magnesium salicylate or salsalate, without increased risk of bleeding. Patients taking anticoagulants such as warfarin can take valdecoxib, which has no effect on warfarin steady-state pharmacokinetics. Valdecoxib (20 mg b.i.d.) has the analgesic potency of combinations of oxycodone (10 mg) / acetaminophen combinations following dental surgery and was found to add to the relief provided by morphine alone in patients undergoing joint replacement. Patients with somatic pain would therefore likely benefit from the addition of one of these agents (Reynolds et al. 2003).

Patients with congestive heart failure, cirrhosis, or chronic renal failure experience increased edema, worsening renal function, or hypertension if treated with either nonselective agents or COX-2 inhibitors, so both should be avoided (DeMaria and Weir 2003).

For patients with mild to moderate somatic or visceral cancer pain refractory to NSAIDs alone, aspirin and acetaminophen are very effective when combined with an opioid. The most commonly used combination pills contain 5 mg of oxycodone along with either 325 mg of aspirin (e.g., Percodan), 325 mg of acetaminophen (e.g., Percocet), or 500 mg of acetaminophen (e.g., Tylox). Unfortunately, patients can take only a limited number of these pills each day because of the toxicities of the acetaminophen and aspirin. Patients who need more opioid can take higher doses of an oxycodone or other opioid preparation along with a safe dose of an NSAID. A patient with uncontrolled bone pain from metastatic breast cancer, for example, might be switched from twelve Tylox a day, which contain 60 mg of oxycodone (5 mg × 12 pills = 60 mg), to, for example, 80 mg of sustained-release oxycodone along with an NSAID.

Ketorolac (e.g., Toradol) is likely to be effective for someone with acute, severe pain. It has the pain-relieving potency of an opioid and is used in situations in which the clinician does not want to prescribe an opioid but the patient needs the level of pain relief an opioid can deliver. For example, ketorolac is frequently given by emergency room physicians who wish to avoid the mental status changes that opioids can induce. In this setting, it is given parenterally (see Table 5.1 for doses and frequency). A 30-mg dose of parenteral ketorolac is equivalent in pain-relieving potency to 15 mg of parenteral morphine. However, ketorolac can impair renal function and is therefore contraindicated for patients with renal insufficiency. And it cannot be used for chronic pain relief because it is associated with a significant incidence of acute renal failure and gastrointestinal side effects.

ROUTES OF ADMINISTRATION

For patients who cannot take oral preparations, aspirin, indomethacin, and naproxen are available by suppository. Suppositories should be inserted base first, to promote retention. Naproxen may be the best choice because it has the longest half-life and 80 percent bioavailability. Either a 500-mg naproxen suppository or 10 to 30 ml of the liquid suspension (125 mg / 5 ml) can be given twice a day. Ibuprofen is not available in suppository form, and the liquid suspensions are available only in pediatric doses (100 mg / 5 ml). A therapeutic dose of ibuprofen would necessitate giving 30 ml rectally (p.r.) every 4 to 6 hours, and this may be difficult for patients to tolerate.

SIDE EFFECTS

The inhibition of prostaglandin synthesis can cause a number of serious abnormalities in platelet and kidney function, as well as in the lungs and the gastrointestinal tract. Because prostaglandins are necessary for normal platelet function, most NSAIDs impair platelet function and predispose the patient to bleeding. And since prostaglandins are also required to maintain renal arterial blood flow, NSAIDs may precipitate renal failure in patients with impaired flow, such as many elderly patients. NSAIDs may also enhance salt and water retention and cause edema to develop in patients with congestive heart failure or cirrhosis.

PRACTICE POINTS: TOXICITY OF NSAIDs

- Avoid NSAIDs for patients older than 70 or for those with renal failure, cirrhosis, heart failure, or asthma.
- Use nonacetylated salicylates (e.g., choline magnesium salicylate or salsalate) for patients taking anticoagulants or with bleeding disorders.
- Consider adding a proton pump inhibitor (e.g., esomeprazole) to prevent gastrointestinal ulceration for patients older than 60 or for those with a history of peptic ulcer disease.
- Rule out salicylate toxicity in a patient taking aspirin or an aspirin/oxycodone combination who develops otherwise unexplained mental status changes, ataxia, or tachypnea, even if there are no complaints of tinnitus.

LIFE-THREATENING TOXICITIES

The side effects described above occur with therapeutic doses of NSAIDs. At toxic blood levels, however, some of the NSAIDs can be life-threatening.

ASPIRIN OVERDOSE.   Aspirin can be particularly dangerous. Aspirin and the nonacetylated salicylates are metabolized by the liver; less than 5 percent is excreted by the kidneys. But the liver can only metabolize a limited amount of aspirin; if a person ingests more than that, the drug accumulates and can rapidly reach toxic levels. Patients who increase their dose of aspirin much above 6000 mg/day can easily develop salicylate toxicity, which manifests as tinnitus, ataxia, hyperventilation, delirium, and even coma.

Few patients would knowingly take that much aspirin, but aspirin can be "hidden" in the combination products mentioned above. It's not hard to imagine that someone could have an exacerbation of her pain, double or triple the amount of Percodan she is taking, and, in consequence, develop an aspirin overdose. Older patients with presbycusis may be at particular risk because they cannot hear tinnitus. Despite my warnings to the contrary, a number of patients have increased their aspirin intake in this way and developed life-threatening salicylism.

The "Drunk" with an Undetectable Alcohol Level

Mr. Lafferty was one such patient. He was taking two Percodan every four hours for his metastatic prostate cancer pain. His wife called to ask our advice because, she said, "He is staggering around and talking out of his head like he used to when he was drunk all the time. But when I took him to the local emergency room they said he couldn't be drunk; there was no alcohol in his blood."

As it turned out, her husband had not been drinking. When she inspected his medication bottle she found that instead of the 12 pills a day he normally took, he had taken 25 Percodan the day before. These contained 8125 mg of aspirin! I asked her to take Mr. Lafferty back to the hospital because he needed immediate medical attention.

When he again arrived in the emergency room, the triage nurse noted that he was still ataxic and confused, and I could understand why she thought he was inebriated. On further evaluation, he was also found to be hyperventilating because of the metabolic acidosis the salicylate induces. An electrolyte panel confirmed the characteristic anion gap acidosis. To minimize the deposition of salicylates in his central nervous system (CNS) and to increase salicylate clearance, the emergency medical staff gave him intravenous sodium bicarbonate. They also avoided any agents that could sedate him because if he stopped hyperventilating, the acidosis would worsen, more aspirin would deposit in his CNS, and he would deteriorate further. Mr. Lafferty responded well to this therapy and was back to his old self within a few days.

ACETAMINOPHEN OVERDOSE. While aspirin toxicity is not uncommon, it would be very difficult for a patient with normal hepatic function to accidentally take enough acetaminophen to induce serious toxicity. This would require an intake of more than 20 g of acetaminophen at one sitting. Even someone taking Tylox, which has 500 mg of acetaminophen per pill, would have to take 40 tablets over one to two hours.

In patients who have chronic liver disease, however, such as that induced by alcohol, liver toxicity can develop even with therapeutic acetaminophen doses, and accidental overdose may occur. If you discover such an overdose soon after the patient ingests the acetaminophen, you can prevent hepatic toxicity with Mucomyst. But if the overdose is recognized late, Mucomyst will be ineffective. Liver transplantation can be life-saving for appropriate patients.

OPIOID ANALGESICS

Although NSAIDs can be useful, opioids are a necessity for the vast majority of cancer patients with pain. Obtaining the appropriate opioid is much easier than it was a decade ago. State Cancer Pain Initiatives, which now exist in all 50 states, are working to induce legislators to remove the legal barriers to prescribing opioids for cancer patients. The Medical Board of California, for example, adopted guidelines for intractable pain in 1994, which it republished in 1996. It states in the 1996 introduction,

> The under treatment of intractable pain is often a more significant problem than over treatment, and one reason among many is the physician's fear that a complaint for over prescribing may put his/her license in jeopardy. The Medical Board of California (MBC) is aware of this dilemma and encourages physicians to apply their best medical judgment when treating the patient, rather than basing their treatment on a fear of discipline by the MBC... The

MBC created these requirements to complement legislation... which established California public policy as supportive of the responsible practice of pain management. Simply stated, the treatment of chronic pain, as is true with any medical treatment, must be consistent with established medical standards that serve the patient's total well-being. These guidelines are being republished to reinforce the MBC's position that the public is best served by a health care environment where physicians are free to exert their own best medical judgment consistent with accepted community standards of care.

In addition, the Medical Board of California requires that, by December 2006, all licensed physicians show proof of six hours of CME in pain management and an additional six hours in end-of-life care.

Availability and cost, once barriers to obtaining effective opioids, have also become less of a problem (see Table 5.2). Increasing numbers of community pharmacies, particularly those that work with home hospice agencies, now carry even potent opioids in stock. For patients receiving the Medicare Hospice Benefit, all drugs that provide comfort care, including opioids, adjuvant agents, and agents that treat side effects, are covered. And for patients with limited financial means, there is a very effective and inexpensive opioid: methadone.

GENERAL GUIDELINES FOR OPIOID USE

The pharmaceutical companies have provided numerous agents in a variety of formulations and now, to a very large extent, we can tailor the drug to the patient's needs. Uncontrolled pain, however, remains one of the major reasons why cancer patients are not able to accomplish their goals. Some of the reasons for this are inadequate pain assessment, physicians' reluctance to prescribe opioids in the appropriate frequency and dose, and patients' reluctance to take them. Physicians also may mistakenly believe that for patients taking opioids, the opioids will interfere with the ability to diagnose the cause of acute pain in the emergency setting. In fact, in a prospective, randomized trial, patients arriving at an emergency room with abdominal pain of unknown etiology were initially (i.e., for the first sixty minutes) given morphine or saline. This study found no occasions when the administration of morphine masked a physical finding or led to a decrease in diagnostic accuracy (Thomas et al. 2003).

Adhering to the following guidelines may help:

Guidelines for Opioid Use

- Give "whatever it takes" to relieve the patient's pain; be sure that the opioid dose is adequate.
- Give opioids often enough to prevent the pain from recurring.
- Use the least invasive route.
- Use adjuvant medications to minimize opioid-induced side effects.

WHAT IS AN "ADEQUATE DOSE?"   An adequate opioid dose is whatever dose is needed to provide pain relief, no matter how high. There is no arbitrary "maximal dose" of any opioid (except for meperidine). If a patient receiving 20 mg/hr of intravenous morphine still has pain and does not have unacceptable side effects, increase the dose until the pain is relieved or intolerable side effects appear. One patient of mine with extensive head and neck cancer whose dose had gradually increased over about a month required 1000 mg/hr of morphine, and dosages of 1500 mg/hr have been reported.

SCHEDULING OF DOSES.   Many advanced-cancer patients whose pain rarely remits should be taking the drugs at regularly scheduled intervals "around-the-clock" rather than as needed (p.r.n.). They need both a long-acting agent or sustained-release formulation of an opioid to relieve their baseline, steady pain and a short-acting, "rescue" agent to relieve unexpected exacerbations. With the variety of available agents, around-the-clock pain control is usually achievable.

Mild to moderate cancer pain may be intermittent, however, and for patients with this kind of pain, p.r.n. dosing may be appropriate. When they are at home, they can give themselves pain medicine whenever they need it. But hospitalized patients can experience significant delays in receiving needed p.r.n. medication. For these patients, instead of ordering opioids "p.r.n." I use a "patient-may-refuse" order. The nurse offers the medication on a regular basis (e.g., Percocet every 4 hours) and the patient has the option to take it or refuse it.

USE THE LEAST INVASIVE ROUTE.   Ninety percent of cancer patients will be able to take opioids orally or apply them transdermally in a skin patch. The drugs can also be given rectally. Even patients who are dying will seldom need intravenous, intramuscular, subcutaneous, or intraspinal opioids.

USE ADJUVANT MEDICATIONS.   More opioid will *always* provide more pain relief, but the higher doses will also cause more side effects.

Dr. Michael Levy, one of the leaders in pain management in the United States, has extended the concept of the therapeutic window to enable us to more easily conceptualize the balance between pain relief and opioid-induced side effects (Levy 1996). The *therapeutic window* of any drug is the range of blood concentrations in which it is effective but not toxic. What Dr. Levy points out is that different patients may have very different therapeutic windows even for the same opioid.

In patients who have normal renal and hepatic function and whose pain is of somatic or visceral origin, the window may be "wide open": that is, they can take the amount of opioid they need with minimal, easily controllable side effects. But in other patients, those with renal, hepatic, or mental impairment or with neuropathic pain, that window may be all but closed. The patient may experience intolerable side effects without being able to achieve satisfactory pain relief.

Dr. Levy suggests we first try to "widen the window" by treating any underlying conditions that would exacerbate an opioid-induced side effect. To minimize sedation, for example, irradiate brain metastases or aggressively treat hepatic encephalopathy. But for patients in whom (to extend the metaphor) the window is stuck, add nonopioids as adjuvant agents to minimize the opioid dose needed for effective pain relief.

Because adjuvants cause their own side effects, add them only when a patient cannot achieve satisfactory pain relief without them. Don't use them simply to lower the opioid dose in a patient whose pain is well controlled with opioids with a minimum of side effects.

Selecting an Opioid Analgesic

PATIENT PREFERENCE.   For my initial choice of drug, I consider patients' preferences, which are influenced by their past experiences with opioids. For example, a patient who has had his wisdom teeth extracted might have had good pain relief from Percodan or Tylox. If he now needs something more long-acting, I can use that same opioid (oxycodone) in a sustained-release preparation.

If, on the other hand, the patient had a serious side effect from an opioid, I know to avoid that agent and, if possible, other agents in the same class. Unfortunately, the immediate-acting potent opioids are all structurally related to morphine. Unless the patient has had a true morphine allergy, you will usually be able to switch to another opioid that is less likely to cause the troublesome side effect. If, for example, a patient has nightmares or hallucinations from morphine, you can switch her to an

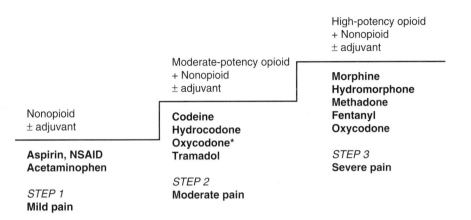

5.1   Analgesic Ladder.   *Oxycodone (5–10 mg) in combination with aspirin, acetaminophen, or NSAID is a step 2 agent; alone, it is a step 3 agent. Adapted from the World Health Organization, *Cancer Pain Relief: With a Guide to Opioid Availability,* 2nd ed., Geneva: World Health Organization, 1996.

equianalgesic dose of hydromorphone. The rare patient with a true morphine allergy can take methadone, which is not chemically related to morphine.

PAIN INTENSITY.   Next, determine the pain's intensity. As I discussed in Chapter 4, pain intensity can be measured using a number of numerical or word scales. In a numerical rating scale, pain ratings of 1 to 4 are considered mild, 5 to 6 moderate, and 7 to 10 severe. The World Health Organization (WHO) has adopted an "analgesic ladder" (Figure 5.1) and guidelines for using it to relieve cancer pain.

In addition to these guidelines, WHO recommends a stepwise escalation that matches the potency of the opioids to the intensity of the pain. For mild pain, start with nonopioid analgesics. Moderate pain should be treated with less potent step 2 opioids (see Table 5.3) and severe pain with the most potent step 3 opioids (see Table 5.4). Nonopioid analgesics and adjuvant medications should be added at any step when indicated.

In addition, if a patient has pain that is unrelieved by the agents recommended for that step, the WHO guidelines suggest moving up to the next step. If a patient with mild to moderate pain, for example, does not get adequate pain relief from a step 2 opioid, a step 3 opioid should be prescribed. The WHO ladder and guidelines have been shown to be very effective, even in dying patients. In one study in which they were used, at the time of death, only 3 percent of patients reported severe pain and no patient died of respiratory depression due to the opioids (Mercadante 1999).

STEP 2 OPIOID AGENTS.   In my experience, cancer pain is rarely if ever mild. For cancer patients with mild to moderate pain, I have found low-dose hydrocodone/acetaminophen combinations (e.g., Vicodin, Lortab) and codeine to be the *least* useful of the step 2 opioids. The dose of hydrocodone in the Vicodin or Vicodin ES preparations is not strong enough, and codeine is often nauseating and causes dysphoria. A higher-dose hydrocodone is available in a combination preparation, Vicodin HP CIII, which contains 10 mg of hydrocodone with 660 mg of acetaminophen per tablet; this should be given orally every 4 hours. There is no parenteral preparation. (See Table 5.3.)

PRACTICE POINTS: SELECTING AN OPIOID

- Consider patient preference when choosing the opioid and the opioid formulation.
- Match opioid agent with pain intensity using the WHO ladder; advance up the ladder if pain persists, even if the patient still characterizes it as "mild" or "moderate."
- Match opioid formulation to the temporal pattern of pain (i.e., continuous, intermittent, or both).
- Except for patients who have previously used codeine with good results, avoid codeine for cancer patients.
- Consider methadone for patients with severe neuropathic pain, or when drug cost is important.

Codeine.   Codeine is problematic in cancer patients, for several reasons. While the side effects of codeine may be helpful in discouraging abuse in people with nonmalignant pain, they are unacceptable in someone with cancer pain. Further, for codeine to provide pain relief, it must be metabolically converted to morphine by a specific hepatic enzyme. Patients who either lack that enzyme or are taking drugs such as cimetidine that inhibit the enzyme's function will get little or no analgesia from codeine.

Oxycodone.   Oxycodone and tramadol are effective step 2 agents for cancer patients. Oxycodone is a very useful oral opioid analgesic for patients with mild to moderate cancer pain. It is listed with both the step 2 and step 3 agents because, in step 2, there are several formulations that combine a low dose (5 to 10 mg) of oxycodone with an NSAID. All provide excellent relief for this degree of pain, often induce slight euphoria, but cause only mild to moderate constipation. Many patients with moderate, intermittent pain due to bony metastases from breast, lung, or prostate cancer respond very well to these agents. For unclear reasons, women have a 25 percent higher blood level of oxycodone than men after ingesting the same dose (Kaiko et al. 1996a). To minimize side effects, therefore, consider using lower initial oxycodone doses for female patients.

Tramadol. Tramadol (e.g., Ultram) is also very useful for cancer patients with mild to moderate pain. It is a centrally acting, nonopioid analgesic that is chemically unrelated to opioids but binds to one of the opiate receptors. Approximately one-third of its analgesic effect is reversed by naloxone. The rest of the analgesia it produces may be due to its ability to decrease reuptake of norepinephrine and serotonin.

Tramadol can relieve mild to moderate somatic or neuropathic pain, including post-herpetic neuralgia (Gobel and Stadler 1995); 100 mg of tramadol is more effective than 60 mg of codeine but is approximately equivalent in potency to 60 mg of codeine plus 650 mg of acetaminophen or aspirin. Side effects are similar to those caused by opioids but, in addition, tramadol may increase the risk of seizures in certain patients. The usual dosage is 50 to 100 mg every 4 to 6 hours; total 24-hour dose should not exceed 400 mg. Doses should not exceed 300 mg for patients over 75 and 200 mg for those with renal insufficiency or cirrhosis. Tramadol is available in Europe in a once-daily formulation that provides pain relief equivalent to that of standard-release capsules taken three times a day (Bodalia et al. 2003).

STEP 3 OPIOID AGENTS. For patients with more severe pain, the more potent, step 3 opioids are needed (see Table 5.4). These include, besides morphine, hydromorphone (e.g., Dilaudid), levorphanol (e.g., Levo-Dromoran), methadone, fentanyl, and higher doses of oxycodone alone (i.e., not combined with an NSAID). Any of these can be safely used for patients with normal renal and hepatic function. All are metabolized by the liver and renally excreted, and they or their metabolites may reach toxic levels in a patient with severe hepatic or renal failure. Morphine has an active metabolite, morphine-6-glucuronide (M-6-G), which is excreted by the kidney. In a patient with hepatic or renal failure, if the doses of the opioid preparations are not properly adjusted, levels of both morphine and M-6-G can easily reach toxic levels.

If the creatinine clearance decreases by half, opioid doses can be reduced or their frequency of administration can be changed accordingly. Since patients usually do not develop toxicity unless the creatinine clearance drops, if monitored closely these patients can receive lower doses of opioids given in immediate-release formulations.

Methadone.   Methadone is not a new drug, but it is being increasingly used for patients with moderate to severe pain. It is by far the least expensive of the opioids and has particular utility for patients with neuropathic pain—the most refractory type of pain.

Methadone is structurally unrelated to morphine and fentanyl, and it can be used in the rare case of true allergy to these agents. It is also helpful when patients are suffering from the neurotoxic side effects of the high doses of other opioids that are often needed to control severe neuropathic pain. Methadone contains d- and l-isomers that act as opioid receptor agonists and NMDA (*N*-methyl-d-aspartate) receptor antagonists (Foley 2003). Both patients with neuropathic pain and patients taking opioids over the long term have increased levels of NMDA receptors in the dorsal horn of the spinal cord. NMDA antagonizes the activity of the opiate receptors, and so blocking the NMDA receptors enhances the analgesic effect of externally administered opioids.

The difficulties with using methadone lie in its biphasic elimination, its metabolism by CYP 3A4 isoenzyme (one of the isoforms of the cytochrome P-450 system), and its controversial equianalgesic dosing range. Because of its initial distribution phase, initial loading with methadone usually requires that it be given every 4 to 6 hours. But methadone has a second, extended phase lasting 36 to 60 hours that causes drug levels to accumulate. By the fifth to sixth day of treatment, methadone usually needs to be taken only twice to three times a day to maintain analgesia and only once a day to prevent withdrawal. After the first few days of methadone therapy, therefore, the dosing interval should be increased to twice or three times a day to minimize the chance of inducing sedation or respiratory depression.

Drugs that inhibit or induce the CYP 3A4 isoenzyme can raise or lower the blood level of methadone, and so patients must be monitored when methadone and one of these drugs are given together. Common drugs used for cancer patients that inhibit the CYP 3A4 system and so raise the blood level of methadone include fluconazole, ketoconazole, itraconazole, all the SSRIs (except venlafaxine), cimetidine, nefazodone, aprepitant, and the antibiotics ciprofloxacin, norfloxacin, clarithromycin, and erythromycin. Inducers of CYP 3A4 include phenytoin, carbamazepine, and phenobarbital and risperidone, and concomitant use can precipitate opioid withdrawal (Tarumi et al. 2002).

THE DANGER OF MEPERIDINE/NORMEPERIDINE. You are probably wondering why meperidine (Demerol) is not included in the lists of step 2 and step 3 agents. Demerol is very useful for postoperative and postpartum pain or to relieve a variety of acute pains, but it is not recommended for patients with cancer pain. It is inconvenient to give, and it can be dangerous.

PRACTICE POINTS: WHY MEPERIDINE (E.G., DEMEROL) IS UNSUITABLE FOR CHRONIC CANCER PAIN

- Meperidine relieves pain for too short a period (about 2 hours, at most).
- Meperidine has poor oral availability (75 mg IV = 300 mg p.o.).
- Meperidine's toxic metabolite, normeperidine, causes seizures; it accumulates rapidly in patients with renal insufficiency.
- Meperidine is contraindicated in patients who are also taking monoamine oxidase inhibitors.

Meperidine provides pain relief for only one to two hours. To provide around-the-clock relief, the patient would have to have ten to twelve intravenous (IV) shots or take six to twelve 50-mg pills at each dose (75 mg intravenous [IV] is equivalent to 300 mg p.o.; 150 mg IV equals 600 mg p.o.) (see Table 5.5). And meperidine is contraindicated for patients receiving monoamine oxidase inhibitors for depression or as part of a chemotherapy regimen. Meperidine has caused hyperpyrexia, seizures, and death in these patients.

Of equal concern are the potentially life-threatening side effects induced by meperidine's toxic active metabolite, normeperidine. At high serum levels, normeperidine causes *seizures*. In patients receiving frequent therapeutic doses of meperidine, high normeperidine levels can be reached rapidly. Normeperidine's half-life is 13 to 24 hours and, since it is renally excreted, its levels build even more quickly when the patient is dehydrated or has any impairment of renal function.

Normeperidine toxicity is easy to diagnose: 36 to 48 hours after beginning the meperidine (100 to 150 mg IV every 2 to 3 hours), the patient complains of not feeling well; he appears agitated and restless and may even manifest myoclonic jerking. If you do not stop the meperidine, the patient will develop seizures. And you cannot reverse the effects of *normeperidine* with naloxone—in fact, naloxone exacerbates these effects and is very likely to precipitate seizures in a normeperidine-toxic patient. Give the patient with toxic effects another opioid for pain relief and hope the normeperidine levels fall before a seizure occurs. If the patient does have seizures, use diazepam to control these. To avoid painting myself into this corner, I do not prescribe meperidine for my cancer patients with chronic moderate to severe pain.

TEMPORAL ASPECTS OF THE PAIN.   To decide which formulation of the opioid to prescribe, consider whether the pain is continuous, intermittent, or both. Most patients whose cancer is far advanced have both types of pain. To treat the continuous pain, I usually prescribe a sustained-release preparation of an opioid with a short half-life (i.e., oxycodone, morphine, hydromorphone, or fentanyl as the active agent). In 2005, Purdue Pharma is scheduled to release a new extended-release formulation of hydromorphone, called Palladone. According to materials submitted to the FDA, Palladone has an 18-hour elimination half-life and is given orally once daily. It is a capsule containing a pellet formulation and will be supplied in doses of 12 mg, 16 mg, 24 mg, and 32 mg. Each capsule has a biphasic absorption, rising to a peak at 2 hours, after which pain control is reportedly maintained for 24 hours. Eating does not affect the peak or the sustained level of pain relief. More rarely, as I discussed above, I start with methadone, an opioid with a 24-hour half-life. Because of this long half-life, it is harder to titrate doses of methadone to the patient's pain level. I therefore generally choose methadone as the initial opioid only when there is a history of allergy to morphine, or when I need to use the least expensive agent.

To treat intermittent pain or brief exacerbations of continuous pain, I prescribe a shorter-acting preparation of oxycodone, morphine, or hydromorphone that can begin to provide relief in about 30 minutes to an hour. I might also prescribe as a rescue dose an immediate-acting preparation of oral transmucosal fentanyl citrate, which can begin to provide relief in as little as 10 minutes. Doses of a short- or immediate-acting preparation given to someone who is taking "around-the-clock" opioids are often referred to as "rescue" doses: they rescue the patient from break-through pain.

ROUTES OF ADMINISTRATION

Once you have chosen an appropriate opioid, you need to decide the route by which it should be taken. Most patients will be able to use the oral route. Those with a feeding tube in place can receive medications through the tube. For cancer patients who cannot take oral medications, the transdermal, rectal, intravenous, or subcutaneous (SQ) route can be used. Step 2 agents (which include oxycodone in fixed combinations with NSAIDs) are available only in oral formulations. Table 5.4 indicates which formulations are available for each of the step 3 opioids listed (including pure oxycodone).

Opioids should not be given intramuscularly for either short- or long-term management of cancer pain. The injections are painful and, since absorption of the opioid is variable, they lead to unpredictable blood concentrations of the analgesic and give suboptimal pain relief.

ORAL ROUTE.   Over 90 percent of patients can achieve effective therapy with oral opioids. All the step 3 agents listed in Table 5.4, except oxymorphone, are available in oral formulations: lozenges, liquids, or immediate- or sustained-release tablets, pills, or capsules. Patients with feeding tubes can safely use crushed tablets of immediate-release hydromorphone or methadone, liquid immediate-release oxycodone or morphine, or morphine in sustained-release pellets (e.g., Kadian, Avinza).

Oral Sustained-Release Agent for Patients with Feeding Tubes or with Difficulty Swallowing Tablets.   Most sustained-release preparations of oxycodone and morphine are designed to provide pain relief for 8 to 12 hours, but they may cause serious side effects if they are cut or crushed, because the full 12-hour opioid dose will be absorbed in an hour or two. There are morphine formulations (Kadian, Avinza) that consist of capsules containing polymer-coated sustained-release pellets from which the morphine is released. Because of this novel formulation, the capsules can be opened and the pellets sprinkled on food or put into a liquid such as orange juice or water and placed into a 16 French or larger gastrostomy tube in 20 ml of liquid. Do not attempt to put the beads through a nasogastric (NG) tube. (Efficacy studies of absorption in patients with feeding tubes are currently in press.) Kadian is effective for

12 to 24 hours and is available in 20-, 50-, and 100-mg capsules. Avinza is effective for 24 hours and is available in 30-, 60-, 90-, and 120-mg capsules.

Oral Agents for Patients without Feeding Tubes but with Difficulty Swallowing Large Volumes of Liquids or at Risk of Aspiration. Concentrated (20 mg/ml) morphine (e.g., Roxanol) or oxycodone solutions (e.g., Intensol), given sublingually or bucally, are very helpful for these patients. The efficacy of these agents is due in large part to their being swallowed and absorbed from the gastrointestinal tract in the same way that larger volumes are absorbed. Only about one-fifth of sublingual morphine solution or about one-third of a sublingual methadone solution is absorbed, even when held under the tongue for 10 minutes (Weinberg et al. 1988). Sublingual buprenorphine tablets can provide relief for mild to moderate pain, but these are not available in the United States.

Transmucosal Agent. An immediate-acting preparation of fentanyl (Actiq) is available in the form of an oral sweetened lozenge containing 200 to 1600 mg of fentanyl citrate, attached to a handle. The fentanyl is easily absorbed transmucosally; it is effective in 75 percent of patients, produces rapid pain relief (in 10 to 15 minutes), and is well tolerated. There is no evidence of decreased effectiveness of this agent over time (median duration of use, 79 days; range, 1 to 423 days).

TOPICAL AND TRANSDERMAL ROUTES. Topical opioids may act through opioid receptors of all classes that are present in peripheral nerve terminals of inflamed tissue. These receptors appear in normal tissue within minutes to hours of the onset of inflammation (Stein 1995). Data demonstrating the efficacy of topical opioids are limited, but two randomized double-blind pilot studies support their use in treating patients with decubitus ulcers (Flock 2003; Zeppetella et al. 2003). Compounding pharmacies can add morphine to the IntraSite gel that is a standard treatment for stage II or III pressure ulcers. The gels are topically applied once to several times a day and covered with a standard dressing. The opioid-containing gels can provide equivalent or better relief of pain and cause fewer side effects than the higher doses of systemic opioids. Case reports suggest they are also useful for patients with open tumor infiltrates of the skin.

The Duragesic patch is a transdermal fentanyl delivery system. It consists of a drug reservoir lined on the bottom by a rate-limiting membrane, which itself is attached to an adherent backing (Figure 5.2). The lipophilic opioid fentanyl is contained in the patch's drug reservoir; once

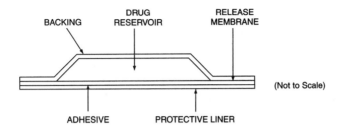

DRUG   RELEASE
BACKING   RESERVOIR   MEMBRANE

(Not to Scale)

ADHESIVE   PROTECTIVE LINER

5.2 Duragesic Patch. After the unit is placed on the chest wall, fentanyl, contained in the drug reservoir, diffuses through the release membrane into the skin. The drug is absorbed from the skin reservoir into the bloodstream. By 14 to 24 hours after the first patch is applied, blood levels of fentanyl are sufficient to provide pain relief. New patches are usually applied every 72 hours. From Janssen Pharmaceutica; with permission.

the patch is attached to the skin, the fentanyl diffuses through the rate-limiting membrane into the fat in the skin. It is then absorbed into the bloodstream from this skin reservoir.

Because fentanyl is very rapidly metabolized by the liver, at least 12 hours are required to build up enough drug in the skin reservoir to establish an adequate blood level. By 14 to 20 hours, an effective, stable plasma concentration is reached and in most patients is maintained for a total of 72 hours. New patches are usually applied every 72 hours, though some patients find they need to replace the patches every 48 hours.

For many patients with stable, chronic pain, transdermal fentanyl patches are useful as the sustained-release component of their pain regimen. The patches are especially helpful for those who are unable to take oral medications, who cannot tolerate other opioids, or who simply prefer a patch to taking pills even once or twice a day. In a randomized crossover study of patients who expressed a preference, significantly more preferred the fentanyl patches over oral sustained-release morphine (Payne et al. 1998).

The patch is not the best choice for managing the chronic pain of some types of patients. Transdermal fentanyl is not recommended for patients under 18 years old who weigh less than 110 pounds. And though I have not seen any studies documenting this observation, I and many of the hospice nurses with whom I work have noticed that older, cachectic patients seem to get less relief using the patch. Also, since the drug takes many hours to be absorbed, the transdermal system is not indicated for someone with acute severe or excruciating pain. In these patients, an opioid drip using morphine, fentanyl, or hydromorphone is more appropriate.

The patch can also be problematic for patients who have recurrent bouts of fever and infection, even simple urinary tract infections. During fevers, more drug is absorbed from the skin reservoir into the bloodstream and the patient may develop a fentanyl overdose. In addition, if the patient becomes acidotic during sepsis, more drug will be liberated from albumin binding sites. This "free" drug can also cause significant toxicity.

If the patient does develop symptoms of overdose, removing the patch will not stop delivery of fentanyl into the bloodstream. Fentanyl continues to pass into the vasculature from the skin reservoir until it is empty. Twenty-four hours after the patch is removed, the amount of fentanyl in the reservoir has decreased by only 50 percent. These patients may require a low-dose naloxone drip until the remaining drug is metabolized. To avoid precipitating a withdrawal syndrome due to the naloxone, use just enough to restore adequate respiration but allow the patient to remain asleep.

PRACTICE POINTS: CLINICAL IMPLICATIONS OF THE TRANSDERMAL FENTANYL DELIVERY SYSTEM

The fentanyl is deposited into a skin reservoir, from which it is absorbed. Therefore,

- Rescue dosing is needed for 12 to 24 hours while the reservoir is accumulating fentanyl.
- Used alone, the patch is not an effective initial treatment for patients with severe pain.
- For patients with severe pain, short-acting drugs should be used to establish the opioid dose that relieves the pain; then a fentanyl patch of appropriate strength can be placed.
- Toxicity can result from increased absorption during febrile episodes.
- In cases of overdose, 50 percent of the fentanyl is still present in the skin reservoir 24 hours after the patch has been removed.

Despite these limitations, for many patients the transdermal system is a very useful way to deliver a steady dose of a potent opioid. It is usually very well tolerated and very effective for patients who are medically stable and whose pain medication requirements do not vary markedly from day to day.

RECTAL ROUTE.   The rectal route of opioid delivery is especially helpful in a patient who is suddenly, unexpectedly unable to take oral pain medication. It is preferable to intramuscular injections and will provide effective relief. Tramadol, codeine, morphine, oxycodone, and methadone can all be given rectally. These drugs are available as commercially or custom-made suppositories, as custom-made gelatin capsules that enclose the oral long-acting formulation (e.g., MS Contin), or as elixirs that can be given as microenemas (i.e., in less than 30 ml of liquid) (Davis et al. 2002).

The sustained-release morphine preparations are as effective given rectally as orally, and the same or higher opioid blood levels are achieved after 24 hours. Hospice nurses suggest that before patients have the sustained-release tablet inserted, they have a soapsuds enema to remove any stool from the rectal vault. The tablet is then placed in the lower part of the rectum. Hospice pharmacies can often prepare customized suppositories containing the oxycodone, methadone, or morphine the patient was previously receiving.

The venous drainage from the rectum flows into a mix of portal and systemic circulation. Since morphine and oxycodone are extensively metabolized by the liver, avoiding the portal system maximizes the active blood levels you can achieve per dose, but minimizes the levels of hepatically created active metabolites such as M-6-G. Unfortunately, colostomies are solely drained by the portal system; opioids placed in colostomies have less than half the bioavailability of those placed in the rectum.

Although placing sustained-release morphine or oxycodone tablets into the rectal vault is not approved by the U.S. Food and Drug Administration (FDA), morphine has been extensively studied and is safe and effective. Doses of rectal sustained-release morphine as high as 900 mg/day have been used. Placing them into colostomies is not recommended, however.

INTRAVENOUS OR SUBCUTANEOUS ROUTES.   Patients with rapidly escalating pain, and those who are not getting relief from a transdermal patch, cannot swallow, do not have feeding tubes, or who have a bowel obstruction, need to have the opioid delivered by the intravenous or subcutaneous route. Opioids can be given by either route continuously (to deal with the chronic portion of the patient's pain) and as bolus doses (to treat acute breakthrough pain).

The members of the Memorial Sloan-Kettering Cancer Center Supportive Care Program have developed guidelines to determine which patients will benefit from parenteral pain management at home.

Guidelines for Recommending Home Parenteral Opioid Therapy*

- Parenteral pain management can be costly. We should discuss the cost/benefit of other routes and verify insurance coverage.
- The infusion can be deadly if not given correctly; we need to determine whether the infusion can be done safely: Who else is present in the home? Can they or the patient be taught how to manage the infusion? If the patient is alone, how will he or she be monitored?
- Do we feel we have adequate knowledge to manage the infusion, or is there a hospice physician available who has agreed to be responsible?
- Will the community hospice or home care system provide skilled personnel, including 24-hour nursing staff, on call for home visits?

Intravenous Route.   Intravenous morphine has the advantage of rapidity of action and ease of dose adjustment. It is often offered as part of a program of patient-controlled analgesia (PCA).

PRACTICE POINTS: ADVANTAGES OF INTRAVENOUS OPIOIDS

- Prompt dose escalation in medically unstable patients with moderate pain who cannot use oral medication
- Rapid, precise, safe dose escalation for rapid relief of severe or excruciating pain
- Patient-controlled analgesia option

You are probably most familiar with PCA in the postoperative patient. These patients usually do not receive a continuous dose of morphine; they simply give themselves bolus doses as needed. A computer regulates the amount of drug given and how often a patient can dose

---

*All guidelines modified from N. Coyle, N. Cherny, and R. Portenoy, Pharmacologic management of cancer pain, in *Cancer Pain Management,* 2nd ed., D. B. McGuire, C. H. Yarbro, B. R. Ferrell (eds), Boston: Jones and Bartlett, 1995.

himself; it records both how often the patient asks for a dose and how much drug he actually receives. For example, the computer may record that the patient requested drug twelve times in an hour but received it only four times, because the device was set to deliver a bolus dose only every 15 minutes. It also records the total 24-hour quantity of morphine delivered.

PCA is also for cancer patients. If I admit someone in severe pain, I set up the intravenous route with PCA because I can escalate doses quickly and precisely. If the patient has been taking opioids at home, I start the intravenous drip at an opioid dose equivalent to what I think she has been taking at home. Patients can also give themselves bolus doses, as needed, every 10 or 15 minutes. An hour later, the nurse reviews the computer record and repeats the pain assessment. I use this information to increase the strength of the bolus and, every 8 to 12 hours, to adjust the continuous-infusion dose (I explain this in detail later in the chapter). The morphine drip rate is increased until the patient's pain is relieved. If the patient was in pain because she was taking much less opioid than I prescribed, that quickly becomes apparent as well, and the drip rate can be lowered accordingly. When the required opioid dose has been determined, if the patient can tolerate oral medications I prescribe oral sustained-release morphine or another oral opioid at an equivalent dose.

For patients with severe or excruciating pain, there is really no safer way to achieve adequate opioid plasma levels quickly. An opioid-naive patient, for example, might present with severe neuropathic pain due to cancer in the brachial plexus. Such patients often require morphine infusions of 10 to 12 mg/hr or more to relieve their pain. This would translate into 360 to 430 mg of sustained-release oral morphine every 12 hours (Table 5.5); that is, 10 mg/hr × 24 hr = 240 mg IV / day = 720 mg p.o. / day; 12 mg/hr × 24 hr = 288 mg IV / day = 864 mg p.o. / day. Using the intravenous route and adjusting as noted above, you will be able to reach the needed 10 to 12 mg/hr within 36 to 48 hours. Using oral morphine alone, reaching a dose of 360 to 430 mg every 12 hours in an opioid-naive patient is likely to take much longer.

The intravenous route is also preferable for medically unstable patients who cannot use oral medications. For the reasons mentioned above, I would not prescribe the transdermal fentanyl patch in these patients. If a patient with good pain control taking oral medications needs to be NPO for surgery, I prescribe a morphine drip at a dose equivalent to his oral dose then place him back on his oral medication as soon as possible.

Rare patients will not be able to tolerate oral medication and will not respond to transdermal fentanyl patches. Most of these patients will be able to use subcutaneous infusions, but some will require continuous intravenous infusions because of the dose of medication needed and the toxicity associated with delivering that dose subcutaneously.

If a patient has been receiving oral medications or using a patch, you simply need to convert the 24-hour oral dose to an intravenous one using the techniques detailed later in the chapter (see also Table 5.5). Many of these patients will already have an implanted vascular access device (e.g., a catheter or port) through which they can receive the infusions. If not, I usually ask the hospice or home care nurse to insert a PICC line (peripherally inserted central venous catheter). Trained personnel can place PICC lines in patients in their home, and the catheters are easily maintained for the remaining two to three months of these patients' lives. Some home care agencies may require a chest x-ray to verify placement.

Subcutaneous Route.   Some patients who cannot take oral medications and whose pain is unrelieved by transdermal fentanyl find subcutaneous opioid infusions effective. Ambulatory patients can use one of a variety of pumps, many of which can provide both continuous infusion (for the chronic pain) and bolus medication (for breakthrough pains). I always check with the hospital's or the hospice's oncology pharmacist to choose a device appropriate to the patient's needs. The pharmacist will be providing the opioid for the infusion and will help the patient with questions about its use.

Morphine and hydromorphone (e.g., Dilaudid) are the most commonly used opioids in the infusions. They are generally nonirritating and are well absorbed. You can prescribe the same doses as for a continuous intravenous infusion. Methadone is less well tolerated subcutaneously and often induces a local reaction.

While most advanced cancer patients need only the equivalent of 400 to 600 mg/day of morphine, about 10 percent will need more than 2000 mg. But even these very high doses can be delivered subcutaneously. One hydromorphone preparation (hydromorphone HP) delivers 10 mg/ml of hydromorphone, and 2 to 5 ml/hr is well tolerated subcutaneously. Using this preparation, you can easily deliver 30 mg/hr of hydromorphone with only 3 ml/hr of solution. This is the equivalent of 200 mg/hr of morphine, or 4800 mg/day of parenteral morphine. If necessary, the pharmacist can prepare even more highly concentrated solutions.

For the subcutaneous infusions, patients have a 27-gauge "butterfly" or Silastic needle inserted subcutaneously, usually on the anterior chest wall or in the abdomen. The site is changed every 5 to 7 days to minimize skin irritation. Many patients or their families are able to insert the needles themselves. Local inflammation is common but rarely is severe enough to warrant discontinuing the infusion. If it is bothersome, the patient can try changing to a different opioid to reduce the concentration or volume of the infusion or to eliminate allergic reactions to preservatives or impurities in the preparation.

SPINAL OPIOIDS (EPIDURAL, SUBARACHNOID).   Spinal delivery of opioids produces pain relief because the exogenous opioids bind to receptors for the natural opiates (e.g., enkephalins) already present in the spinal cord. Nerves containing endogenous opiates are present in the same area of the spinal cord that contains the synapses between afferent neurons and spinal interneurons. When exogenous opioids bind to those receptors, they prevent the spinal interneuron from transmitting the signal. Since the cortex does not receive a pain signal, the person does not experience pain. And because they are delivered locally, epidural opioids are effective at one-tenth of the doses required for the same opioid given peripherally. Subarachnoid opioids are effective at one-hundredth of the systemic doses. Even though spinal opioids are absorbed into the systemic circulation, the side effects from the lower doses are usually milder.

Spinal opioids can be used alone or with anesthetics, alpha-adrenergic agents, or baclofen to improve their efficacy or to minimize the opioid-induced side effects. They can be delivered via either temporary epidural catheters or permanent epidural or subarachnoid catheters. Patient-controlled epidural analgesia (PCEA) is available for either temporary or permanent infusions. As with PCA, in which the patient can self-administer a bolus of systemic opioids, PCEA allows patients to give themselves, as needed, extra spinal opioids or extra doses of the opioid/anesthetic mixture.

Implantable Intrathecal Drug Delivery Systems.   A randomized trial comparing implantable intrathecal drug delivery systems (IDDS) with conventional medical management delivered by an expert pain team demonstrated some surprising findings (Smith et al. 2002, 2003). This trial enrolled 202 patients who were taking at least the equivalent of 200 mg of oral morphine a day and were unable to achieve satisfactory pain relief with standard therapy, even when managed by pain experts, or who were taking <200 mg oral morphine equivalent per day but were suffering intolerable side effects from what otherwise was satisfactory relief of their pain. If the conventional management was ineffective, an IDDS was offered. Significantly more of the patients given an IDDS had a >20 percent reduction in their pain and in side effects related to the treatment (38 vs 58 percent), particularly fatigue and sedation. These differences likely resulted from the lower systemic opioid doses required to control the pain. More unexpected, however, was that patients with IDDS lived longer! The patients were more alert, less fatigued, and in less pain, and perhaps they had increased mobility; all these may have contributed to the documented increase.

Anesthesiologists and their teams typically place and manage both temporary and permanent epidural and intrathecal infusions. I offer below a general overview of the use of these routes. More detailed discussions of the devices used, the insertion techniques, and the management of the catheters are provided in the bibliography at the end of the chapter.

PRACTICE POINTS: ADVANTAGES OF SPINAL OPIOIDS

- Treatment of refractory neuropathic pain resulting from injury to peripheral nerves.
- Opioids, anesthetics, alpha-adrenergic agents (e.g., clonidine), and other drugs are infused.
- Temporary infusions can be used to
  —Help patients regain sensitivity to lower systemic opioid doses.
  —Determine whether the epidural route provides effective pain relief. If so, a permanent catheter may be placed.
- Patient-controlled epidural analgesia is available.

Indications.   Spinal opioids benefit those patients whose neuropathic pain syndrome is not responding to systemic opioids, or who require such high systemic opioid doses that, despite the use of appropriate adjunctive agents, the side effects are intolerable.

Temporary infusions or boluses of epidural opioids are most commonly used to manage postoperative or obstetric pain. Temporary catheters are placed before surgery and opioid solutions are given as a bolus or infused (e.g., Duramorph). The infusions or boluses are repeated as needed in the next several days, then the catheter is removed.

Temporary opioid/anesthetic or opioid/alpha-adrenergic agent (such as clonidine [e.g., Duraclon]) infusions are used in a rare cancer patient to enable him to regain sensitivity to lower doses of systemic opioids. Even in these patients, systemic opioids usually are not stopped entirely, because many patients would develop opioid withdrawal. To prevent this, clonidine patches (0.1 to 0.3 mg) can be placed and systemic opioid doses then reduced gradually. The systemic opioid dose is maintained at 50 percent of the previous dose, and the remaining 50 percent of the systemic dose is replaced by the epidural opioids. The systemic dose is then decreased by 20 percent per day as the equianalgesic epidural dose is increased by 20 percent per day. Once the patient is comfortable on epidural opioids alone, he is switched back to the oral route. Patients usually can get adequate pain relief receiving about half their previous systemic opioid dose. The temporary catheter can then be removed. The spinal opioid infusion is considered a success if the dose of systemic opioid can be lowered enough that the associated side effects become tolerable.

Other patients, such as (but not limited to) those with bilateral severe neuropathic pelvic pain due to recurrent colorectal, bladder, or gynecologic cancers, receive temporary catheters to determine whether opioids given via the epidural route will provide satisfactory pain relief. If the temporary infusion reduces the patient's pain by at least 50 percent, she

---

NEURAXIAL DRUG-DELIVERY SYSTEMS

- Temporary (1 to 4 weeks): Percutaneous epidural or intrathecal catheter.
  —Taped to patient's back (for diagnostic infusions).
  —Tunneled 1 to 2 inches from insertion site (for therapy).
- Intermediate (1 to 2 months).
  —Tunneled and attached to implanted injection port.
- Permanent (years): Implanted epidural or intrathecal catheter.
  —Attached to totally implanted pump.
  —Attached to totally implanted programmable pump for intrathecal infusions.

is considered to be a good candidate for insertion of a permanent epidural Silastic catheter for pain management.

For those who do benefit, a permanent catheter is placed, with infusion systems that vary from simple external mechanical syringe-drivers to totally implantable delivery systems with programmable infusion pumps. Because of the cost associated with the implantable infusion systems, it is recommended that they be inserted only in patients who are expected to live at least three months.

Epidural versus Subarachnoid Catheter Placement. Anesthesiologists can place permanent catheters in either the epidural or subarachnoid spaces. The choice of the subarachnoid site over the epidural for a permanent catheter depends on the experience of the clinician, the needs and life expectancy of the patient, and the expertise of the home care teams. Extensive preoperative education of the patient and the family is required before any permanent catheter is inserted.

Subarachnoid catheters have a number of advantages over epidural catheters. Subarachnoid opioids act more quickly and for a longer time. In addition, only 10 percent as much opioid is needed as in the epidural space. Because of the lower opioid doses required, patients experience fewer systemic opioid-induced side effects. The implanted pumps require no maintenance and their reservoirs require infrequent (usually monthly) drug refills.

PRACTICE POINTS: COMPARISONS OF SUBARACHNOID (SA) AND EPIDURAL CATHETERS

Advantages of SA Catheters	Disadvantages of SA Catheters
• Smaller drug volume	• Increased incidence of meningitis
• Fewer systemic side effects	• Cost of totally implanted system
• Lower incidence of fibrosis if used for 3 to 6 months	

Subarachnoid catheters are also considered when a patient is expected to live more than six months, because, over time, epidural catheters are more frequently obstructed by fibrosis. They are also indicated for patients who cannot tolerate the volume of epidural infusion that they would need for pain relief.

While the subarachnoid site can be beneficial, it also has its disadvantages. Though subarachnoid catheters allow access to the spinal fluid for sampling, infections of subarachnoid catheters can more easily induce meningitis. And their insertion requires a totally implantable delivery system with a subcutaneous infusion pump, which alone can cost more than $20,000.

Drugs Used in Spinal Infusions. Morphine or hydromorphone are the agents most commonly used in epidural and intrathecal infusions. They are hydrophilic drugs, not very lipid soluble, and take quite a while to diffuse across the meninges and into the cord. But they also remain in the cerebrospinal fluid (CSF) and are bound to the spinal cord opioid receptors for a long time. And because they migrate to other spinal segments, the spinal catheter does not have to be placed directly over the affected segment for the infusion to be effective.

More lipid-soluble agents such as fentanyl or sufentanil are also used in spinal infusions. They are potent spinal analgesics, but because they don't migrate in the CSF, their effectiveness depends on precise catheter placement.

The dose of the epidural opioid is calculated from the daily amount of intravenous opioid the patient has been receiving. For epidural infusions, one-tenth of the total daily parenteral opioid dose is given over 24 hours; for intrathecal infusions, only one-tenth of the *epidural* dose is required. For a patient on a 10 mg/hr morphine drip, the calculation would be as follows:

10 mg/hr parenteral morphine = 240 mg / 24 hr parenteral morphine
(240 mg / 24 hr)/10 = 24 mg over 24 hours for the epidural dose
(24 mg / 24 hr)/10 = 2.4 mg over 24 hours for the intrathecal dose

The morphine is given as a continuous infusion (i.e., 1 mg/hr epidural or 0.1 mg/hr intrathecal infusion).

Local anesthetics (e.g., bupivacaine), alpha-adrenergic agonists (e.g., clonidine), and baclofen (e.g., Lioresal) are also given by spinal infusion. Infused alone or added to opioid solutions, bupivacaine and clonidine can provide pain relief for patients who do not get relief from opioids alone, and they can minimize the side effects of the opioids by decreasing the doses needed for pain relief. Bupivacaine is the most commonly used anesthetic agent; the starting dose of intrathecal bupivacaine is 3 mg/day and it is escalated as needed. Rarely, epidural infusions of 0.125 to 0.150 percent bupivacaine cause sensory or motor impairment. Baclofen is very effective in relieving neuropathic pain and spasticity, with few associated side effects compared with oral administration. Doses used are 100 to 1000 times less than oral doses. More rarely, somatostatin, octreotide, calcitonin, ketamine, or midazolam are infused.

Side Effects of Spinal Opioids and Anesthetics. Opioid-naive patients who receive epidural opioids for pain relief after surgery experience pruritus, nausea, vomiting, urinary retention, constipation, and more rarely, respiratory depression. Most cancer patients, however, are not opioid-naive and they rarely develop these side effects. If they do, small doses of naloxone (a 40-µg bolus followed by a continuous infusion starting at 5 µg/kg/hr) can reverse the side effects without eliminating analgesia. Compared with the opioid-naive patient with nonmalignant pain, cancer patients usually require much higher spinal opioid doses. As these doses are absorbed into the circulation, the patient may become sedated. Very high subarachnoid opioid doses can cause the patient to develop myoclonic jerking.

PRACTICE POINTS: SIDE EFFECTS AND DRUG- AND CATHETER-RELATED COMPLICATIONS OF NEURAXIAL INFUSIONS

- Pruritus, nausea, vomiting, and urinary retention are rare in patients taking systemic opioids.
- Depending on the dose infused, patients may have typical opioid-related side effects.
- Anesthetic may induce hypotension.
- Placement-related complications include superficial bleeding (or, very rarely, hematomas compromising the cord or the cauda equina), abdominal or retroperitoneal organ or lung perforation, nerve root damage, seromas, post-spinal headache in up to 20 percent of patients receiving subarachnoid catheters.
- Catheters become dislodged, tear, kink, or become plugged by fibrosis or catheter-related granulomas.
- Patients may underdose or overdose as a result of errors in refilling or programming.
- CNS or skin infection may occur.

The side effects caused by anesthetics used intraspinally are due to the sympathetic blockade they induce as well as their systemic absorption. Depending on the location of the catheter, patients may become hypotensive initially, so they are usually given concomitant intravenous fluids when the infusion is begun. In animal studies, bupivacaine caused both systemic and local toxicities, including seizures, cauda equina syndrome, and impaired sensation. But in clinical trials, while patients might experience dose-dependent local toxicities, systemic effects were rarely seen, possibly because the bupivacaine is so highly protein-bound. The neurologic side effects are not reported for bupivacaine doses of less than 25 mg / 24 hr (Du Pen et al. 1992).

Catheter-Induced Complications. The most common complications of spinal infusions arise during implantation or from the catheters themselves. Permanent catheters are inserted following administration of local anesthesia and tunneled subcutaneously to an implanted injection port. During implantation, bleeding can occur superficially or, very rarely, in the epidural space, where it can cause an epidural hematoma, spinal cord compression, or a cauda equina syndrome that may require emergency neurosurgery. Other surgery-associated problems include perforation of an abdominal or retroperitoneal viscus or lung by the tunneling needle, or damage to nerve roots or the cord by the needle or the catheter itself. Patients also may develop pump pocket seromas, which usually require no specific therapy.

Catheters can become dislodged, kink, or tear. They can also cause epidural fibrosis when in place for several months, which occasionally leads to cord compression. The fibrosis can also restrict the migration of the drug and decrease its efficacy. Catheters may even have to be repositioned.

Fibrosis is not a problem with catheters in the subarachnoid space, but there can be catheter-associated granuloma. Post-spinal headache due to CSF leaks occurs in up to 20 percent of patients with intrathecal catheters. If the headaches persist, epidural blood patching is necessary.

Other Complications. Errors in refilling or programming the continuous-infusion pumps can lead to serious or even life-threatening complications. Anesthesiologists minimize this risk by ensuring that only properly trained individuals perform these tasks and that they check their work meticulously. If an error is discovered that might cause an overdose, the patient is immediately hospitalized for observation and treated symptomatically (e.g., naloxone for respiratory depression, anticonvulsants for seizures). Underdosing can result in recurrence of severe pain.

With very long-term use, patients can develop impotence (reversible with testosterone), amenorrhea, and other endocrine abnormalities. Edema of the hands and feet also occurs and is only partially responsive to elevation and diuretics.

Infection is the most serious complication. Implanted epidural catheters have an infection incidence of 8 percent, but the infection is usually limited to the skin around the injection port and the subcutaneous track of the catheter. If the injection port and catheter are removed promptly, the infection rarely progresses to an epidural abscess.

Contraindications. Certain medical and social situations preclude the use of spinal opioids. Patients with bleeding diatheses or active septicemia cannot have the catheters placed. Diabetics and immunocompromised patients have higher rates of septicemia, but these are not absolute contraindications. Epidural metastases can lead to CSF obstruction, but catheters can be placed rostral to the obstructing lesions.

As with continuous-infusion opioid therapy, cost and maintenance issues must be addressed. Will the patient or family be able to care for the catheter? Can they afford the devices and the home care services required or can a source of financing be identified? Are physicians available to manage the infusions and the catheters?

Caring for Patients Receiving Spinal Opioids. Anesthesiologists along with specially trained nurses care for patients with spinal catheters as both inpatients and outpatients. They work with the patients' families and with the home care and hospice services that are helping patients and their families maintain the catheters at home.

Patients usually receive spinal medications as continuous infusions, but bolus doses may be given. If boluses are planned, a simple port (like that in a Port-a-cath used for intravenous access) is implanted when the catheter is placed. Bolus dosing provides adequate analgesia with less dose escalation and may therefore be preferable to the more costly programmable continuous-infusion pumps.

For bolus dosing, family members or specially trained nurses inject preservative-free morphine two to four times a day into the reservoir in the subcutaneous port. If the bolus becomes ineffective and pain relief is not reestablished after the catheter is repositioned, continuous infusions of opioid alone or combined with a local anesthetic (e.g., bupivacaine) and/or an alpha-adrenergic agent (e.g., clonidine) are instituted. In those who have not had a programmable pump inserted, the infusion can be given by connecting an external infusion pump to the subcutaneous port with a specially adapted needle. Patients receiving opioid alone have the option of patient-controlled epidural boluses along with the continuous infusion. The infusion pumps are refilled either at the hospital or by the home care nurse about every two weeks. Alternatively, a fixed-flow implantable pump can be inserted.

Summary. Spinal infusions add significantly to the quality of life of those rare patients who need them. I have seen patients with severe thoracic or bilateral lower abdominal or pelvic pain, unable to tolerate systemic therapy, experience a marked improvement in their day-to-day existence on receiving the spinal opioid/anesthetic/± clonidine combinations. I urge you not to hesitate in referring patients who might benefit from this treatment to anesthesia pain specialists or neurosurgeons.

PREVENTING AND RELIEVING SIDE EFFECTS OF OPIOIDS

For many patients, especially older ones, it is not enough that opioids relieve their pain. Over 75 percent of patients are concerned that if they take opioids, they will develop constipation, nausea, drowsiness, or confusion. Even side effects that seem minor to us can persuade patients that these drugs are not for them.

Searching for a Natural Solution

Mr. Samuels, a former longshoreman, was such a patient. He was suffering from recurrent rectal cancer that involved the nerves in his perineum. As you can imagine, his pain was excruciating, and we hospitalized him to bring it under control as quickly as possible. After a few days of escalating doses of intravenous morphine, he told us that his pain control was satisfactory. We switched him to the equivalent dose of an oral sustained-release preparation, which, in his case, was 90 mg of morphine every 8 hours, and discharged him.

When we saw him a week later, his pain was again excruciating. He told us that he didn't like the "artificial laxative" we had prescribed (lactulose syrup) and therefore he did not take any of it. When he became constipated, he quite accurately attributed his constipation to the opioids, and he stopped taking them as well. He said he preferred the pain to being constipated—that a daily bowel movement was very important to him. It was only when we discussed the fact that a more "natural" laxative was available, and he purchased some senna from a health food store, that he agreed to resume his opioids.

Other opioid-induced side effects can be equally troublesome and can similarly prevent patients from taking enough medication to control their pain. Nausea, sedation, and various manifestations of delirium such as nightmares and hallucinations must be treated aggressively.

CONSTIPATION

Constipation is the most common side effect of opioid therapy, occurring in almost everyone who takes opioids, even in those with colostomies. In my experience, the only exceptions are patients with total gastrectomies or those with gastric or jejunal feeding tubes whose diet consists mainly or entirely of liquid enteral nutrition.

Even patients taking step 2 opioids develop constipation. In one hospice study (Bruera et al. 1994), for example, 40 percent of those not receiving opioids, 63 percent of those on step 2 opioids, and 87 percent of those taking step 3 opioids required laxative therapy. Unfortunately, constipation is one side effect that usually does not diminish with time. The gut does not accommodate or return to its normal pattern. I strongly recommend, therefore, that you prescribe routine, not p.r.n., laxatives for any patient beginning opioid therapy.

A number of factors may contribute to constipation in cancer patients with pain. Inactivity, lack of a private place to defecate, poor food or fluid intake, hypercalcemia and hypokalemia, peritoneal studding with cancer, bowel obstruction, as well as damage to the spinal cord, cauda equina, or peroneal nerve plexus can induce constipation even in patients not receiving opioid pain medications. So can a number of drugs, including anticholinergics, calcium-containing antacids, calcium channel blockers, diuretics, opioid adjuvant agents such as tricyclic antidepressants and phenothiazines, and serotonin antagonists used as antiemetics (e.g., granisetron).

Unfortunately, the lifestyle changes and medications we normally recommend to patients with constipation who are not taking opioids are not likely to be effective for patients who need opioids. Increased water intake, increased activity, fiber therapies, or disodium disuccinyl docusate (e.g., Colace) are generally fine for people who are constipated, but won't work for patients on opioids; fiber may even exacerbate the problem. Even if the patient is able to take the amount of water needed and get some exercise, the slowed intestinal transit time makes fiber therapy much less effective in this population. And patients often feel bloated or "full," further impairing what may be an already diminished appetite.

MECHANISM.   The difference lies in the effect of the opioids on intestinal motility. The bowel normally empties through coordinated waves of peristaltic movements that are more frequent in the first half of the day. Inactivity itself reduces these waves and increases the colonic transit time from the normal 2 to 3 days to between 4 and 12 days.

In contrast, the bowel of a patient on opioids is in a state of muscle "fibrillation"; the intestinal muscles are unable to produce the normal coordinated peristalsis, colonic mucosal secretions are decreased, and colonic transit time and the time for water to be reabsorbed from the stool are prolonged. Although the gut has opiate receptors, it is unlikely that these effects are due entirely to the local receptors. Patients taking parenteral opioids also suffer from constipation, and switching from oral to parenteral opioids does not completely reverse the problem. In addition, opioids increase the tone and decrease the sensitivity of the anorectal sphincter, which then does not relax appropriately. This side

---

PRACTICE POINTS: TREATING OPIOID-RELATED CONSTIPATION

- All patients taking step 2 or 3 opioids need routine (not p.r.n.) prophylactic laxatives.
- Fiber should not be increased and may need to be decreased if the patient is bloated.
- Give osmotic agents (e.g., lactulose, polyethylene glycol) or agents that stimulate the myenteric plexus (e.g., senna).
- Increase the laxative dose as the opioid dose increases.
- In patients taking opioids without laxatives, diarrhea or urinary incontinence suggests impaction.
- Opioid bowel syndrome may respond to motility agents (e.g., metoclopramide) or to oral opioid antagonists (naloxone or methylnaltrexone).
- If the syndrome does not respond to motility agents, methylphenidate and clonidine can prevent withdrawal while the opioid dose is lowered.

effect further predisposes older patients, who already have decreased sphincter sensitivity, to opioid-induced constipation.

THERAPY.   A number of bowel regimens have been published but none has been studied in a controlled fashion. (Sources for a number of these are provided at the end of the chapter.) Table 5.6 indicates the drugs most commonly used to prevent or treat constipation, along with their mechanism of action, recommended doses, and frequency of administration.

Agents that stimulate the myenteric nerve plexus such as senna (e.g., Senokot) and bisacodyl (e.g., Dulcolax), and osmotic agents such as magnesium hydroxide (e.g., Milk of Magnesia), magnesium citrate, lactulose/sorbitol, and polyethylene glycol (e.g., Miralax), are the most effective agents. Senna is usually given at a starting dose of two tablets twice a day and can be increased to three to four tablets two or three times a day as needed. Bisacodyl is started at two tablets at bedtime, to be repeated in the morning if necessary. It can be increased to two to three tablets two or three times a day if needed. Lactulose is given at much lower doses than are needed for patients with hepatic encephalopathy. It is effective at 15 to 30 ml at bedtime, but can be increased to 60 ml every 6 hours as needed. Polyethylene glycol (Miralax) is started at 17 g in 4 to 8 oz of liquid once a day. All the stimulants are of course contraindicated in a patient with bowel obstruction.

In my practice, I have found a combination of senna and an osmotic agent (sorbitol, lactulose, or polyethylene glycol) to be very effective and very well tolerated by patients on opioids. When I first prescribe a preparation that contains even a low dose of opioid (e.g., Tylox, Percodan, or Percocet), I also prescribe a bedtime laxative, such as one or two senna tablets per day. I explain to the patients that to maintain regular bowel movements, they must take the laxatives daily, even if they have had a bowel movement that day.

Patients taking step 3 opioids such as sustained-release morphine or oxycodone or transdermal fentanyl may need as many as 12 senna tablets in divided doses, along with a bedtime osmotic agent as needed (e.g., one or two tablespoons of lactulose or 17 g of polyethylene glycol). Generally, the more opioid, the more laxative a patient needs. My goal is for patients to have one soft bowel movement every one or two days.

If a patient becomes obstipated, adding magnesium hydroxide (e.g., Milk of Magnesia) (30 to 60 ml) plus mineral oil (15 to 30 ml) daily or twice a day, magnesium citrate (8 oz), or enemas, or increasing the dose

---

PRACTICE POINTS: LAXATIVE ESCALATION

- Initial regimen:
  —Senna (e.g., Senokot + Colace or Senokot-S) ± lactulose or poly-
  ethylene glycol h.s.
     or
  —Bisacodyl h.s. ± lactulose/polyethylene glycol
- If ineffective:
  —Escalate doses of initial agents (e.g., three senna tablets b.i.d. or
  t.i.d. plus 30 to 60 ml of lactulose or 17 to 34 g of polyethylene
  glycol).
- If patient is obstipated:
  —Add Milk of Magnesia + mineral oil or magnesium citrate
     or
  —Increase lactulose up to 60 ml q.i.d. or increase dose of polyeth-
  ylene glycol.
- If patient is impacted:
  —Lubricate rectum, disimpact, and give enemas until clear.
  —Institute appropriately aggressive prophylactic regimen.

---

of lactulose (30 to 60 ml) or polyethylene glycol to two to four times a day may be needed, but these agents are less well-tolerated and are not usually needed as part of a routine regimen. For paraplegic patients a cup of polyethylene glycol two to three times a day is usually effective.

If your patient is hospitalized, you need to be careful that the house staff have not written the laxative order as "p.r.n." Patients in pain do not think to ask for a laxative. They only realize that there's a problem when, a week or so later, they have not had a bowel movement.

IMPACTION.   Fecal impactions can occur when patients do not take the prescribed laxatives. Older patients, especially those who are confused, are particularly susceptible to this problem because their decreased rectal sensitivity allows a large mass of stool to form. These impactions may be difficult to diagnose, as patients and their families may not be aware of them. Rather than complain of constipation, the patient may instead complain of symptoms caused by the pressure of the fecal mass: urinary incontinence or diarrhea, which is actually stool passing around the impaction through a sphincter that has become incompetent.

Since 90 percent of impactions occur in the rectum, they are easily diagnosed by digital rectal examination. They are readily treated by lubricating the rectum and doing a manual disimpaction, followed by saline rectal lavage or enemas. Glycerine suppositories or mineral oil enemas may be required to soften the impaction. After the impaction is cleared, you can institute one of the prophylactic regimens outlined above.

OPIOID BOWEL SYNDROME. A very small minority of patients develop the so-called opioid bowel syndrome. Unlike impaction, this syndrome is caused by a functional, not a mechanical, bowel obstruction. Patients with this syndrome experience nausea, vomiting, abdominal distention, and mild abdominal pain. The pain will exacerbate if higher opioid doses are used to treat it.

If there is no mechanical bowel obstruction, you will often be able to reverse the syndrome with an agent that increases bowel motility, such as metoclopramide (e.g., Reglan) or oral opioid antagonists. Naloxone given orally (4 mg b.i.d. to t.i.d.) is usually effective but can produce an explosive result. Methylnaltrexone, a peripheral opioid receptor antagonist, is also effective within one to two hours and causes no increased pain or evidence of withdrawal (Table 5.6). For patients who cannot take oral medications, metoclopramide can be given subcutaneously or intravenously.

On occasion I have found that the syndrome would not reverse until I lowered the dose or even totally discontinued the opioid. If you must discontinue the opioid, consider intravenous ketorolac. As I discussed earlier in this chapter, 30 mg IV ketorolac is equivalent to 15 mg IV morphine and it can be given every 6 hours. You will also need to prevent opioid withdrawal. Withdrawal symptoms after chronic opioid use are mediated in part by increased activity of noradrenergic neurons, which can be blocked by clonidine or lofexidine. Clonidine has been successfully used at 0.1 to 0.2 mg (p.o.) every 4 hours for heroin users, tapered after day 3 for a total of 10 days. Cancer patients may be treated with a clonidine patch, 0.1 to 0.2 mg / 24 hr. If insomnia or muscle cramps appear, chlordiazepoxide is recommended. Lofexidine, 0.2 mg titrated up to 1.2 mg twice daily, can also be used (Kosten and O'Connor 2003).

NAUSEA

Nausea is also a very common side effect of certain opioid agents. If no antiemetics are given, one-half to two-thirds of patients who take oral codeine or morphine for the first time will develop nausea or vomiting. These patients may mistakenly think that they are "allergic" to the opioid. If you don't warn them about this side effect, you may not be able to convince them to continue taking these agents even if they have been effective in relieving the pain.

To prevent nausea in opioid-naive patients, I consider adding prophylactic prochlorperazine (e.g., Compazine) (10 mg p.o. t.i.d. or q.i.d.). If I do not prescribe this initially, I warn patients and their families that nausea may develop, that it is likely to last only a few days, and that I can relieve it with prochlorperazine. Some patients require as much as a week of therapy, but most patients do not experience nausea for more than seven days despite continued opioid therapy.

PRACTICE POINTS: TREATING NAUSEA IN PATIENTS TAKING OPIOIDS

- Eliminate other contributing factors (constipation, gastritis, peptic ulcer disease, gastric outlet or bowel obstruction, hypercalcemia, hyponatremia, hepatic or renal failure, CNS disease).
- Warn opioid-naive patients about transient nausea or prescribe a prophylactic antiemetic.
- Consider lowering the opioid dose for patients who develop nausea after receiving other treatments to eliminate the painful condition (e.g., radiation therapy).
- Give a different opioid agent.
- Add neuroleptics (e.g., prochlorperazine) for patients with nausea and vomiting.
- Consider a gastric motility agent (e.g., metoclopramide) for patients with nausea, vomiting, early satiety, or bloating after eating.
- Give antivertigo agents (e.g., meclizine) if nausea is induced by movement.

If patients taking opioids develop nausea later in the course of their treatment, other etiologies must be eliminated. Other common causes of nausea in cancer patients include chemotherapy, radiation therapy, constipation, gastritis or gastric ulcer disease, gastric outlet or bowel obstruction, hypercalcemia, hyponatremia, hepatic or renal failure, or disease of the CNS. If the nausea is due to one of these problems, it will usually be relieved if you can eliminate the cause. Constipation, for example, is a very common, easily reversible cause of nausea in these patients.

If none of these problems is present, late-developing nausea in a patient taking opioids may be an indication that the patient's pain is diminishing and his opioid dose should be lowered. Consider, for example, a patient who is receiving radiation therapy for a painful bony metastasis and has been taking an opioid to relieve the pain until an adequate radiation dose could be given. Weeks later, although the pain from the metastasis has diminished significantly, the patient is still taking the same opioid dose and, as a result, develops nausea. In such a case, I simply lower the dose of the opioid agent. The nausea usually disappears promptly, and the pain relief remains satisfactory.

Other patients being treated with opioids will develop nausea as they begin to take a higher dose of opioid to treat an increased intensity of pain. In these cases, if you substitute a different opioid agent the nausea often disappears. If the patient has been receiving morphine, for example, substitute an equianalgesic dose of hydromorphone (e.g., Dilaudid) or fentanyl.

THERAPY.   If none of the maneuvers described above is effective, try to determine the mechanism by which the opioid is producing nausea and use the agent(s) most efficacious in reversing the problem (see Table 5.7). Treatment of chemotherapy- and radiotherapy-induced nausea is reviewed in Chapter 7.

Patients who have nausea without vomiting are likely suffering from opioid stimulation of the chemoreceptor trigger zone in the medulla (the area in the brain that is responsible for chemotherapy-induced nausea). They may benefit from neuroleptics such as haloperidol (1 to 2 mg p.o. every 8 to 12 hours or 0.5 to 1 mg parenterally every 8 to 12 hours), prochlorperazine (10 mg p.o. t.i.d. to q.i.d. or 25 mg p.r. every 12 hours), or olanzapine (Zyprexa, Zydis) (2.5 to 5 mg p.o. h.s. or b.i.d.).

Delayed gastric emptying is likely to be responsible for the nausea and vomiting, early satiety, or bloating after eating experienced by other patients taking opioids. Metoclopramide, with its dual sites of activity (blocking the chemoreceptor trigger zone and enhancing gastric emptying) is the agent of choice for these patients.

Metoclopramide is very effective even in low doses (10 to 20 mg b.i.d. to q.i.d. or 1 to 3 mg/hr IV). It can also be given rectally at the oral dose, either by suppository (if available) or through rectal administration of the tablets or liquid drug. At these low metoclopramide doses, diarrhea, acute dystonic reactions, and akathisia are unusual. These side effects are more commonly seen in patients receiving the much higher doses of metoclopramide needed to prevent chemotherapy-induced emesis. Ondansetron, an agent that is very effective in chemotherapy- or radiotherapy-induced nausea, may be efficacious in any type of opioid-induced nausea (4 to 8 mg p.o. b.i.d. or t.i.d.). Corticosteroids, also effective in chemotherapy-induced emesis, have not been studied in the treatment of opioid-induced nausea.

Patients taking opioids who complain of nausea along with movement-induced vertigo usually benefit from agents such as scopolamine (transdermal patch or 0.3 mg t.i.d. p.o. or SQ) or meclizine (Bonine, Antivert) (25 mg t.i.d. p.o.).

SEDATION

Sedation can be an important dose-limiting side effect in patients taking opioids. It can lead patients to limit the opioids they will take, even though their pain remains uncontrolled. Like nausea, sedation is most prominent when the patient first begins taking opioids and lessens within a few days, even if the dose remains the same. I caution patients not to drive for the first two weeks after they begin taking sustained-release opioids. Studies have shown that, after this time, no psychomotor impairment remains and it is safe for patients to drive again (Fishbain et al. 2003; Vainio et al. 1995).

In fact, a comprehensive, structured, evidence-based review indicates that for patients taking long-term opioids, there is moderate to strong consistent evidence for lack of impairment of psychomotor abilities, even immediately after taking a usual dose of opioids (Fishbain et al. 2003). The review also found no higher incidence of accidents or motor vehicle violations, and no impairment as tested in on- or off-road driving simulations. Evidence on cognitive impairment, however, was inconclusive. Unless local statutes or state legislation prohibit it, patients taking a stable dose of chronic opioids should be allowed to continue driving. They should be cautioned, however, not to drive if they feel sedated, if they have taken alcohol or other sedating medications, or, as noted above, for a week or two after beginning opioids or after an increase in opioid dose.

PRACTICE POINTS: MINIMIZING SEDATION

- Advise patients to avoid driving for 2 weeks after opioids are initiated or dose is increased.
- Don't mistake "catch-up" sleep for oversedation.
- Give sustained-release agents for baseline pain control, immediate-release agents for exacerbations.
- When possible, eliminate contributing factors (e.g., medical causes or medications).
- Change the opioid dose or agent.
- Add a psychostimulant (e.g., methylphenidate).
- Consider referral to an anesthesia pain specialist.

In some patients, what may look like excessive sleepiness is simply a natural effect of pain relief in someone who has been sleep-deprived. Patients who have just begun opioid treatment often have experienced days to weeks of severe to excruciating pain before coming to see you, and the pain has deprived them of much-needed sleep. Be careful not to mistake this natural "catch-up" sleep as oversedation. Leave the opioid dose the same for the first few days, and if the patient then complains of excessive drowsiness, lower it.

PRESCRIBE BOTH IMMEDIATE- AND SUSTAINED-RELEASE FORMULATIONS. A simple way to minimize sedation, which I use for almost all my patients, is to take advantage of the lower peak opioid levels induced by long-acting or sustained-release opioids (i.e., methadone, transdermal fentanyl, or the sustained-release morphine or oxycodone preparations). But sustained-release preparations are not flexible enough to meet the patient's changing pain needs. What works best for most patients, therefore, is a combination of a sustained-release preparation to keep the pain at a satisfactory level most of the time, along with an immediate-acting agent for "rescue" dosing.

CONTRIBUTING CAUSES. If sedation persists beyond the first few weeks, I try to determine in appropriate patients whether a new medical problem is contributing to the somnolence. Before obtaining a CT scan or MRI to determine whether the patient has developed an unsuspected brain metastasis or a subdural hematoma, I check for hypercalcemia and hyponatremia. Hyperglycemia, if it is causing sedation, is usually clinically apparent, as are uremia or hepatic failure, which also are likely to exacerbate the sedating effects of opioids.

In immunocompromised patients, I search for CNS infections, such as viral encephalitis, toxoplasmosis, or tuberculous or cryptococcal meningitis. Carcinomatous or lymphomatous meningitis usually manifests as headaches and cranial nerve abnormalities rather than sedation.

If none of these conditions is present, review the patient's other medications, because a number of them can exacerbate opioid-induced sedation. Cimetidine, anticholinergic drugs, alcohol, and drugs that decrease glomerular filtration, such as NSAIDs and some ACE (angiotensin converting enzyme) inhibitors, all increase drowsiness in patients taking opioids. Sleep medications are the most often implicated.

Benzodiazepines with long half-lives, such as clonazepam (e.g., Klonopin) or diazepam (e.g., Valium), may induce daytime somnolence in patients taking opioids. To minimize daytime sedation, use agents with shorter half-lives such as oxazepam (e.g., Serax) (15 to 30 mg p.o.), lorazepam (e.g., Ativan) (1 mg p.o.), temazepam (e.g., Restoril) (7.5 to 30 mg p.o.), or zolpidem (Ambien) (5 to 10 mg p.o.).

CHANGE THE OPIOID DOSE OR THE AGENT.   If sedation persists when the contributing factors are eliminated, try decreasing the dose of the sustained-release opioid by 10 to 25 percent and monitoring the patient's use of rescue medication. If the patient doesn't use more rescue doses, you can assume the pain relief is still satisfactory.

Alternatively, substitute a different opioid agent at an equianalgesic dose (I discuss how to do this later in the chapter). Just as opioids differ in how often they induce nausea, morphine, hydromorphone, fentanyl, and the other agents differ in the frequency with which they induce sedation. You may be able to achieve equivalent pain relief with less sedation simply by using a different agent.

PSYCHOSTIMULANTS.   If none of these measures is successful, consider adding a psychostimulant, such as an amphetamine. Some effective psychostimulants and their usual starting doses are listed in Table 5.8. Amphetamines have been shown to reduce drowsiness, and to enhance mood. They are contraindicated for patients with arrhythmias, delirium, or psychosis, and some patients cannot tolerate either the cardiac or the psychological side effects after starting the drugs. Even patients who can tolerate these agents may need an increased dose to maintain their pain-relieving, antisedating, and mood-enhancing effects after three to four weeks.

For selected patients, however, psychostimulants can be very effective and the benefits can persist for periods of 6 months or more. I most often prescribe methylphenidate (e.g., Ritalin). It is a CNS stimulant that increases concentrations of dopamine at the synapse by preventing its reuptake, affects norepinephrine reuptake, and binds to the serotonin transporter. Its effects peak 2 hours after it is taken, and the immediate-release form lasts up to 6 hours. The sustained-release formulation has its peak effect 4 to 7 hours after it is taken, and lasts approximately 8 hours.

There have not been any large randomized and controlled trials that demonstrate the effectiveness of methylphenidate in relieving the somnolence induced by opioids, but numerous trials of cancer patients with impaired cognition (e.g., with brain tumors) have demonstrated that this drug is effective and safe. Patients should begin with 2.5 to 5 mg of immediate-release methylphenidate once a day; you can add a noontime dose if necessary, and escalate to no more than 1 mg/kg/day in divided doses (Rozans et al. 2002). Modafinil (Provigil) (100 to 400 mg/day p.o.), a nonamphetamine psychostimulant, is an agent approved for treatment of patients with narcolepsy. Patients with brain tumors or with sedation from opioids may find it increases their alertness.

If a patient needs an extra degree of mental acuity for a special event, such as a wedding, an important meeting, or an anniversary party, beginning the psychostimulant a week or so before the event and adjusting its and the opioid's dose can often provide the perfect degree of pain relief and mental alertness for the important day.

ANESTHESIA PAIN SPECIALISTS.   If all these techniques are ineffective and the patient remains unacceptably sedated, you might consider referring her to an anesthesia pain specialist, whose contributions I discuss elsewhere in the chapter.

Delirium

Delirium can be a frightening side effect for both patients and their families. The first manifestation may be something as mild as nightmares, but the process can rapidly progress with the patient developing hallucinations and even frank psychosis.

As reviewed in Chapter 4, delirium from all causes shares the same manifestations: agitation, hallucinations, paranoid ideation, disordered thinking and perception, delusions, labile mood, and what is termed "psychomotor behavior"—picking at bed sheets, for example. Even delirious patients who seem withdrawn share the same mental disturbances as those who appear agitated.

For some patients, lowering the opioid dose resolves the problem without impairing pain relief. For others, a change of opioid may be needed. I now routinely ask my patients who take opioids whether they have begun having nightmares and, if so, I switch them to another opioid agent.

The cause of the delirium induced by opioids is not known, but it is unusual for a full-blown delirium to be due to an opioid alone. Contributing factors include structural brain lesions, hypoxia, metabolic abnormalities such as renal or hepatic failure, electrolyte imbalance, nutritional deficiency (especially of B vitamins), infections, and drugs.

DRUG-INDUCED DELIRIUM.   Drugs other than opioids and psychostimulants can induce delirium. Corticosteroids can cause delirium either immediately or weeks to months after they are instituted. Benzodiazepines, particularly lorazepam (e.g., Ativan), can paradoxically cause extreme agitation or delirium.

PRACTICE POINTS: MANAGING DELIRIUM (PART 1)

- Change the opioid or lower the dose.
- Evaluate appropriate patients for contributing medical conditions (e.g., brain lesions, electrolyte imbalance, hypoxia, infection, nutritional deficiency, renal or hepatic dysfunction).
- Discontinue contributing medications (e.g., acyclovir, amphotericin B, anticholinergics or agents with anticholinergic side effects, antiemetics, psychostimulants, short-acting benzodiazepines, steroids).
- Review the recent antineoplastic drug regimen (asparaginase, bleomycin, carmustine, cisplatin, cytosine arabinoside, etoposide, 5-fluorouracil, hexylmethylmelamine, ifosfamide, interferon, interleukin-2, methotrexate (high-dose), procarbazine, vinblastine, vincristine).

Anticholinergic agents (H_2 blockers [e.g., cimetidine] and tricyclic antidepressants), especially when combined with drugs with anticholinergic side effects (such as diphenhydramine [e.g., Benadryl] or hydroxyzine [e.g., Atarax, Vistaril]), can cause a "cholinergic crisis," a life-threatening syndrome that includes high fevers and delirium.

Identifying the Cause of Delirium

A combination of drugs induced a delirium in Mr. Martinez, a patient with metastatic pancreatic cancer. Mr. Martinez's family complained to his oncologist, Dr. Greenleaf, that his pain medications were "making him act funny." They wanted them stopped. Over the past week, they said, he had become intermittently confused and agitated. He occasionally appeared to be having hallucinations, and he sometimes accused his family of being "out to get him." Mr. Martinez's pain was still well controlled by a 100 μg/hr Duragesic (transdermal fentanyl) patch, though he needed twice daily Dilaudid (hydromorphone) for rescue.

Dr. Greenleaf evaluated Mr. Martinez and thought he might be becoming delirious. She agreed with the family that the fentanyl and hydromorphone might be contributing, but felt that Mr. Martinez needed opioids of some type to control his pain. She asked me to recommend several agents that she could safely prescribe, contacted Dr. Blair, a psychiatrist, and admitted Mr. Martinez for observation and therapy.

Dr. Greenleaf told me that Mr. Martinez, like many patients with pancreatic cancer, was depressed and that for four months before this incident he had been taking amitriptyline. His response to the amitriptyline had been excellent: his mood was much improved and he was getting much more pleasure out of life. Two weeks earlier Dr. Greenleaf had added cimetidine and Atarax (hydroxyzine) for gastritis and severe pruritus due to biliary obstruction. His family confirmed that Mr. Martinez had been taking most of these medications as prescribed, but that one week prior to his change in behavior he had doubled his Atarax dose when his pruritus worsened.

I thought it was possible that the opioids were causing Mr. Martinez's delirium, but both Dr. Blair and I were more concerned that the combination of amitriptyline, cimetidine, and an increased dose of Atarax had precipitated a cholinergic crisis manifesting as delirium.

On our recommendation, Dr. Greenleaf discontinued all the drugs that could be contributing, removed the Duragesic patch, and substituted a different opioid, intravenous morphine, for pain management. Dr. Blair suggested haloperidol and lorazepam to control Mr. Martinez's agitation and disordered mentation. Ten days later Mr. Martinez's mental status had greatly improved and he no longer required lorazepam or haloperidol. Because we could not be sure the fentanyl and hydromorphone had not contributed to the delirium, I advised Dr. Greenleaf to treat Mr. Martinez's pain with sustained-release oral morphine and immediate-release oral morphine for rescue. Since Dr. Blair and I thought the delirium was a manifestation of a cholinergic crisis, we also advised her to replace the cimetidine and hydroxyzine with omeprazole and Questran (cholestyramine), respectively. However, because he had not developed the crisis when taking amitriptyline and opioids alone, and because amitriptyline had been of significant benefit, we thought it could safely be restarted.

We explained to Mr. Martinez and his family why the delirium had developed and why it was safe for him to continue taking opioids and amitriptyline. On this regimen, he was able to maintain excellent symptom control without recurrence of a cholinergic crisis until his death two months later.

THERAPY.   I always consult a psychiatrist for patients with delirium and, when the patient's condition permits, I initiate treatment for the underlying cause. It is fortunate, however, that the initial episode of delirium reverses in 50 percent of patients, even when the cause remains unknown (see Table 5.9). Subsequent episodes reverse only 25 percent of the time (Lawlor et al. 2000). Dr. Eduardo Bruera, a noted hospice physician, educator, and researcher, was able to identify an etiology for the delirium in only half of his terminally ill patients. But he and others have identified some simple but effective measures: asking a nurse, friend, or family member to sit with the patient to decrease his anxiety and help with orientation; moving the patient to a well-known favorite room; leaving the light on; and placing a clock and a calendar within sight, along with favorite, familiar objects (Ingham and Caraceni 2002).

PRACTICE POINTS: MANAGING DELIRIUM (PART 2)
- Obtain a psychiatric consultation for all patients with delirium.
- Begin therapy directed at reversing the underlying etiologies whenever possible.
- Surround the patient with the familiar (people, objects, and sounds).
- Frequently reorient the patient to place, day, date, and time.
- Give haloperidol, 0.5 to 1.0 mg IV or 1 to 2 mg p.o., and repeat q6h with 1 to 2 mg q2h p.r.n. until either the agitation resolves or 20 mg has been given within 24 hours.
- For refractory patients who can take oral medication, give olanzapine, 2.5 to 5 mg p.o. b.i.d., and 2.5 mg q4h p.r.n.
- For very agitated patients, consider adding lorazepam (0.5 to 1 mg).

If these techniques do not work, pharmacologic therapy often does. Haloperidol (Haldol), (1 to 2 mg p.o. every 6 hours and every 2 hours p.r.n.; do not exceed 20 mg in 24 hours) will diminish the patient's agitation, clear her sensorium, and improve her ability to think clearly. If the haloperidol is not effective and the patient can take oral medications, give olanzapine (Zyprexa, Zydis) (2.5 to 5 mg p.o. b.i.d. plus 2.5 mg p.o. every 4 hours p.r.n.). If the delirium was induced by corticosteroids, opioids, or metabolic abnormalities (e.g., hypercalcemia), the patient is likely to respond even though the precipitating cause is still present.

For patients requiring parenteral therapy, chlorpromazine (e.g., Thorazine) (25 to 100 mg IV or p.r. b.i.d. to q.i.d.) is effective, but haloperidol (e.g., Haldol), a butyrophenone, is less sedating and has a lower incidence of anticholinergic and cardiovascular side effects. Start with 0.5 to 1 mg of intravenous haloperidol, depending on the patient's size. The parenteral dose is approximately twice as strong as the oral dose. To avoid inducing the neuroleptic malignant syndrome (NMS), I do not exceed doses of 20 mg in 24 hours. Patients who receive higher doses and develop NMS appear rigid and develop a high fever, encephalopathy, and widely fluctuating pulse and blood pressure, and are likely to die from it.

Repeat the haloperidol dose every 6 hours with additional doses every 2 hours as needed until the agitation resolves, the patient falls asleep, or the maximum dose is reached. Continue it four times a day for several days at whatever dose was effective, and then taper it over several weeks, as tolerated. The patient's mental status may not return to normal for several days, but her agitation and fear usually resolve within one or two days.

For a patient experiencing an agitated delirium, adding lorazepam to the haloperidol may control the delirium more rapidly. Oral, rectal, or parenteral lorazepam (e.g., Ativan) is used in doses of 0.5 to 1.0 mg every 1 to 2 hours. It can be given to patients with renal or hepatic impairment, is relatively inexpensive, and in the parenteral form is 80 percent bioavailable when given rectally. The parenteral form of diazepam (e.g., Valium) is also well absorbed rectally. Unfortunately, studies show that more than half of patients treated with rectal diazepam experienced a sensation of rectal burning lasting up to 15 minutes (Warren 1996). Clonazepam has been shown to be absorbed rapidly from the rectum in normal adults, so it, too, can be considered in treating agitation.

The treatment of delirious patients who are actively dying is reviewed in Chapter 8. Home hospice teams can administer medications that help both the patient and the family find peace during the patient's last days.

RESPIRATORY DEPRESSION

Respiratory depression is a very unusual side effect of opioids when given to treat cancer pain, as long as the opioid dose is titrated to the degree of pain and the patient's renal and hepatic functions remain stable (Legrand et al. 2004). Opioids do marginally decrease the brain's sensitivity to carbon dioxide levels and are associated with a slight, usually clinically insignificant, degree of hypoventilation.

It is sometimes difficult to determine whether a patient's respiratory depression is due to the opioid or to something else. If an opioid is responsible, the patient will also be confused and somnolent, because opioid-induced respiratory depression is due to general depression of the central nervous system. If the patient is anxious or agitated, however, something other than opioids must be causing the respiratory depression.

PRACTICE POINTS: MANAGING OPIOID-RELATED RESPIRATORY DEPRESSION

- Respiratory depression in an agitated patient is unlikely to be due to the opioid.
- Respiratory depression may indicate worsening of renal or hepatic function, hypothyroidism, persistence of drug in the bowel because of obstruction, or sepsis.
- Induce evacuation of residual opioid from the gut and remove any opioid-containing skin patches.
- If respiratory rate is dangerously low, infuse a dilute solution of naloxone until the rate returns to a safe level. Do not give enough to awaken the patient or to induce opioid withdrawal.

Occasionally, patients have underlying medical conditions that make them more susceptible to these depressive effects of opioids. Hypothyroid patients or those whose obstructive lung disease causes them to retain carbon dioxide are in this category. Hypothyroid patients with coronary artery disease and angina can be particularly problematic; they can develop respiratory arrest with even the 1 or 2 mg of morphine they receive for pain in the emergency room. For patients with chronic obstructive pulmonary disease, I find that I can safely prescribe opioids if I start with very low concentrations (e.g., morphine 0.25 mg/hr), increase the doses very slowly, and monitor the patient carefully.

Other patients, especially those taking a sustained-release preparation, can develop respiratory depression because the metabolism of the opioid suddenly changes (e.g., sudden renal or hepatic failure) or more drug is absorbed (e.g., a bowel obstruction). Those wearing transdermal fentanyl patches can develop toxicity if they become febrile (which increases the drug's absorption from the skin reservoir) or septic (as acidosis increases the free fraction of the drug).

In such cases, you may find yourself caring for a patient whose pain control depends on opioids and who also has CNS and respiratory depression. It is very important even in this situation that you *resist* the temptation to use an undiluted injection of naloxone to reverse the effects of the opioid completely. If you do administer undiluted naloxone, you may precipitate a severe withdrawal syndrome and the patient may wake up in excruciating pain that you will have a very hard time bringing under control, even if you reinstitute opioids.

If the patient is breathing normally but cannot be aroused, simply withholding further opioid doses is sufficient. If significant respiratory depression has occurred you will need to administer a dilute solution of naloxone. The low dose of naloxone enables the patient to reestablish normal respirations and wake up gradually without experiencing withdrawal.

Dilute naloxone can be given as either a slow intravenous "push" or a continuous infusion. For patients whose respiratory rates are between 10/min and 12/min, who are just mildly oversedated, and whose renal, hepatic, or gut function can be expected to normalize quickly, I suggest the following: dilute the 1 ml containing 0.4 mg of naloxone into 10 ml of normal saline, then infuse as much of this dilute naloxone as is necessary to establish a normal respiratory rate but not enough to awaken the patient. The dose can be repeated as needed.

For patients whose opioid levels are likely to be elevated for a prolonged period, I suggest you begin an intravenous infusion of naloxone and adjust the rate so that normal respirations are established but the patient does not wake up suddenly. Patients who have developed toxic effects from the fentanyl of a transdermal fentanyl patch, and those who have been taking sustained-release morphine or oxycodone and develop hepatic or renal failure or an ileus, are likely to require naloxone drips.

In addition to the naloxone drip, it is wise to institute measures that will stop the patient from aspirating and from absorbing additional amounts of the opioid. Laxatives, oral or intravenous motility agents (e.g., metoclopramide), and enemas all help the patient eliminate the remaining sustained-release opioid from the gastrointestinal tract. Unfortunately, as mentioned earlier in this chapter, even after the transdermal fentanyl patch is removed, the patient will be absorbing fentanyl from the skin reservoir for 12 to 24 more hours. As the patient begins to wake up, reduce the naloxone infusion gradually to match the residual opioid level. Patients will awaken safely, without withdrawal; as pain reappears, appropriate opioid therapy can be resumed.

MISCELLANEOUS SIDE EFFECTS

Myoclonic jerking (multifocal myoclonus) indicates opioid-induced neurotoxicity. It can be seen in patients taking high doses of any opioid, but is most common in patients receiving frequent, repeated therapeutic doses of meperidine. In its earliest stages, patients only experience the muscle jerking as they are falling asleep. With increasing opioid doses, family members or patients themselves may report muscle spasms or involuntary movements. The spasms may be severe enough to exacerbate the distress from an already painful limb. Patients receiving moderate to high doses of other opioids who develop renal insufficiency or dehydration may develop myoclonus, possibly related to increased levels of opioids and their metabolites.

Changing to another opioid often relieves the problem. But if myoclonus persists and the patient would prefer not to change opioids, baclofen or dantrolene can reduce the spasms. For patients with severe myoclonus or for those too close to dying for a trial of opioid rotation, benzodiazepines such as clonazepam, lorazepam, or midazolam are usually needed. Rarely, patients can either be resistant to the benzodiazepine or have a history of increased agitation after receiving one. For these patients, I use a barbiturate infusion, usually with pentobarbital. In Chapter 8, I review how to use both midazolam and pentobarbital.

Opioid-induced *urinary retention* is also troublesome, especially for older patients or those with underlying bladder outlet obstruction. Discontinuing any agents with anticholinergic side effects is often effective, but some patients may require finasteride (e.g., Proscar) (5 mg/day p.o.) to diminish the outlet obstruction, or bethanechol (e.g., Urecholine) (10 mg p.o. t.i.d., to a maximum of 50 mg p.o. t.i.d.) to relax the bladder smooth muscle that is being stimulated by the opioid.

Pruritus, which most commonly occurs in opioid-naive patients receiving epidural or intrathecal opioids, may be caused by activation of spinal opiate receptors, by opioid-induced release of histamine from mast cells, or by disinhibition of itch-specific neurons (McNicol et al. 2003). Pruritus may resolve with a change in opioid, but you may need to add ondansetron (4 mg p.o. or IV); paroxetine (Paxil) (10 to 20 mg p.o.) (Zylicz et al. 1998); or nalmefene (10 to 25 µg IV) or nalbuphine (1 to 5 mg IV) (Hough et al. 2003).

SUMMARY

Constipation, nausea, sedation, delirium, respiratory depression, myoclonus, urinary retention, and pruritus are treatable side effects that can often be prevented. They can discourage patients from taking the doses of opioid therapy they need to achieve satisfactory control of their pain. For patients with complicated pain syndromes, you may need to prescribe a number of agents to prevent or control side effects, and the patient may need to try two or three different opioids before achieving satisfactory pain control with tolerable side effects. By using these strategies you will be able to reverse or ameliorate those problems that do occur and markedly increase the comfort of your patients.

ADJUVANT ANALGESIC TREATMENTS

Adjuvant analgesics are drugs that are used primarily for other indications but which also produce pain relief. They are of particular value for patients with neuropathic pain, including patients with spinal cord compression (see Tables 5.10 and 5.11) or bone pain (see Table 5.12). In the sections that follow, I describe how to use a variety of adjuvant analgesics for the treatment of neuropathic pain, including corticosteroids, anticonvulsants, and psychotropics. I also review agents useful for bone pain, neuroleptics, and skeletal muscle relaxants.

Adjuvant analgesic agents are usually given orally or parenterally, but occasionally rectal administration is preferable. Unfortunately, while there is good information about the rectal use of opioids and NSAIDs, we have less information about administering adjuvant medications via this route.

ADJUVANT TREATMENTS FOR NEUROPATHIC PAIN

Opioids can relieve both central and peripheral neuropathic pain syndromes (Rowbotham et al. 2003), but side effects can limit the doses that

are tolerable. When a peripheral nerve is injured, inflammatory mediators are released that cause changes in the sodium channel activity of the
nerves at that site and at the dorsal root ganglion, and new calcium
channels appear. These changes cause "peripheral sensitization," which
is both a lowering of the threshold for nerve firing and a spontaneous firing of the nerves. Unlike opioids, drugs that can modify the ion channels, such as corticosteroids, gabapentin and the other anticonvulsants,
tricyclic antidepressants, local anesthetics, and clonidine (see Table 5.10),
can provide the extra analgesia needed for satisfactory relief of the discomfort that comes from peripheral and central sensitization (Beydoun
and Backonja 2003).

"Central sensitization" refers to changes in the spinal cord that occur
after peripheral nerve injury. Substance P and neurokinin A released
into the spinal cord by injured peripheral nerves cause changes in the activity of the calcium channels and a lowering of the threshold for firing
of spinal cord neurons. These neurons also begin to respond not only to
signals from the nerves that enter at their level of the cord but also to signals from nerves synapsing above and below them. In addition, more
spinal cord NMDA receptors appear. These receptors inhibit the ability
of opioids to relieve pain. Given all these changes, patients with central
sensitization usually need treatment with agents that affect the activity
of calcium channels (such as gabapentin, discussed later in this chapter),
and may need agents that affect the activity of the sodium channels
(such as tricyclic antidepressants) or that can inhibit the activity of the
NMDA receptors (such as methadone or ketamine; ketamine also is discussed later in the chapter).

CORTICOSTEROIDS. Corticosteroids are effective both for patients
with malignant bone pain and for those with malignant neuropathic
pain, such as that caused by compression of the spinal cord by tumor. By
inhibiting synthesis of prostaglandins and by decreasing firing from injured nerves, corticosteroids diminish transmission of the pain signal
from the periphery to the spinal cord or from the spinal cord to the brain.
By decreasing capillary permeability, they reduce edema and thereby
relieve the pain of brain metastases or tumor infiltration of nerves or
nerve roots. There are also clinical reports of corticosteroids relieving
esophageal or gastroduodenal obstruction, but no controlled studies
have been done to confirm their efficacy in these conditions.

Corticosteroids can be given epidurally, intravenously, or orally.
Epidural corticosteroids have been studied only in patients with non-

malignant pain syndromes, but their success in some patients with radiculopathies (e.g., from disk disease) suggests that they might be beneficial as adjuncts for those with malignant epidural disease who cannot tolerate systemic corticosteroid therapy.

PRACTICE POINTS: CORTICOSTEROIDS AS ADJUVANTS
- Corticosteroids decrease pain due to peripheral nerve injury (e.g., acute herpes zoster or metastases to the brachial or lumbosacral plexus), spinal cord compression, and brain metastases.
- Corticosteroids also decrease bone pain.
- Onset of pain relief is often rapid.
- To minimize side effects:
   —Give the minimal effective dose.
   —Consider prophylaxis for oral and esophageal candidiasis and for gastritis/ulcer disease.
- Be alert for mood changes (euphoria or depression) and delirium.

Corticosteroid therapy is indicated for all patients with radiologic evidence of cord compression. Corticosteroids decrease cord edema and pain and help preserve neurologic function and overall outcome after specific therapy (i.e., radiation, surgery, or radiation followed by surgery). Intravenous corticosteroids can induce very rapid pain relief. Patients who receive high doses of intravenous corticosteroids for cord compression, for example, often experience a significant decrease of back pain within hours. There is controversy, however, about the dose that should be used. For patients treated with radiotherapy, high-dose dexamethasone (100 mg IV bolus followed by 24 mg p.o. q.i.d. for 3 days, then tapered over 10 days) is recommended. More patients remained ambulatory after receiving both radiotherapy and this high-dose dexamethasone than after receiving radiotherapy alone (81 percent vs 63 percent) (Sorensen et al. 1994). (Selected patients with little epidural disease and contraindications for corticosteroid therapy have been shown to tolerate radiotherapy safely without corticosteroids.) Patients usually receive lower doses of dexamethasone (10 mg IV bolus, then 4 mg IV q.i.d., then tapered over 14 days), but in one study these lower doses had no significant effect on patient mobility. The group of patients who received lower-dose dexamethasone remained ambulatory at the same rate as the group not given any dexamethasone (57.1 percent vs 57.9 percent) (Heimdal et al. 1992). The lower dose of dexamethasone (10 mg) does, however, provide as much pain relief as the higher dose (100 mg).

Corticosteroid therapy is also indicated as an adjuvant for all patients with radiologic evidence of cord compression while they are being evaluated for decompressive surgery. Surgery was formerly reserved for patients without a diagnosis of cancer with a reasonable life expectancy, with tumors that were very unlikely to respond to radiation, or with disease that progressed despite radiation therapy. Recent data from a randomized trial suggest, however, that patients treated with surgery followed by radiation therapy either remained ambulatory longer or were more likely to become ambulatory than patients who received radiation therapy alone (Patchell et al. 2003). If you are interested in more information about assessing and treating patients with spinal cord compression, please refer to Chapter 4 and to the reviews included in the bibliography at the end of this chapter (Abrahm 2004; Loblaw et al. 2004; Schiff 2003).

For patients with brain metastases or impending but not actual cord compression, consider starting with the lower-dose corticosteroid regimen, tapering to 4 or 2 mg every 6 hours during the second week of radiation treatments. If you choose the 100-mg dose, be sure it is given over at least 15 to 30 minutes; if given more rapidly it is likely to cause a severe, though transient, perineal burning sensation. After the radiation is completed, switch to oral corticosteroids and taper the dose as the patient tolerates. Reinstate a higher dose if back pain, headache, or other symptoms of cord or CNS edema return.

Corticosteroids are also effective adjuvants for patients with peripheral nerve injuries, such as those with tumor infiltrating the brachial plexus (typically lung or breast cancer) or the lumbosacral plexus (typically recurrent colorectal cancer). To the opioid therapy, add 4 to 6 mg of dexamethasone orally two to four times a day or 50 mg of prednisone twice a day. In responding patients the pain diminishes significantly by 48 to 72 hours. To minimize the corticosteroid-induced side effects, taper the dose rapidly, watching for reemergence of unacceptable pain. In many cases, patients have been able to maintain effective pain control with alternate-day corticosteroid dosing.

Corticosteroids alone have been shown to decrease the acute pain associated with herpes zoster infections, but there is no long-term benefit. Similarly, adding acyclovir (800 mg five times a day for 21 days) to prednisone (60 mg/day for 7 days, 30 mg/day for the next 7 days, and 15 mg/day for the last 7 days), while leading to quicker resolution of neuritis, return to uninterrupted sleep, return to usual daily activities, and cessation of analgesics, does not prevent post-herpetic neuralgia (Wood et al. 1994; cancer patients were excluded from this study).

Oral corticosteroids have also been used to increase patients' appetite and sense of well-being, but results of controlled studies of their efficacy have been conflicting. Increases in appetite in the short run (about one month) were consistently noted. In some studies, improvement in the amount of food eaten and patients' sense of well-being or quality of life was also seen, but neither weight nor survival time increased. The patients who showed the most improvement were those with neuropathic pain. For selected patients with advanced cancer, for whom appetite or sense of well-being is a significant issue, consider a course of corticosteroids, expecting at least a short-term benefit.

The limitation to using corticosteroids is the significant incidence of corticosteroid-induced side effects. Many of these can be prevented and others readily managed, but some of the most serious ones occur unpredictably. The corticosteroid-induced side effects and recommended treatments are described below.

Gastrointestinal Disorders.   Corticosteroids alone probably do not cause ulcers. Patients taking corticosteroids along with an NSAID (other than acetaminophen), however, do have a higher incidence of ulcers than those taking the NSAID alone. Therefore, consider prescribing a proton pump inhibitor (e.g., omeprazole (20 mg/day) for patients taking both corticosteroids and NSAIDs.

Candidiasis.   One of the most common corticosteroid-induced side effects, especially in patients who are debilitated or otherwise immunocompromised, is oral or esophageal candidiasis (thrush). These conditions can be very distressing and may seriously decrease your patient's oral intake. It is therefore important to carefully describe to the patient and his family the signs and symptoms of oral and esophageal candidal infections (the painful, burning red tongue and the esophageal pain syndrome described below). They will then be able to call you promptly and receive appropriate therapy should an infection develop.

If you plan a prolonged corticosteroid course, you might consider starting prophylactic antifungal therapy with oral fluconazole (200 mg on day 1 followed by 100 mg/day). For patients expected to require only a short-term course of corticosteroids, consider oral prophylaxis with topical antifungals such as clotrimazole troches (e.g., Mycelex) given three times a day. But patients will need to be monitored for esophageal candidiasis because these agents do not prevent it.

Esophagitis causes a very distinctive pain syndrome. Even though the infection usually involves only the lower esophagus, the pain can be experienced in the mid or even upper esophagus. You have probably experienced esophageal pain if you have swallowed a fish bone that "got stuck" or have drunk a very hot liquid too quickly. As you may remember, a few seconds after you swallow, when the wave of peristalsis passes the injured area, the pain appears. Patients with this problem will grimace a few seconds after swallowing, when they experience the pain. You can treat esophageal candidiasis effectively with oral ketoconazole or fluconazole; patients usually experience significant pain relief within 48 hours.

Mood Changes. Corticosteroid-induced delirium is more common in people with a previous psychiatric history, and high-dose corticosteroids should be used with caution in such patients. For most patients the mood changes are less marked. In some, a euphoria occurs that can be quite enjoyable. The commonly associated insomnia can be prevented by instructing the patient to take the corticosteroids before noon. Other patients develop a severe corticosteroid-induced depression, which may respond to lowering the corticosteroid dose or to discontinuing it altogether. Antidepressant drugs are not usually required.

Miscellaneous. Corticosteroid-induced *glucose intolerance* is usually easily managed with insulin. For patients with impaired mental status, the visiting nurse or hospice team can be of great assistance in regulating and administering the insulin doses. Prophylaxis for pneumocystis is needed for patients on prolonged steroid therapy.

Proximal muscle weakness can be quite disabling and very refractory to therapy. Home physical therapy or, for those who can tolerate it, hydrotherapy can preserve some muscle function, but many patients will need assisting devices such as lift chairs to keep them independent in their daily activities. Others may require wheelchairs and support devices such as shower chairs.

ANTICONVULSANTS. The anticonvulsants—gabapentin (Neurontin), phenytoin (e.g., Dilantin), carbamazepine (e.g., Tegretol), lamotrigine (Lamictal), topiramate (Topamax), and oxcarbazepine (Trileptal)—are important adjuvant agents for patients with neuropathic pain that is "burning," "sharp," "cutting," or "like an electric shock" (Table 5.10). The mechanism by which these agents relieve such pain has not yet been determined.

Gabapentin is the most commonly used agent with the fewest side effects. It has demonstrated efficacy in patients with post-herpetic neuralgia and peripheral neuropathies resulting from diabetes or chemotherapy, and is empirically used for patients with neuropathic pain of any etiology. To minimize sedation, especially in older patients, use low doses initially and raise the dose every 3 to 4 days (or weekly in older patients) as tolerated. Start at 100 mg orally, three times a day, or, for patients with difficulty sleeping, 100 mg in the morning and evening and 300 mg at bedtime. The dose for patients with renal insufficiency is 100 to 200 mg twice a day. Give patients with renal failure who are undergoing dialysis a 300–mg loading dose, and then 200 to 300 mg after each dialysis. The minimal effective dose is usually 300 mg orally, three times a day, but if some pain relief is produced, the doses can be increased to improve pain relief, up to 3600 mg/day in divided doses. Sedation and peripheral edema are the usual dose-limiting side effects. If the gabapentin does not provide sufficient relief alone, try adding (in succession) lamotrigine (150 to 500 mg/day in two divided doses), topiramate (25 to 400 mg/day in two divided doses), or oxcarbazepine (300 to 2400 mg/day in two divided doses) to improve the pain control. Other active agents include divalproex (150 to 3000 mg/day in three divided doses), zonisamide (100 to 400 mg/day in two divided doses), and the benzodiazepine clonazepam (1 to 10 mg/day in two divided doses) (Farrar and Portenoy 2001; Rowbotham et al. 1998).

For patients with lancinating, electric shock–like pain that does not respond to any combination of these agents, discontinue the gabapentin and try phenytoin (100 to 300 mg/day) or carbamazepine (100 to 1600 mg/day, in two to four divided doses). Although carbamazepine has most often been shown to be effective, as, for example, in trigeminal neuralgia (tic douloureux), consider beginning with phenytoin. You can reach therapeutic levels of phenytoin within a day and complete a therapeutic trial in one or two weeks. If by that time the pain has not improved, discontinue the phenytoin and begin carbamazepine, increasing doses slowly (i.e., incrementally every week or two) until therapeutic levels are reached. This may take as long as a month but may help selected patients.

Except for gabapentin, the anticonvulsants cause a number of side effects and require careful monitoring. Patients taking phenytoin may develop ataxia, nausea, vomiting, or visual problems if the dose exceeds the therapeutic range; they may also develop allergic reactions involving the skin or liver. Carbamazepine causes hypotension in ambulatory patients if the dose is escalated too rapidly, and it can (rarely) cause severe neutropenia. Lamotrigine commonly causes fatigue, dizziness, headache, rash, mental status changes, blurred vision, and nausea and vomiting, and, rarely, causes serious allergic skin reactions and cytopenias and hepatic failure. Begin by giving 25 mg/day orally for 2 weeks, increasing to 50 mg/day orally for 2 weeks and then to 100 mg/day orally for 1 week, as tolerated. The maximum dose is 200 mg/day orally.

Topiramate commonly causes dizziness, somnolence, fatigue, mental status changes, and depression, and, rarely, causes kidney stones, acute angle-closure glaucoma, oligohydrosis and hyperthermia, cytopenias, psychosis, and severe allergic skin reactions. Begin topiramate doses at 25 to 50 mg/day orally, and increase by 25 to 50 mg/day each week. Doses above 400 mg are rarely more effective than lower doses.

Oxcarbazepine commonly causes dizziness, somnolence, confusion, diplopia, fatigue, nausea/vomiting/abdominal pain, abnormal gait, nystagmus, and, rarely, severe allergic skin reactions, cytopenias, angioedema, and hyponatremia. Oxcarbazepine doses should begin at 300 mg orally twice a day and increase by 300 mg every 3 days as tolerated, to a maximum of 2400 mg/day orally.

Levetiracetam (Keppra) is particularly difficult for patients to tolerate, as it commonly causes somnolence that does not remit with continued therapy. It also commonly causes asthenia, dizziness, ataxia, agitation, anxiety, emotional lability, behavior changes, and anemia. Begin at 500 mg orally every 12 hours, for 2 weeks and increase by 1000 mg/day every 2 weeks to a maximum of 3000 mg/day.

TRICYCLIC ANTIDEPRESSANTS.   Tricyclic antidepressants are also prescribed as adjuvant analgesics for patients with neuropathic pain (see Table 5.11), but their anticholinergic side effects (e.g., dry mouth, dry eyes, blurred vision, constipation, hypotension, urinary retention, and sedation) limit their usefulness. At doses far below those needed for an antidepressant effect, nortriptyline, which has the least of these side effects, is well tolerated and effective. Neuropathic pain is often worse at night, so give the nortriptyline at bedtime, starting at 10 mg orally. Patients taking gabapentin can also take this low dose of nortriptyline to improve the therapeutic effect while keeping side effects to a minimum.

I have found that, to avoid misunderstandings, before a patient begins taking an adjuvant antidepressant I need to be sure the patient and family understand how the medication fits in the pain-relief regimen. I don't want patients to assume that because I'm using an antidepressant to treat their pain, I think the pain is "all in their mind."

PRACTICE POINTS: ADJUVANT AGENTS FOR NEUROPATHIC PAIN

- Gabapentin is the most useful anticonvulsant for neuropathic pain. It is effective and has the fewest side effects.
- Carbamazepine is best studied for tic douloureux–like pain, but consider giving phenytoin to achieve therapeutic levels rapidly.
- Consider adding low-dose nortriptyline to enhance pain relief with minimal additional side effects.

BACLOFEN.   Baclofen, a GABA (gamma-aminobutyric acid) antagonist, acts primarily at the spinal cord level and is normally used to relax spastic limbs of patients with CNS disease. It is also useful for cancer patients who have developed spasticity after spinal cord injury. Baclofen also relieves trigeminal neuralgia pain and so may help those patients with cancer of the head and neck who develop a neuropathic pain syndrome similar to that of trigeminal neuralgia.

Baclofen is usually given orally, three times a day, but it can be given intrathecally if necessary. Doses begin at 5 mg three times daily and are escalated every 3 days by 5 mg at each dose to a target of 40 to 80 mg/day. This gradual dose increase minimizes the drowsiness, dizziness, hypotension, nausea, and confusion that the drug can induce. If the patient needs to discontinue baclofen, it is important that you taper it gradually to prevent the patient from developing psychiatric disorders, hallucinations, or seizures.

CLONIDINE.   Clonidine, an alpha-2-adrenergic agonist usually used to treat hypertension, is also able to relieve pain and will prevent opioid withdrawal in patients who must discontinue opioids following development of opioid bowel syndrome. Used either transdermally or in intrathecal infusions, clonidine is also helpful in some patients with postoperative pain, post-herpetic neuralgia, and other types of neuropathic pain.

KETAMINE.   Ketamine is a pure NMDA antagonist that is typically used as an anesthetic but can be helpful for selected patients with neuropathic pain that is resistant to the combinations of agents discussed above. Ketamine is particularly helpful for patients with central sensitization who cannot get pain relief without sedation, and who wish to be awake. Patients who are taking ketamine describe being "dissociated" from their pain. They know it's there, but it's not theirs. Unfortunately, they can also be more generally dissociated, and for some this can be frightening, as can the strange dreams and even daytime hallucinations that sometimes occur. Benzodiazepines (e.g., diazepam 1 mg) are effective in reversing these side effects (Mercadante et al. 2000).

Two randomized controlled trials, methodologically sound, found that ketamine (intrathecal [Yang et al. 1996] or IV [Mercadante et al. 2000]) allowed a reduction in the use of morphine and a significant improvement in pain control for patients with neuropathic cancer pain (Bell et al. 2003). Dr. Perry Fine, a professor of anesthesiology at the University of Utah Health Sciences Center and national medical director of VistaCare hospice in Scottsdale, Arizona, has used ketamine for his patients for many years and has published his experience (Fine 1999). I

PRACTICE POINTS: KETAMINE FOR REFRACTORY PAIN

- Inform the patient that he is likely to experience a "dreamlike" state.
- Give a ketamine bolus of 0.1 to 0.2 mg/kg IV or 0.5 mg/kg SQ, monitoring vital signs.
- If there is no change in the pain, double the dose of ketamine at 15 minutes (for IV dosing) or 45 minutes (for SQ dosing).
- Repeat step 3 [doubling of dose] until pain relief is achieved, and then begin a continuous IV or SQ drip to deliver the equivalent amount. For example, a patient who required a total of 12 mg of ketamine in 60 minutes should be started on a drip of 12 mg/hr. Increase the drip as needed and tolerated.
- If a decrease in opioid dose is desirable because of opioid side effects (e.g., myoclonic jerks), decrease the opioid dose initially by 50 percent when the ketamine drip is begun, and halve again every 24 hours as tolerated.
- Excess salivation may require additional therapy. Scopolamine (Transderm Scōp), hyoscyamine (e.g., Levsin), or glycopyrrolate.

(From Fine 2003)

have used his protocol (published in the *American Academy of Hospice and Palliative Medicine [AAHPM] Bulletin* in 2003) and found it very effective. Ketamine administration has been successfully converted to the oral route, but dosing is affected by the drug's active metabolite, norketamine. Levels of norketamine are two to three times higher with oral dosing of ketamine than when given parenterally, so the oral ketamine dose is about one-third the parenteral dose (Fitzgibbon et al. 2002).

Adjuvant Treatments for Bone Pain

External beam radiation is the longest-lasting palliative treatment for bone pain, and radiopharmaceuticals (e.g., strontium chloride 89) enhance its effectiveness and are also effective used alone. In addition, NSAIDs, corticosteroids (see Tables 5.1 and 5.10), bisphosphonates, and calcitonin can serve as pharmacologic adjuvants to opioids for patients with bone pain (Table 5.12).

external beam radiation and radiopharmaceuticals.   External beam radiation is an important palliative tool for treating localized bone metastases (Janjan 2001). It provides pain relief for over 70 percent of patients, and the relief usually lasts about three months. Palliative radiation given in a single large fraction produces pain relief just as fast and for just as long as the more conventional treatments involving ten fractions.

Systemic radiopharmaceuticals, such as strontium chloride 89, samarium-153 lexidronam (Serafini et al. 1998), rhenium-186 HEDP (hydroxyethylidenediphosphonate), and rhenium-188 HEDP, are used for patients with diffuse bony metastases. These agents are beta-particle emitters that localize in osteoblastic metastases. They provide pain relief in about 70 to 80 percent of patients with bony metastases from prostate or breast cancer (McEwan 1997; Palmedo et al. 2000, 2003). Pain relief usually begins within 1 to 3 weeks and is maintained for 3 to 6 months. Strontium chloride 89 can prolong the pain relief induced by external beam radiotherapy (Janjan 2001; Porter et al. 1993).

Repeat doses can also be effective. Patients treated with repeat doses of rhenium-188 HEDP had superior pain relief and lived longer than patients receiving a single dose in a randomized phase II study (Palmedo et al. 2003). Radiopharmaceuticals may also play a role in anticancer therapy for patients with prostate cancer (McCready and O'Sullivan 2002; Porter et al. 1993).

PRACTICE POINTS: TREATING PATIENTS WITH BONE PAIN

- For patients with localized bone metastases, consider recommending strontium chloride 89 along with external beam radiation to decrease the need for repeat courses of radiation.
- Consider systemic radiopharmaceuticals for patients with diffuse bone pain due to multiple metastases.
- Give zoledronic acid (Zometa) or pamidronate for pain due to lytic bone metastases. Both can also decrease pathologic fractures in patients with metastatic breast cancer or multiple myeloma. Use pamidronate for patients with renal insufficiency.
- For patients over 60 years old or with congestive heart failure, renal disease, asthma, or a history of gastrointestinal bleeding, the risks of NSAIDs (used as opioid adjuvants for bone pain) probably exceed the benefit.

Strontium-89 is chemically similar to calcium and is deposited in bone preferentially to calcium. It may therefore exacerbate hypercalcemia and should not be given to hypercalcemic patients. Strontium chloride 89 is given by slow intravenous push in the outpatient setting by a nuclear medicine physician. For 48 hours after the injection, patients should flush twice after using a toilet and should avoid using urinals and bedpans if possible. Families should be cautioned to wear disposable gloves while handling any items contaminated with the patient's urine, feces, or blood. Patients and families should also be warned that 5 to 10 percent of patients will suffer a "flare" (i.e., an increase in bone pain) 2 to 3 days after the injection, which will remit in 7 to 10 days; flares occur more often in patients with breast cancer than in those with prostate cancer.

Myelosuppression occurs in most patients; platelet and leukocyte counts usually fall 25 to 40 percent. Strontium chloride 89 is therefore contraindicated for patients with platelet counts of $<60,000/mm^3$ or leukocyte counts of $<2400/mm^3$. Initial blood counts and previous irradiation of marrow do not predict the extent of the subsequent reductions in blood counts. Life-threatening thrombocytopenia, however, has been noted in patients with low-grade disseminated intravascular coagulation (DIC) or rapidly falling platelet counts, and some researchers suggest obtaining DIC screens for such patients prior to strontium chloride 89 therapy. The nadirs occur at 4 to 8 weeks and counts are somewhat recovered by 12 weeks.

Samarium-153 lexidronam is also excreted intact in the urine, and the excretion is complete within 12 hours. Patients and families should exercise the same precautions as they would if the patient had received strontium. Pain relief, however, is more rapid. Seventy percent of patients have pain relief, and it occurs within 1 to 2 weeks. Patients should be monitored for opioid toxicity, therefore, and doses lowered as needed. Hematologic recovery is also more rapid and is usually complete within 8 weeks.

Hemibody radiation is as effective as strontium chloride 89 for patients with prostate cancer but is more toxic (Janjan 1997). Hemibody radiation can relieve pain in the lower spine, pelvis, and femora in as many as 80 percent of prostate cancer patients, with 30 percent obtaining complete relief. The relief begins as early as 48 hours after treatment but lasts a median of only 15 weeks. A randomized study indicated that patients treated with fractionated rather than single-dose regimens experienced longer durations of response (8.5 vs 3 months) and a decreased need for retreatment (13 percent vs 70 percent). Hemibody radiation, however, is not often chosen as the initial therapy for patients with bony metastases, because of technical difficulties in delivering the radiation, side effects of the therapy, and concerns about toxicity to viscera and bone marrow in the treatment field.

BISPHOSPHONATES.   These drugs inhibit osteoclast activity and can provide immediate relief of pain due to bony metastases or bone lesions of multiple myeloma. Pamidronate (Aredia) (60 to 90 mg IV over 2 to 4 hours) and zoledronic acid (Zometa) (4 mg IV over 15 minutes) have been shown to decrease pain or the need for pain-relieving medications. If the pain returns, repeat doses 3 to 4 weeks apart are often effective. Both drugs have the added benefit of slowing the growth of some tumor metastases and, when given monthly, of preventing fractures from lytic bone metastases in patients with myeloma (Berenson et al. 1998) and breast cancer (Hortobagyi et al. 1998). Both can cause renal toxicity. Renal function should be monitored in patients who have baseline impairment or are at high risk for dehydration (Johnson et al. 2003; Kloth et al. 2003). Vitamin D-deficient patients can become hypocalcemic.

CALCITONIN.   Calcitonin (100 to 200 IU), which also inhibits osteoclast activity, can be considered in the treatment of bone pain, but it must be taken subcutaneously or nasally twice daily for several weeks and can cause symptomatic hypocalcemia.

VERTEBROPLASTY/KYPHOPLASTY. Pain from benign or malignant compression fractures can be very difficult to treat, especially in older patients who develop confusion and marked worsening of constipation while using the opioid doses they need, even when they are taking NSAID adjuvants. For selected patients (those with very localized intense pain from a new or progressing fracture) (Papaioannou et al. 2002), vertebroplasty or kyphoplasty may be the answer. In both procedures, bone "cement" (polymethylmethacrylate + antibiotics + an opacification agent) is injected under fluoroscopic guidance into the collapsed vertebra to stabilize it; in kyphoplasty, the endplates of the vertebral body are elevated by inflatable bone tamps before the cement is injected. Both procedures can be done in the outpatient setting by the interventional radiologist, neurosurgeon, or orthopedic surgeon.

Case reports suggest that these procedures are successful in relieving pain for 70 to 100 percent of patients with compression from osteoporosis (Watts et al. 2001) or malignancy (Jensen and Kallmes 2002), producing short-term documented improvement in pain and disability, mental function, and quality of life (Zoarski et al. 2002) and long-term (1 to 1.5 years) improvement in pain (Jensen and Kallmes 2002; Zoarski et al. 2002). Patients with malignancies are most often also treated with radiation, so it is difficult to assess the long-term contribution of the vertebroplasty, but case reports indicate pain relief within 48 hours that is most likely due to the procedure (Jensen and Kallmes 2002).

The mechanism of the relief is not clear, although some authors have postulated that the injection of the cement causes destruction of nerve endings in the local tissue or necrosis of the tumor (Jensen and Kallmes 2002). Side effects are related to extravasation of the cement, which can cause transient increased pain as well as damage to the spinal cord or nerve roots from heat or pressure.

NEUROLEPTICS

Neuroleptic agents include the butyrophenones, such as haloperidol (e.g., Haldol), and the phenothiazines, such as chlorpromazine (e.g., Thorazine). In cancer patients, these agents are most useful in treating patients with delirium, though chlorpromazine can also help those with intractable hiccups. While most butyrophenones and phenothiazines are not useful in relieving pain, there is some evidence that the butyrophenone pimozide has analgesic activity. Pimozide may be useful for patients with pain syndromes that resemble trigeminal neuralgia, but results of studies are conflicting.

SKELETAL MUSCLE RELAXANTS

Skeletal muscle relaxants include agents such as carisoprodol (e.g., Soma), chlorzoxazone (e.g., Parafon Forte DSC), cyclobenzaprine HCl (e.g., Flexeril), methocarbamol (e.g., Robaxin), and orphenadrine citrate (e.g., Norflex, Norgesic). Used alone, they are no more effective than NSAIDs, but they do add to the efficacy of NSAIDs for patients with acute muscle injury and spasm. And carisoprodol, orphenadrine, and methocarbamol are available in preparations that include aspirin.

Skeletal muscle relaxants are not as effective for patients with chronic nonmalignant pain as for those with acute pain, and they have not been studied in patients with cancer pain. Because they are metabolized by the liver and excreted by the kidneys, skeletal muscle relaxants are relatively contraindicated for patients with renal or hepatic dysfunction. In addition, they have the potential for abuse, and patients who stop them suddenly may experience a withdrawal syndrome.

Muscle relaxants cause significant side effects. Drowsiness is especially problematic and is likely to limit their use in someone receiving other sedating agents such as opioids. They can also cause dizziness, headaches, blurry vision, agitation, confusion, hallucinations, and convulsions. More rarely, patients have developed abdominal pain, nausea, vomiting, or anorexia when taking these drugs. Cyclobenzaprine HCl is related chemically to tricyclic antidepressants, and orphenadrine citrate is related to diphenhydramine; they share the anticholinergic and antihistaminic side effects of these agents.

For cancer patients who develop an acute muscle injury or muscle spasm and who do not need opioid analgesics, one of these combination NSAID / skeletal muscle relaxants may be beneficial. Because of the serious side effects they can induce, I do not prescribe them for prolonged periods of time. I also alert my patients to the side effects they can expect, and if they occur, I have a low threshold for changing to a combination of NSAID and oxycodone.

A *benzodiazepine* such as diazepam (e.g., Valium) can help cancer patients who have muscle spasms, even those induced by spinal cord injury, but it is no more effective than the other skeletal muscle relaxants or baclofen. The side effects of this long-acting agent limit its usefulness, especially for patients who require concomitant opioid therapy. Patients who have been using diazepam chronically for an anxiety or seizure disorder are likely to tolerate the combination of an opioid and the diazepam. Other patients are likely to develop intolerable somnolence.

ANESTHETIC METHODS OF PAIN RELIEF

Anesthetics and anesthetic techniques play a select but valuable role in relieving pain for certain cancer patients. They are most helpful in the less than 10 percent of patients with significant neuropathic pain that has not been relieved by any of the techniques discussed thus far. They are available in topical and oral formulations as well as the parenteral forms that are needed to numb or ablate peripheral or spinal somatic or autonomic nerves, or to block transmissions from the spinal cord.

The parenteral agents are indicated for patients with significant neuropathic cancer pain that has not been satisfactorily relieved by combinations of oral or transdermal opioids, adjuvant agents, and topical or oral anesthetics. They are delivered by specialized anesthesiologists who practice pain management both in free-standing and in hospital-based pain clinics. These anesthesiologists are often leaders of multidisciplinary teams involved in research, education, and clinical care of patients with neuropathic pain. Very few cancer patients will ever need to be referred to these specialists, but for those who do, the quality of their remaining life can be greatly improved.

In what follows, I provide an overview of these techniques and a description of the types of patients they can help. As I am not an anesthesiologist, I do not feel qualified to describe the techniques themselves in detail, but references are provided at the end of the chapter.

TOPICAL ANESTHETICS AND PARENTERAL LIDOCAINE
Topical anesthetics are of limited general utility in cancer patients with pain, but they can be helpful in certain selected instances. The preparations available include a combination of lidocaine and prilocaine (EMLA), lidocaine alone (e.g., ELA-Max), and capsaicin (Table 5.13).

EMLA.   This cream includes a mixture of two anesthetics, lidocaine 2.5 percent and prilocaine 2.5 percent. It anesthetizes the skin to a depth of about one-quarter inch (5 mm) and is used, for example, before venous catheter insertion, lumbar puncture, or bone marrow aspirations or biopsy. The majority of studies have taken place in children, but adults may also benefit from its use. The anesthesia provided by EMLA can be helpful, for example, for patients undergoing placement of a peripherally inserted central catheter (a PICC line).

An hour to 90 minutes before the planned procedure, the nurse, the patient, or a family member places a mound of EMLA cream over the area to be anesthetized, using about half of a 5-g tube. Being careful to maintain a thick layer of cream, the mound is covered with a semipermeable dressing such as Opsite or Tegaderm. Immediately before the procedure, the dressing and cream are removed and the area is prepared as usual. The skin anesthesia will remain for up to 4 hours.

Side effects of EMLA are minimal. The prilocaine in the anesthetic mixture can cause increases in methemoglobin, but when EMLA is used as recommended, methemoglobinemia has not been a problem, even in children as young as 3 months old. The only other consistent findings are changes of skin color to red or white; this rarely lasts longer than 4 hours.

LIDOCAINE GEL/OINTMENT/PATCH.   Topical lidocaine gel (5 percent) was shown to be more effective than placebo in relieving pain in a double-blind controlled trial in patients with post-herpetic neuralgia (Rowbotham et al. 1995). Lidocaine ointment (5 percent and 10 percent) is also available and can be used along with capsaicin for post-herpetic neuralgia or alone for peripheral sensory neuropathy. ELA-Max, a cream containing 4 percent lidocaine, is now available over the counter as an alternative to EMLA cream. Because it does not contain prilocaine, there is no risk of methemoglobinemia.

Lidocaine patches (e.g., Lidoderm) are lidocaine-impregnated dressings that adhere to the skin and deliver anesthesia to the skin surface. They can be placed on skin that is so hyperesthetic that even the touch of clothing is uncomfortable. Hyperesthesia can occur in patients with post-herpetic neuralgia or in those with nerve injury from surgery (e.g., post-thoracotomy or post-mastectomy) or from tumor invasion of either peripheral nerves or dorsal root ganglia. The patches should be applied to intact skin for up to 24 consecutive hours a day, and can be cut to size. As many as four patches can be used concurrently. Systemic concentrations of lidocaine do not reach a level at which they would affect cardiac function. Lidocaine patches should not be used where the skin is broken or over skin directly in the radiation port when the patient is receiving radiation therapy. The patch is FDA approved for use in post-herpetic neuralgia, and has been reported to be effective in patients with other chronic neuropathic pain syndromes, such as diabetic neuropathy and post-mastectomy and post-thoracotomy pain.

Intravenous lidocaine is a rarely used but effective neuropathic pain adjuvant. Case reports of patients with post-herpetic neuralgia suggest giving doses of 5 mg/kg intravenously over 30 minutes (Rowbotham et al. 1991). Ferrini (2000) reported on the experience of the San Diego Hospice Corporation with prolonged lidocaine infusions for hospice patients with intractable pain. The infusion was initiated in the inpatient hospice unit, titrated down to the lowest effective dose, and then continued in the patients' homes. Lidocaine doses were lower in these patients. The protocol called for 1 to 3 mg/kg intravenous loading over 20 to 30 minutes, with careful supervision by a physician, registered nurse, or nurse practitioner, and recording of vital signs every 15 minutes, with assessment of pain and side effects. If the bolus was effective, the infusion was continued at a rate of 0.5 to 2 mg/kg/hr, with a range of 10 to 80 mg/hr. Lidocaine concentration was 8 mg/ml. Ferrini urges caution in using lidocaine for patients with severe hepatic insufficiency or heart failure, but low doses may be tolerable and effective. You can give the lidocaine subcutaneously, but prolonged subcutaneous infusions may result in erythema and induration of the infusion site.

In Ferrini's study, lidocaine serum levels were tested in the first 24 to 72 hours and were not drawn again unless there were dose escalations or toxic side effects. Adverse effects such as lightheadedness, perioral numbness, a metallic taste in the mouth, tinnitus, and blurry vision occur within the therapeutic range of lidocaine, which is a serum range of 2 to 6 µg/ml. When this range is exceeded, patients can develop hallucinations, dissociation, myoclonus, and hypotension (at ~8 µg/ml). Stop the infusion immediately if any of these occur, monitor the airway, and consider adding a benzodiazepine, or a fast-acting barbiturate if benzodiazepines are contraindicated. With higher blood levels of lidocaine, seizures, coma, and respiratory or cardiac arrest may occur.

CAPSAICIN. Capsaicin cream (0.025 percent, 0.075 percent) (e.g., Zostrix, Capzacin-P) has been approved by the FDA for arthritis pain, for post-surgical neuropathic pain, and for treatment of post-herpetic neuralgia, where it can be used along with gabapentin. It is also a useful addition to NSAIDs for patients with pain from bony metastases.

Capsaicin provides analgesia by depleting substance P, a peptide that is an important transmitter of nerve impulses from peripheral nerves to the spinal cord. Capsaicin is found in the seeds of hot peppers and is what causes the intense burning and numbness you've experienced if you've made the mistake of eating one.

Unfortunately, capsaicin cream is expensive and it usually provides only partial pain relief, being effective in about half the patients with post-mastectomy and other post-surgical neuropathic pains who were surveyed, and in up to one-third of patients with post-herpetic neuralgia. Repeated applications (four times a day) for at least 4 weeks are needed.

Further, capsaicin's utility in relieving neuropathic pain is limited by the significant burning it causes in the skin where it is applied. Patients with post-herpetic neuralgia experience more discomfort using the cream than those with post-mastectomy pain, but it occurs in both populations and was the most common reason patients stopped using capsaicin. Some patients have found that applying a 5 percent or 10 percent lidocaine ointment prior to the capsaicin cream diminished the burning sensation; others, even with the lidocaine pretreatment, could not tolerate this agent (Watson et al. 1988).

Capsaicin may be causing intense burning in these patients because their nerves are injured and their skin is hyperesthetic. Patients with normal skin who use capsaicin cream for arthritis or deep muscle pain tolerate it very well. They rub it into the skin over the painful area once to three times a day. The area sometimes becomes warm if it is exposed to water or to sun, but not painfully so. Though I have not seen any studies in this area, I recommend topical capsaicin for patients whose cancer has caused painful muscle spasm or bony pain, with the caution not to use a heating pad or heat wrap over the area.

LOCAL ANESTHETICS TAKEN ORALLY

Mexiletine, a local anesthetic available in pill form, is an effective adjuvant for certain patients with refractory continuous or lancinating neuropathic pains (Table 5.13). It is usually reserved for patients with refractory neuropathic pain that has not responded to the agents discussed above.

Mexiletine use for patients with neuropathic cancer pain has not been studied extensively, but it is the most often used oral local anesthetic for patients with nonmalignant neuropathic pain. It is relatively safe even for patients with a cardiac arrhythmia or receiving drugs to prevent one. The initial recommended dose is 150 mg/day orally, and it can be escalated if tolerated to doses of 300 mg orally three times a day. Dyspepsia and diarrhea may limit its tolerability.

NEURAL BLOCKADE AND NEUROABLATION

Neural blockade and neuroablation are the province of interventional radiologists and anesthesiologists who specialize in pain management. These techniques are often employed as initial therapy for post-thoracotomy syndrome, acute pain from herpes zoster (neural blockade alone), post-herpetic neuralgia, or pain from pancreatic cancer, but they are otherwise used only when the therapies mentioned elsewhere in this chapter have been ineffective.

The only patients with refractory neuropathic pain who are unlikely to benefit from neuroablative procedures are those with *deafferentation* pain. Deafferentation pain is a poorly localized, deeply aching, and distressing sensation that occurs when a peripheral nerve is "disconnected" from the spinal cord surgically or by any other process that injures a nerve. Patients with injury to the spinal cord from cancer or with tumor invading the brachial or lumbosacral plexus can develop deafferentation pain. Though such patients might experience temporary relief from a local anesthetic block, a neurolytic procedure is unlikely to be of benefit.

NEURAL BLOCKADE.   Neural blockade is a regional anesthetic procedure that can include blocks of spinal and peripheral somatic nerves and of the sympathetic nervous system. Injections of local anesthetics such as lidocaine or bupivacaine along with a corticosteroid are used for diagnosis, prognosis, therapy, and pain prevention.

A *diagnostic* nerve block can determine which nerve is mediating the pain and whether it is a somatic or sympathetic nerve. The anesthesiologist can then plan the appropriate therapeutic block or neurolytic procedure. The patient's response to this block will also allow the anesthesiologist to predict the likely outcome and the side effects of a more permanent procedure (e.g., neuroablation).

To minimize ineffective procedures, the American Society of Anesthesiologists' Task Force on Pain Management, Cancer Pain Section (Ferrante et al. 1996), recommends that *prognostic* blocks always precede a planned neuroablative procedure; if anesthetizing the nerve does not relieve the pain, the anesthesiologist does not proceed. Unfortunately, the converse is not true: a positive result from a block does not always predict a positive outcome from the neuroablative procedure.

Sometimes, *therapeutic* nerve blocks are sufficient, and a neuroablative procedure will not be needed. Interestingly, their effectiveness may outlast the known half-life of the anesthetic agent that was injected. Anesthetics, in combination with a glucocorticoid, can be injected into the spinal space or nerve roots affected by tumor, and the relief can last from days to weeks. *Trigger point injections* can help with myofascial pains, such as those associated with the post-mastectomy syndrome. A local anesthetic is usually injected into the trigger point, though dry needling or local instillation of saline or a corticosteroid are also used. Before adding systemic opioids to NSAIDs for patients with myofascial pain, I often suggest trigger point injections.

Subcutaneous administration of local anesthetic plus corticosteroids is often helpful for the somatically mediated acute pain of herpes zoster and for prevention of post-herpetic neuralgia. Because these injections are so often effective and have so few associated side effects, I refer patients with these syndromes to an anesthesia pain specialist before I begin treating them with opioids or an adjuvant such as gabapentin.

RADIOFREQUENCY ABLATION. Radiofrequency ablation (inducing coagulation necrosis by heating tissues to ~100°C) has been used to ablate focal tumors, and to treat patients with trigeminal neuralgia (tic douloureux) by destroying the trigeminal nerve ganglion. This technique is now being used to treat painful focal tumors in bone, skin, or viscera (Goetz et al. 2004; Patti et al. 2002). Controlled trials are currently underway.

Sympathetic nerve blocks of the celiac plexus or the stellate or gasserian ganglia are usually done as diagnostic and prognostic procedures in patients with pancreatic cancer or with cancer of the head and neck, respectively. A chemical neurolytic procedure or radiofrequency lesioning is performed if anesthetic blockade of the relevant sympathetic structure results in remission of the pain.

Sympathetic nerve blocks are also often used for patients suffering from causalgia, which arises from injury to sympathetic nerves due to trauma, scarring, or direct invasion by a malignancy. The patient complains of burning pain in the arm or leg, and the limb becomes hyperalgesic and allodynic (i.e., even clothing touching the skin causes a burning pain). The skin may be edematous, red or pale, may manifest decreased sweating and increased warmth, and, over time, will become atrophic. You may note such changes in the arms of patients with infiltration of the brachial plexus due to cancers of the breast or superior sulcus of the lung, or those who have received radiation to the brachial plexus. In some cases the causalgia will respond to a blockade alone, but in others chemical destruction of involved ganglia or surgical rhizotomy (i.e., selective ablation of the affected ganglia) is needed.

NEUROLYTIC PROCEDURES.   Neurolytic procedures (i.e., ablation of the nerve) are indicated for patients who are expected to live only a short time, whose neuropathic pain is well localized, and whose pain has not responded to other measures. Pain mediated by spinal, peripheral somatic, and sympathetic nerves can be treated by these techniques.

Neuroablation can be achieved surgically, but at present, thermal and chemical means are more commonly used. Thermal techniques include radiofrequency ablation, as discussed above, and cryoanalgesia. Chemical agents include glycerol (which is used to block the trigeminal ganglion), phenol, and ethanol. Phenol, unlike ethanol, has local anesthetic as well as lytic effects and is therefore painless when injected. Ethanol injections are so painful that they must be preceded by injections of local anesthetic, and the patient must be sedated. The usual clinical doses of phenol or ethanol are unlikely to cause side effects from systemic absorption. If phenol is injected intravascularly by accident, however, it can cause convulsions, CNS depression, and cardiovascular collapse.

Spinal Neurolytic Procedures.   Patients suffering from recurrent gynecologic, colorectal, or bladder cancers may experience severe bilateral pelvic pain in a "saddle" distribution. Systemic opioids or a spinal opioid/anesthetic infusion usually provide these patients with satisfactory pain relief. For over 60 percent of the very few who still have intolerable pain, subarachnoid neurolytic blockades may provide good pain relief for several months; rarely, pain relief lasts up to a year. The pain relief may be so complete that the patient abruptly discontinues all oral opioid therapy. To prevent patients from experiencing withdrawal, they are instructed before the procedure on how to taper their opioids safely.

Saddle blocks are considered when a spinal catheter cannot be used or its insertion is problematic, as can be the case for patients with frequent infections, lack of home care coverage, or a family situation too unstable to assure safety of the epidural catheter. Patients with, for example, a rectovaginal fistula or burning perineal pain from locally advanced pelvic cancers (e.g., colorectal, bladder, cervical, or endometrial cancer) may benefit from these blocks. Phenol, which is hyperbaric, is placed intrathecally and sinks to the level of S2–S4 nerves. Patients usually continue to be mobile, but the block may cause bowel and bladder incontinence. Usually, however, patients who need this block for pain relief already have diverting colostomies, ureters diverted into Indiana pouches, or renal stents to relieve obstruction caused by the tumor. Side effects (e.g., leg weakness) and pain relief depend on the concentration of phenol used. Higher concentrations of phenol can be given to patients with urinary diversions. Generally, patients have at least a 50 percent pain reduction and clearer thinking, because systemic agents can be markedly reduced. Relief usually lasts for a month, but it sometimes lasts for two months and, rarely, can persist for as long as six months.

Subdural and epidural neurolysis is used for pain in the cervical region, an area in which subarachnoid blockade is not effective. It can be helpful to patients with refractory pain due to cancer of the ear, nose, throat, or lung, or for those with bony cervical metastases.

Ablation of Peripheral Somatic Nerves.   Neuroablation of intercostal nerves can relieve the post-thoracotomy syndrome, especially when performed within six months of its onset. This procedure can also relieve the pain of a pathologic rib fracture in someone who is not a candidate for radiation therapy. Because neuroablation is often so effective and has so few associated side effects compared with the doses of systemic opioids or neuropathic adjuvant agents that would be needed, I ask patients with these pain syndromes to consult with an anesthesia pain specialist as soon as possible.

Sympathetic Nerve Ablation.   Some patients' neuropathic pain syndromes are caused by injury to the sympathetic nervous system. The in-

---

PERIPHERAL NEUROABLATIVE PROCEDURES

Target	Indications
• Sacral nerves	Perineal pain
• Intercostal nerve	Post-thoracotomy syndrome
• Sympathetic ganglia:	
—Celiac plexus	Upper abdominal pain
—Inferior mesenteric (impar)	Perineal, rectal pain
—Stellate	Head and neck pain
—Gasserian	Tic douloureux-like pain
• Hypogastric plexus	Pelvic pain
• Percutaneous dorsal rhizotomy	Causalgia of upper extremity

jury can be to ganglia or to the sympathetic fibers in a nerve plexus such as the brachial or lumbosacral plexus.

The most commonly used and most effective sympathetic neurolytic blocks for cancer patients have been blocks of the celiac plexus. This plexus contains sympathetic ganglia that mediate pain from upper abdominal organs. Celiac plexus blocks have been found to relieve the pain of half to three-quarters of patients with pancreatic cancer. Because they are so effective, some surgeons will resect the celiac ganglion or inject it with alcohol or a phenol solution at the time of definitive or palliative surgery.

A celiac block may also relieve pain due to cancer of the stomach, liver, small bowel, proximal colon, or abdominal metastases if it resembles the pain caused by pancreatic cancer. I refer patients who develop such pain syndromes to an anesthesia pain expert as soon as they require opioids for pain relief. Anesthesiologists can perform the neuroablation percutaneously with fluoroscopy or CT guidance.

The common side effects caused by destroying the celiac plexus result from interruption of the sympathetic innervation to the upper abdominal organs. They include temporary orthostatic hypotension and diarrhea due to increased gut motility. Rarely, the neurolytic solution will spread to the lumbosacral plexus or nerve roots and cause radicular pain or, very rarely, paraparesis or paraplegia.

Rectal pain/tenesmus and perineal pain respond to blockade of the ganglion impar, located anterior to the sacrococcygeal ligament. Complications include puncture of the rectum and bladder, local infection, and abscess. Spinal anesthesia and intravascular injection may rarely occur.

Sympathetic blockade of the *stellate ganglion* with local anesthetics can reduce the incidence of post-herpetic neuralgia in the upper extremity and face if used within two weeks of the onset of the herpes zoster. Some researchers have found that it can be effective if used within the first two months of appearance of the lesions.

Selected cancer patients with pain in the arms or in the head and neck or with Pancoast tumor will benefit from neuroablation of the stellate ganglion. Chemical neuroablation is rarely done, because of the damage that may be caused to nearby nervous, vascular, and brain structures by the lytic agents.

In the past, injection of the *gasserian ganglion* with alcohol was used for patients with benign or malignant causes of tic douloureux. More recently, however, for patients with pain refractory to carbamazepine or baclofen, injection of the ganglion with glycerol, thermogangliolysis, or surgical rhizotomy is used.

Chemical neuroablation of the *superior hypogastric plexus* is very effective in the treatment of selected patients with pelvic cancer pain, such as that caused by gynecologic or recurrent colorectal cancer. Relief can last as long as six months. The older procedure, chemical lumbar sympathectomy, has also been shown to be effective for pelvic pain, but the blockade is less selective.

Some patients with injury to the brachial plexus have causalgia that does not respond to anesthetic blockade. For these patients, *percutaneous surgical dorsal rhizotomy* is considered preferable to a chemical rhizotomy because it rarely has to be repeated.

THE ANESTHETIC TECHNIQUES REVIEWED ABOVE are often crucial to providing effective therapy for the less than 10 percent of patients for whom opioids and adjuvant agents have caused intolerable side effects or have failed to relieve their neuropathic pain. By recognizing neuropathic pain when it occurs, using the topical and oral agents judiciously, and referring appropriate patients to anesthesiologists who are experts in pain management, you may enable your patients with very refractory pain syndromes to experience significant relief.

RELIEVING PAIN IN OLDER PERSONS

ASSESSMENT

Staff in long-term care facilities, community nurses, and even hospice nurses underestimate intense levels of persistent pain in elderly patients and consequently undertreat them. Dementia is estimated to occur in about 5 percent of patients over 65, rising to more than 40 percent in patients over 85, and cognitively impaired patients pose a particular challenge. (Ideally, you will be able to collaborate with either the geriatrician or the geriatric psychiatrist caring for the patient.) Inadequate supplies of potent opioids, lack of trained staff to perform the assessments, and lack of expertise among physicians responsible for these patients all contribute to inadequate pain management in this setting. Even the pain of cancer patients living in nursing homes is undertreated. Most receive no opioid analgesia or only a step 2 agent for their pain.

It is often difficult to assess the degree of pain that older cancer patients experience. They have pain as frequently as younger patients and are able to describe its location and qualities (sharp, dull, etc.) just as accurately, but older patients less often report their pain. This may be because they ascribe any new pain to a co-morbid condition such as arthritis and don't realize that it may be due to the cancer. Alternatively, they might just be more stoic, expecting to experience more pain as they age and not wanting to distress those around them.

Pain assessment in either the frail older patient or in patients who are cognitively impaired requires some modification of the techniques described in Chapter 4. Try to determine how well the patient performs the usual activities of daily living, and gauge the success of the treatment by improvements in functional measures. If you use a pain assessment tool, choose one that the patient finds easy to use, such as a *word scale* (mild, moderate, severe, excruciating), a *pain thermometer,* or a *face scale.* Also, refer to pain behaviors, such as those listed in Table 5.14. For patients with advanced dementia, use the PAINAD scale, which is a validated tool for assessing pain in this population (Warden et al. 2003).

The key to achieving pain control in cognitively impaired patients seems to be frequent assessment. Repeated questioning is needed because, while these patients accurately report the pain they are currently experiencing, they are often unable to recall previous pain intensity. To adjust opioid doses in cognitively impaired patients, assess the intensity of their pain before they received pain medication, then repeat the assessment an hour or two later.

MANAGEMENT CONSIDERATIONS

Once you understand the nature of the pain an older patient is experiencing, there are two other important factors to consider: (1) the role of family members in caring for older patients and (2) the pharmacokinetic and pharmacodynamic differences between the metabolism of pain-relieving drugs in older persons and that in younger persons.

FAMILY MEMBERS.   Family members are often the key to success in managing the pain of older patients. But physicians need to recognize how difficult this may be for caregivers, especially if they are elderly themselves. They spend a great deal of time taking care of the person in pain, often relinquishing their own jobs or accustomed routines in the home. The caregivers are often sleepless and exhausted, and feel inadequate to the task and helpless as they watch the suffering of their loved one. They may fear addiction from potent opioids as much as the pain itself. Supporting and educating them is crucial to the well-being of the entire family.

PRACTICE POINTS: PAIN MANAGEMENT IN OLDER PERSONS

- Assure patients and their families that you want to hear about each of the patient's pains.
- Identify a pain scale they understand and can use.
- In cognitively impaired patients, pain *now* is more accurate than remembered pain.
- Involve caregivers and home nursing services in monitoring the effectiveness of the regimen and the occurrence of side effects.
- Avoid NSAIDs. If they are used, monitor carefully for side effects and exacerbations of congestive heart failure, cirrhosis, hypertension, or renal insufficiency. Consider gastrointestinal prophylaxis.
- Give lower initial doses of benzodiazepines, gabapentin, and opioids. Increase doses slowly.
- Give drugs with short half-lives that are the least sedating and have the fewest anticholinergic side effects.
- Institute aggressive regimens to prevent constipation.

Home nursing and home hospice services are invaluable in helping ease the family's physical and psychological burdens. The nurses provide expert evaluation and management of the patient's symptoms, along with patient and family education and guidelines on when to contact the physician. The social workers and chaplains can address the psychosocial and spiritual needs of both the patient and the caregiver. And home health aides and volunteers can give the older caregiver a much needed break—either by doing some of the patient care or by sitting with the patient so that the spouse can rest or take a walk.

The Burden of Caregiving

The burden of the caregiver's responsibility was brought home to me by Mr. O'Hara, a 79-year-old man with metastatic bladder cancer and complete ureteral obstruction that required bilateral stents. He lived with an older sister who was dying of multiple noncancerous medical problems. Because of his own physical deterioration, Mr. O'Hara had agreed to receive home hospice services from the same visiting nurse agency that was helping his sister. They received health aide services for as much as 8 hours a day, but for the remaining 16 hours Mr. O'Hara was the sole caregiver for his sister. And he maintained that role until her death.

After she died, he moved into a community home for older people. About a month later, the hospice coordinator got in touch with me. It seemed that Mr. O'Hara was doing so well that they wanted to discontinue the hospice services! What we had attributed to progressive cancer was actually the exhaustion and debilitation caused by caring for his dying sister. In the month after her death, he had gained weight, had less pain, and seemed to need no services from the hospice staff. It has now been two years since the services were stopped, and he is still going strong.

As there was no one else to help him and his financial resources were limited, we were unable to provide all the support Mr. O'Hara needed. But even when there are people who will pitch in, family caregivers are often reluctant to let them. One of my major challenges, in fact, is to convince the spouse or other person primarily caring for the patient to let others help as much as possible—to involve willing family and friends and accept community services. Primary caregivers need to accept that their own health may be endangered if they shoulder the burden alone and that, if they fall ill, there will be no one left to care for the patient at home. Accepting help may be the only solution.

PHARMACOKINETIC AND PHARMACODYNAMIC ALTERATIONS IN OLDER PERSONS.   Both the pharmacokinetics (the absorption, metabolism, and excretion of the drug) and pharmacodynamics (the effects of the drug at various serum levels) of NSAIDs, adjuvants, and opioids are different in older patients. Older persons have less muscle and more fat than younger persons, and their renal and hepatic functions are often mildly to moderately impaired, leading to less rapid hepatic and renal drug clearance. Older patients often suffer from concomitant medical illnesses, and they are more sensitive to opioid-induced sedation and confusion.

NSAIDs can be particularly problematic in the older patient. Of the choices available for mild to moderate pain, acetaminophen, the COX-2 inhibitors (e.g., Bextra, Celebrex), and the nonacetylated salicylates (e.g., Trilisate, Salsalate) are probably the safest agents. But very few clinical trials have included patients older than 65.

Other NSAIDs are likely to cause significant toxicity in older patients. These drugs are highly protein-bound, and older, ill patients may have low levels of serum albumin. Older patients are likely to have higher serum levels of free NSAID than do younger patients receiving the same NSAID dose, and they develop more side effects. Older patients with congestive heart failure or cirrhosis are particularly susceptible.

Older patients taking NSAIDs may develop dizziness, confusion, and excessive salt and water retention. Since NSAIDs may exacerbate hypertension and can induce significant hyperkalemia and renal toxicity in this population, electrolytes and renal function must be checked a week or two after NSAID treatment is started. To minimize gastrointestinal toxicity, prescribe low-dose ibuprofen. But for patients requiring higher doses of this agent, or whose pain is well controlled only by NSAIDs with a higher risk of inducing gastrointestinal toxicity, consider adding a proton pump inhibitor such as omeprazole (20 mg) and periodically monitor the patient with occult blood testing.

Despite its side effects, ketorolac (e.g., Toradol) can, with a few modifications, be used safely in older patients. It should not be given intramuscularly (because of the muscle wasting and decrease in fatty tissue) and, for patients over 65, the initial dose should be reduced by 50 percent and the total daily dose should not exceed 60 mg. Alternatively, consider giving it every 8 hours instead of the usual every 6 hours, monitoring to ensure that the pain is still controlled. Even at the lower dose, ketorolac should not be given for more than five days, and some clinicians recommend stopping it after 48 hours.

Other adjuvants also may cause significant side effects in older patients. Do not use diazepam (e.g., Valium). The increased body fat in these patients can prolong the half-life of lipid-soluble agents, such as diazepam and lead to excessive sedation or delirium. Local anesthetics are also associated with a higher incidence of delirium in the elderly. Avoid using tricyclic antidepressants. They can cause orthostatic hypotension, cognitive changes, and atrial arrhythmias, which can themselves be problematic or may lead to falls. If the patient does not tolerate gabapentin (Neurontin), try desipramine (Norpramin), which has the least anticholinergic side effects. The anticholinergic side effects of the tricyclic antidepressants, the antiemetics, and the antihistamines (used to control opioid-induced pruritus) can be very troublesome. They include constipation, dry mouth, blurred vision, urinary retention, and sedation. Older opioid-naive patients, therefore, should not receive prophylactic phenothiazines.

OPIOIDS.　In general, because of the alterations in metabolism noted above, older patients are more likely to have significant side effects from the usual doses of both immediate- and sustained-release opioids. Given the same dose of opioid, older patients will have significantly higher plasma concentrations than younger patients. In addition, they are more sensitive to the peak effect of the immediate-release preparations, and they can develop excessive respiratory depression, sedation, confusion, and even paradoxical agitation. With either immediate- or sustained-release formulations, the drugs last longer, their metabolites accumulate, and toxicities increase in these older patients.

Even immediate-release opioids, such as immediate-release morphine, have long-lived active metabolites that may cause problems. Avoid meperidine (e.g., Demerol). Older patients are particularly prone to the side effects of normeperidine, the active metabolite of meperidine, which causes dysphoria, myoclonus, and seizures. Hydromorphone (e.g., Dilaudid) or immediate-release oxycodone, which have short half-lives and pose less of a problem with metabolites, are better choices.

To prevent excessive toxicity, "start low; go slow," and reassess frequently. Begin with a dose that is 25 to 50 percent less than the dose you would give to a younger adult. Rescue doses, which should be about 10 percent of the total daily dose in younger patients, initially should be no more than 5 percent in the older patient. Rescue medication, moreover, should probably be taken no more often than every 4 hours, rather than the every 2 hours recommended for younger patients.

Avoid using agents with long half-lives such as methadone and agents with mixed agonist/antagonist properties such as pentazocine and buprenorphine. The former cause excessive sedation, and the latter, hallucinations, agitation, and delirium. Use lower doses of transdermal fentanyl in well-nourished older patients, because there is a marked increase in the transdermal delivery rate of the fentanyl. This may result from the higher fat-to-water ratio in the elderly person's skin, and more fentanyl may deposit in the skin reservoir than in that of younger patients. Be sure the patch is placed over a fat-containing area, not a bone.

For short-term, acute pain relief, patient-controlled analgesia can be used as successfully in older patients as in younger persons. As in younger patients, the oral or transdermal routes are preferred for treating chronic cancer pain. If parenteral opioids are needed, it's best to avoid bolus injections because of the enhanced toxicity associated with the "peak effects." Continuous infusion via subcutaneous or intravenous routes is preferred. Intraspinal opioids can also be given safely. Older patients are less likely than younger patients to develop nausea or vomiting after an epidural injection.

Some special consideration must be given to opioid-induced side effects in older patients. As you might expect, older patients are more susceptible to the constipating effects of opioids. They are less active than younger patients, drink less fluid, and are more often taking other medications that exacerbate constipation. It is therefore essential that older patients start a prophylactic bowel regimen along with opioid therapy.

Older patients are also prone to urinary retention due to the effects of opioids on the urinary sphincter. Urinary retention can be an important problem for patients with prostatic hypertrophy or those taking other drugs with anticholinergic side effects. Initially, these patients may require bladder catheterization to relieve discomfort, but the retention usually disappears after one to two days on opioid therapy. Rarely, patients with prostatic hypertrophy will require either a trial of finasteride or an agent that produces smooth muscle relaxation, such as terazosin (1 mg p.o. at bedtime, increased gradually to 2 to 5 mg as tolerated and as needed).

RELIEVING PAIN IN SUBSTANCE ABUSERS

ACTIVE ABUSERS

The cancer patient who has severe pain but is actively abusing opioids, cocaine, or alcohol poses very difficult management problems. It is hard to trust the patient's report of pain intensity if you know he is actively abusing drugs, and you may be reluctant to prescribe a high opioid dose because you don't know whether you are relieving his pain or acting as his dealer.

But consider how Dr. William Breitbart, who has extensive experience working with substance abusers in pain, views this issue: "I've treated about 500 patients with AIDS-related pain and a history of substance abuse, and I've been fooled a good dozen times. But if I had allowed that experience of being manipulated and fooled to influence me, I would not have been able to help those other 488 patients" (personal communication). I share his sentiments; I would hate to miss the opportunity to help so many people for fear that a few would be "using me" in ways I don't approve of.

I realize it is particularly hard to apply the assessment and management principles discussed thus far to this patient population. Unfortunately, we have no other way to assess or treat patients with severe pain: we must believe their reports of pain and try our best to bring it under control, even if they are actively abusing drugs.

To work with these patients, I borrow the techniques used by the drug abuse professionals. Whenever possible, I involve a team of clinicians to manage the case, including the patient's primary physician (or physician assistant or nurse practitioner), psychiatric clinicians, and drug abuse professionals. You might consider also involving a pain specialist.

PRACTICE POINTS: OPIOID THERAPY FOR ACTIVE DRUG ABUSERS

- Control the environment.
- Establish the therapeutic opioid dose.
- Institute a regimen that minimizes the chance of abuse.

INPATIENTS.   It is particularly important to control the environment of active drug abusers whenever they are admitted to an inpatient site. The patient should be in a private room and restricted to that room or, in some cases, to the floor. Patients should wear hospital, not street, clothing. Visitors (even family) should be restricted, and patients' possessions and packages should be searched by nursing staff. Arrange for daily psychiatric and substance abuse counseling, and try to have the same nurse responsible for the patient throughout the hospital stay (so-called primary nursing).

During the hospitalization, substitute therapeutic opioid doses for the opioids the patient was taking "on the street." I have found that some patients, unable to get relief from a physician, use street drugs to self-medicate their severe pain. My first task with such patients is to demonstrate to them that I can relieve their pain with appropriate prescription agents and that they do not need the illegal substances for symptom control.

Finding the correct opioid dose may be particularly difficult in patients who are actively abusing opioids, both because you may not trust their reported pain level and because they often require very high levels of opioids (e.g., the equivalent of grams of morphine) for pain relief.

These patients may not complain about a euphoric or sedating side effect of a dose of opioids that is higher than needed to relieve the pain. But you and the other members of the care team will often be able to determine whether patients are "high" or somnolent, then decrease the opioid doses accordingly.

When you have brought the acute pain under control, you need to convert the patient to a regimen that minimizes the chance of abuse. Long-acting oral agents such as levorphanol (e.g., Levo-Dromoran) or sustained-release preparations of morphine, hydromorphone (e.g., Palladone), transdermal fentanyl, or methadone are recommended. Avoid immediate-release hydromorphone (e.g., Dilaudid), combination agents (e.g., Percodan, Percocet, Tylox), immediate-release morphine, and sustained-release oxycodone for patients who are active drug abusers.

OUTPATIENTS. After discharge, patients will need to continue to work with the psychiatric and substance abuse counselors to maximize compliance and to prevent recurrence of active abuse. The counselors can also provide education for the patients about the dangers of mixing the therapeutic opioids with alcohol.

As I did when they were inpatients, I detail my expectations of how patients are to work with me and with our team. Substance abuse is an illness that frequently relapses, and weekly urine checks are needed to identify recurrent substance abuse. Current technology can distinguish among a wide variety of opioid metabolites using both quantitative and qualitative methods. When we write prescriptions for the long-acting opioids, we give only a week's supply at a time. And we warn the patient to keep the medications in a safe place, as we will not replace that supply if it is accidentally "flushed down the toilet" or "spilled down the sink." If, despite all the support and repeated warnings, a patient continues to actively abuse opioids or other drugs, we refer the patient to another clinician who may be able to establish better rapport.

Rehabilitation in Remission: Mr. Salat

Initially, I do not even raise the subject of detoxification or drug rehabilitation programs. I have, however, worked with several substance abusers who entered rehabilitation programs after their cancer was in remission. Mr. Salat was such a patient. At the time I first saw him, he was 35 years old and had widely metastatic testicular cancer with lesions the size of grapefruits in his retroperitoneum and lung. He was actively abusing heroin, which he said helped him control the severe back pain caused by his retroperitoneal lesions. With ongoing support from his counselor and our office staff, he maintained pain relief throughout his treatment using only the opioids we prescribed.

When it was clear that his tumor was responding to treatment, I told Mr. Salat that when he was in complete remission, he was unlikely to need opioids for pain. I began to address his opioid dependence and my hope that he would be able to work with a drug counselor to avoid returning to his heroin use. He did not disappoint me: he entered a methadone maintenance program and was still doing well ten years later.

PATIENTS ON METHADONE MAINTENANCE

Patients on methadone maintenance present a less difficult compliance problem because they often have well-established, successful relationships with counselors. In addition to their methadone maintenance doses, however, they often require large doses of other opioids to relieve their pain.

PRACTICE POINTS: OPIOID THERAPY FOR PATIENTS ON METHADONE MAINTENANCE

- Don't use methadone as the pain-relieving opioid. Leave the methadone dose unchanged and titrate other opioids to achieve pain control.
- Be aware that large opioid doses may be required for patients on significant doses of methadone.
- Maintain an ongoing relationship with the patient's drug counselor.

You'll need to explain to the hospital staff or your office staff that these patients' reports of pain are just as reliable as those of nonabusers and that you plan to escalate the medications until their pain is relieved, whatever that takes.

I find it works best to leave the methadone dose the same and to use other agents for pain relief. This seems to allow patients to separate their drug abuse issues from their pain issues and helps them provide me with accurate pain assessments. And the other agents are easier to titrate than methadone. If financial restraints require it, I use methadone alone.

FORMER ABUSERS

People who have formerly abused opioids are often very reluctant to take opioids, even for excruciating pain. They and their families remember the mess drug addiction made of their lives. They are terrified that if they take opioids to relieve their pain, they will again find themselves living that nightmare.

PRACTICE POINTS: OPIOID THERAPY FOR FORMER ABUSERS
- Be sensitive to the patient's and family's concerns about using opioids even for pain relief.
- Maintain an ongoing relationship with the patient's drug counselor.
- Monitor for signs of recurrent drug abuse.

Psychological support from a counselor familiar both with drug abuse issues and with opioids for pain management may be crucial to enabling patients to accept the pain medications they need for relief. Former abusers are very sensitive to being perceived as "addicts," and staff need to receive careful instruction in how to work with these patients to help them relieve their pain. While relapse is uncommon in former abusers who suffer from cancer pain, they should still be monitored for signs indicating they have relapsed, such as "losing" medication, escalating doses without consulting you, obtaining medications from other physicians, or committing prescription fraud.

PHYSICIANS CAN RELIEVE THE PAIN of people who are actively abusing opioids, who are on methadone maintenance, or who formerly abused drugs. Patients will usually understand the need for the limits we set, or will at least comply with them in order to get pain relief. The teams we set up to support them may make it possible for them to "stay with the program." As long as we are aware of the potential pitfalls, and are vigilant, we will be able to prescribe opioids for substance abusers just as we do for nonabusing patients: to free them from disabling pain.

COMMON CLINICAL SITUATIONS

STARTING A PATIENT ON OPIOIDS

As discussed in Chapter 2, starting patients on opioids can be unexpectedly difficult. Most patients and their families, at least initially, resist accepting a prescription for opioids. To overcome their objections, I recommend conducting at least a ten-minute discussion in which you accomplish the following:

- Assume that patients and families are harboring the common fears and misconceptions about opioids, and dispel these fears.
- Explain the difference between tolerance and addiction, and affirm that they will not become "addicts." Addicts use opioids "to get out of life"; patients use them to get back into their lives.
- Reassure them that taking medication now does not jeopardize achieving pain relief if the pain worsens ("there is plenty more where that came from").
- Using an analogy of the treatment of diabetes or heart failure, remind patients how opioids can help them reach their personal goals.
- Explain the likely side effects (e.g., constipation, sedation, nausea) and how you can prevent or treat these:
  —They may feel somewhat sleepy for the first two or three days, but the drowsiness will pass and the pain relief will remain.
  —Constipation will persist as long as they continue to take opioids, and it requires ongoing therapy. Advise them to replace any fiber laxatives with the laxatives you prescribe, to take them whether or not they have had a bowel movement that day, and to take more laxatives if they need them.
  —Nausea is not a sign of opioid allergy. It resolves over four to seven days and can be treated during that time if it is troublesome.

INITIATING A TREATMENT REGIMEN FOR MILD (LEVEL 1 TO 4) TO MODERATE (LEVEL 5 TO 6) PAIN.   Step 2 agents (e.g., Tylox, Percocet, or Percodan) are indicated for patients with mild to moderate somatic or visceral pain, such as from bony metastases. For moderate pain (level 5 or 6 on a 0 to 10 scale), treat as follows:

- Start with two pills orally every 4 hours as needed, along with one or two senna tablets twice a day (or choose another laxative from Table 5.6).
- Identify a pain scale that the patient and family feel comfortable using. Ask the patient to record, at least twice a day, her pain level before and about one hour after she takes the drug, along with any side effects.
- The day after each opioid dose change, check with the patient to determine whether the pain relief is now satisfactory.

- If the pain relief is satisfactory but the patient has developed side effects, treat them as described earlier in this chapter.
- If the pain is only relieved for one or two hours and pain recurs before the next dose, start an equivalent amount of a sustained-release (SR) preparation, adding an immediate-release (IR) form for pain between regularly scheduled doses ("rescue" doses). The rescue dose should be 10 percent of the total daily opioid dose (5 percent initially in older patients). It is sometimes necessary to "round up" or "round down" the calculated opioid dose to accommodate the dosages available in SR or IR preparations. If appropriate, add an amount of NSAID equivalent to the amount in the combination tablet that the patient formerly took.

TREATING PAIN THAT RECURS BEFORE THE NEXT DOSE

Converting from a combination product to acetaminophen or NSAID + a sustained-release form of the same opioid (oxycodone):

- Initial combination agent: oxycodone + acetaminophen, 12 tablets per 24 hours (2 tablets every 4 hours).
- Total oxycodone dose: 5 mg/tablet × 12 tablets = 60 mg.
- Equivalent SR oxycodone: 30 mg every 12 hours.
- Add opioid rescue dose (10 percent of 24-hour dose): 10 percent of 60 mg ≈ 5 mg of IR oxycodone.
- Add acetaminophen or NSAID if needed.

- If the pain relief was never satisfactory despite maximum doses of a step 2 agent, replace it with a step 3 opioid at a dose 50 percent higher than the patient previously received (e.g., a higher dose of oxycodone alone or hydromorphone or morphine). I review how to change opioid agents later in this chapter. The example given below (Treating Pain That Is Unrelieved by a Step 2 Agent) uses the same opioid, oxycodone.

INITIAL OPIOID REGIMEN FOR OPIOID-NAIVE OUTPATIENTS WITH SEVERE (LEVEL 7 OR HIGHER) PAIN. The step 3 opioids are indicated for initial therapy of patients with severe pain. They include hydromorphone (e.g., Dilaudid) for older patients or for patients with renal or hepatic failure, as well as oxycodone, morphine, and fentanyl. Patients and their families can provide important input into whether an oral or transdermal preparation can best provide the continuous portion of pain relief.

TREATING PAIN THAT IS UNRELIEVED BY A STEP 2 AGENT

Converting from a combination agent to a sustained-release preparation containing the same opioid (oxycodone) at a higher dose:

- Initial combination agent: oxycodone + acetaminophen, 12 tablets per 24 hours (60 mg of oxycodone) (2 tablets every 4 hours).
- Increase the oxycodone by 50 percent: 60 mg + (60 mg × 50 percent = 30 mg) = 90 mg of oxycodone ≈ 40 mg of SR oxycodone every 12 hours.
- Adjust rescue dose of oxycodone: 10 percent of 80 mg ≈ 10 mg; rescue dose: 10 mg of IR oxycodone every 2 hours p.r.n.
- Add acetaminophen or NSAID if needed.

Whichever opioid you choose, prevention of constipation is crucial. Prescribe, for example, two Senokot-S or two senna plus two Colace twice daily with an osmotic agent (e.g., one tablespoon of lactulose or 17 g of polyethylene glycol [Miralax]) at bedtime; exclude the osmotic agent if it causes diarrhea. Instruct all patients to take the laxatives even if they have had a bowel movement that day.

Similar principles apply if transdermal fentanyl is used. In that case, rescue dosing is even more important because fentanyl blood levels will not be adequate to relieve pain until 12 to 24 hours after the patch is applied. Rescue dosing is calculated by determining 10 percent of the equivalent 24-hour morphine dose (Table 5.5).

For patients with moderate to severe neuropathic pain, add to the opioid gabapentin taken three times a day (e.g., 100, 100, 300 mg p.o.). If this is well tolerated, increase the dose over several weeks until pain relief is improved or the patient has a dose-limiting side effect. If the gabapentin alone is ineffective, add to it another of the anticonvulsants listed in Table 5.10.

CHANGING OPIOID DOSE, OPIOID AGENT, OR ROUTE OF DELIVERY

ADJUSTING THE DOSE.   The initial dose of opioid is, unfortunately, no better than an educated guess. Doses often need to be adjusted upward or downward both during the first few weeks of therapy and later in the patient's course of treatment, as the disease process advances. If patients and their families want immediate pain relief regardless of the side effects, I tend to err on the high side with the initial dose. If they express a great deal of concern about the potential side effects, I am more con-

---

INITIAL ORAL OPIOID FOR OPIOID-NAIVE PATIENTS WITH SEVERE PAIN

- Hydromorphone 4 to 6 mg p.o. every 4 hours for elderly patients or patients with renal or hepatic failure.
- IR option: IR morphine or oxycodone every 2 hours p.r.n. for 24 hours; then give total daily dose in SR form.

Example.

7.5 mg IR morphine (½ of a 15-mg tablet) × 12 doses = 90 mg of morphine.

SR dose: 45 mg q12h SR morphine with 10 mg IR morphine rescue (e.g., 0.5 ml of a 20 mg/ml morphine solution).

Example.

5 mg IR oxycodone × 10 doses = 50 mg oxycodone.

SR dose: 20 mg q12h SR oxycodone with 5 mg IR oxycodone rescue (alone or in combination with aspirin, acetaminophen, or NSAID).

- SR option

Example.

Morphine SR 30 mg p.o. q12h or oxycodone SR 20 mg q12h with 5 mg IR oxycodone rescue (alone or in combination with aspirin, NSAID, or acetaminophen).

INITIAL TRANSDERMAL FENTANYL FOR OPIOID-NAIVE PATIENTS WITH SEVERE PAIN

- Initial dose of transdermal fentanyl: 25 µg/hr patch, which is approximately equivalent to 50 mg of morphine every 24 hours.
- Add rescue doses of 10 mg of IR morphine or oxycodone (0.5 ml of a 20 mg/ml solution) every 2 hours p.o. or sublingual p.r.n.
- Patients should expect to use rescue doses until fentanyl blood levels are adequate (i.e., for at least the first 12 to 24 hours after receiving the patch).

---

servative with the initial dose, but I supply rescue medication, carefully monitor the patient, and raise the dose until the relief of the constant portion of the pain is satisfactory. Ideally, patients with constant, not intermittent, pain only need to use rescue doses of IR opioids once or twice a day; the bulk of the pain relief should be provided by the SR opioid. Patients without constant pain, whose pain is intermittent, incident pain, will benefit most from taking IR opioids when they have pain. SR opioids may cause excessive sedation in these patients.

USING RESCUE DOSES TO INCREASE SUSTAINED-RELEASE OPIOID DOSE FOR PATIENTS WITH CONSTANT PAIN

Example. A patient taking 45 mg of SR morphine every 12 hours took six rescue doses, 10 mg each, of IR morphine (0.5 ml of a 20 mg/ml morphine solution).

Total morphine dose taken in 24 hours: 90 mg + 60 mg = 150 mg. New SR morphine dose: 75 mg every 12 hours; rescue dose: 15 mg IR morphine.

To safely escalate the opioid dose in a patient with constant pain after the patient has been taking an SR preparation for 24 to 48 hours,

- Ask the patient to record all rescue doses he takes.
- If the total amount of drug he takes as a rescue dose is more than 25 percent of the total SR dose, increase the SR dose by the amount in the rescue doses.

CHANGING OPIOID AGENTS.   It is not at all uncommon for a patient to need to change opioid agents because of intolerable side effects. Use of an equianalgesic table (Table 5.5) will enable you to change agents safely while maintaining adequate control of the patient's pain. In Table 5.5, the columns indicate the equianalgesic oral and parenteral opioid doses for the listed drugs. For example, 30 mg of oral IR morphine equals 20 mg of oral IR oxycodone or 7.5 mg of oral hydromorphone (e.g., Dilaudid). And 10 mg of parenteral morphine equals 1.5 mg of parenteral hydromorphone.

Some patients will not achieve pain relief from the patch. The patient may be very thin, or the patches may appear not to be sticking, because of skin oils or sweat. If you wish to change the treatment to an oral or intravenous opioid, the safest way to do this is to assume the patient was not absorbing any of the fentanyl and to base your calculation on the amount of rescue dose she has taken. But because the patient might be absorbing fentanyl from the skin reservoir, it is safer to give only immediate-release rescue opioid as needed for the first 6 hours after the patch is removed. For the next 6 hours, you can give standing parenteral or oral SR opioids at a dose that is only 50 percent of the full calculated dose. After 12 hours, you can give the full calculated opioid dose.

For example, consider a patient who is not getting adequate relief from a 200-µg/hr fentanyl patch and has used 24 mg of IV hydromorphone in the previous 24 hours for pain relief. After taking off the patch, I would give that patient 2 to 3 mg of IV hydromorphone or 12 to 16 mg of oral hydromorphone every 2 hours p.r.n. for the next 6 hours. I would then start a hydromorphone drip at 0.5 mg/hr for the next 6 hours or continue the oral hydromorphone. Twelve hours after the patch was removed, I would increase the drip to 1 mg/hr or begin 160 mg every 12 hours of sustained-release oxycodone.

Some patients may develop an allergy to the adhesive in the patch. If such patients were taking fentanyl because they poorly tolerated other

---

CONVERTING FROM SUSTAINED-RELEASE MORPHINE TO SUSTAINED-RELEASE OXYCODONE

Example.

Current SR morphine dose: 60 mg p.o. every 12 hours (total dose: 120 mg/24 hr).

Equivalent SR oxycodone dose: 40 mg every 12 hours (total dose: 80 mg/24 hr).

$\frac{2}{3} \times 80$ mg = 55 mg

New SR oxycodone dose: 30 mg every 12 hours; rescue dose: 5 mg IR oxycodone.

CONVERTING FROM SUSTAINED-RELEASE MORPHINE TO EXTENDED-RELEASE HYDROMORPHONE

Example.

Current SR morphine dose: 60 mg p.o. every 12 hours (total dose: 120 mg/24 hr).

Equivalent p.o. hydromorphone (e.g., Dilaudid) dose: (120 mg/30) × 7.5 = 30 mg.

$\frac{2}{3} \times 30$ mg = 20 mg

New hydromorphone dose: 24 mg extended-release p.o. every 24 hours (or 4 mg IR every 4 hours); rescue dose: 2 mg IR hydromorphone.

opioids, the fentanyl can be given as an SQ or IV infusion at the same rate as the patch (Hough 2003).

At the bottom of Table 5.5 the data apply only to equivalencies between fentanyl (delivered by transdermal fentanyl patch in micrograms per hour) and the total amount of parenteral or oral morphine taken in 24 hours. For example, the equivalent morphine dose for a patient with a 50 μg/hr fentanyl patch is 33 mg of intravenous morphine in 24 hours, or 100 mg of oral morphine in 24 hours. Similarly, the equivalent fentanyl dose for a patient on an intravenous morphine drip of 4 mg/hr (i.e., 96 mg in 24 hours) is 150 μg/hr.

Unfortunately, except when converting from fentanyl to morphine or vice versa (Table 5.5), it is not sufficient simply to calculate the equianalgesic dose of the new opioid. Patients who take an opioid for several weeks become tolerant to many of the side effects that opioid induces, but they may not be as tolerant to the side effects caused by the new drug. If their pain is well controlled and they take a full equianalgesic dose of the new opioid, they may develop significant sedation or respiratory depression. To take into account this incomplete cross-tolerance, prescribe about *two-thirds* of the calculated equianalgesic dose of the new opioid. However, if the pain is not adequately relieved, give the full equianalgesic dose of the new agent. In all cases, 10 percent of the 24-hour dose of the new opioid becomes the new rescue dose. For very large doses of oral opioid, reduce the starting dose of the other agent by half.

CHANGING AGENTS WHEN THE OPIOID DOSE IS HIGH

Example. A patient takes 600 mg of sustained-release oral morphine every 12 hours (1200 mg every 24 hours).

Hydromorphone:
> Equivalent: (1200 mg/30) × 7.5 = 300 mg. New dose: 300 mg/2 = 150 mg/24 hr.

SR oxycodone:
> Equivalent: (1200 mg/30) × 20 = 800 mg. New dose: 800 mg/2 = 400 mg/24 hr.

Transdermal fentanyl (extrapolation from available data):
> Equivalent: 600 μg/hr. New dose: 300 μg/hr transdermal fentanyl patch.

It is much more difficult to convert patients safely to methadone, especially from high doses of other opioids. The equianalgesic ratios change as the non-methadone opioid dose increases. Values range from a ratio of 4:1 at morphine equivalents of <100 mg daily, to 20:1 at morphine equivalents of >1000 mg daily. Using the literature cited at the end of this chapter, we and our anesthesia pain colleagues created a table for converting patients from another opioid to methadone. First, we determine the morphine equivalent of all the opioids the patient has taken daily for the previous 2 days. We use this "morphine equivalent" dose to determine the methadone dose using the following ratios:

Oral Morphine Equivalent (mg/24 h)	Morphine:Methadone Ratio
<100	4:1
101–300	8:1
301–600	10:1
601–800	12:1
801–1000	15:1
>1000	20:1

After using this table to calculate the equianalgesic dose of methadone, we decrease that calculated dose by 50 percent, because of methadone's inhibition of the NMDA receptor (see discussion on page 162), and give it in divided doses, usually three times a day. If you have questions about this conversion procedure, consult a palliative care or pain specialist.

Some authors advise a three-day conversion to methadone: on the first day, reduce the dose of the old opioid by one-third, and give one-third the calculated dose of methadone; on the second day, reduce the dose of the remaining opioid by one-half, and give methadone at 2.5 to 10 percent of the total daily methadone dose every 4 hours only if the patient complains of pain; on the third day, discontinue the old opioid and adjust the standing dose of methadone to reflect full amount taken on day 2 (Bruera and Sweeney 2002).

CHANGING THE ROUTE OF DELIVERY.   Even changing from the oral to the parenteral route of the *same* agent necessitates a change in opioid dose. A large proportion of an oral opioid dose is metabolized in its first pass through the liver, and these metabolites cannot cross the blood-brain barrier to provide pain relief.

House staff need to be reminded that it's very important to specify the

CHANGING FROM MORPHINE TO METHADONE

Example. A patient takes 600 mg of sustained-release oral morphine every 12 hours (1200 mg every 24 hours)

Morphine to methadone ratio: 20:1

Equianalgesic methadone dose: 1200 mg/20 = 60 mg of methadone

Conversion method 1:

Decrease calculated methadone dose by 50 percent because of NMDA activity of methadone:

   30 mg methadone

   New dose: 10 mg p.o. q8h, beginning day 1

Conversion method 2:

Day 1: Give 400 mg of sustained-release morphine and 10 mg of methadone q12h

Day 2: Give 200 mg of sustained-release morphine and 20 mg of methadone q12h and 120mg MSIR as needed q4h if the patient complains of pain.

   Patient takes three 5-mg doses during the 24 hours.

Day 3: Give 20 mg of methadone p.o. q12h and 5 mg methadone q4h p.r.n. For moderate or severe pain increase dose of methadone q12h or give 15 mg methadone q8h.

SOME COMMON ORAL-TO-PARENTERAL OPIOID CONVERSIONS

Morphine: ratio of oral dose to parenteral dose = 3:1

   Example.

   Oral dose: 360 mg q 12 hours; 24-hour total dose = 720 mg p.o.

   Equivalent IV/SQ dose: 720 mg p.o./3 = 240 mg/24 hr IV (i.e., 10 mg/hr).

Hydromorphone: ratio of oral dose to parenteral dose = 5:1

   Example.

   Oral dose: 12 mg every 4 hours; 24-hour total dose = 72 mg p.o.

   Equivalent IV/SQ dose: 72 mg p.o./5 ≈ 14 mg/24 hr IV or SQ (i.e., 2.3 mg IV every 4 hours or 0.6 mg/hr).

route by which the opioid should be given. I was once called by the nurses because a house officer had written an order for "6 mg of Dilaudid IM or p.o. q4h." The patient had been taking the oral Dilaudid dose, but was going to be NPO for surgery. Luckily, the nurses did not give the 6-mg intramuscular shot; if they had, the patient would have received the equivalent of 30 mg of oral Dilaudid.

Converting from Multiple Oral to a Single Parenteral Agent. While converting from an oral to a parenteral route of the same opioid is fairly straightforward, other conversions can be more challenging. Not infrequently, when admitted to the hospital patients are taking several different oral opioids, and these must be converted to a single parenteral medication. To start a drip using morphine, I calculate the patient's total daily oral opioid dose in morphine equivalents, reduce the doses of other opioids by one-third to adjust for incomplete cross-tolerance, and then give a third of the total as the intravenous morphine dose.

For example, a patient with myeloma broke her femur and needed to have a pin placed before she received radiation. She would be NPO in the perioperative period. She had been taking 60 mg of SR morphine every 12 hours, with two Percocet every 4 hours as needed for breakthrough pains. Since the fracture, she had in fact taken twelve Percocet a day in addition to the morphine, and her pain relief was satisfactory.

CONVERTING FROM IR OXYCODONE PLUS SR MORPHINE TO AN EQUIVALENT PARENTERAL MORPHINE DOSE

- Calculate oral morphine equivalents taken in the past 24 hours and decrease doses of other opioids by one-third to adjust for incomplete cross-tolerance.

Current Medications	Oral Morphine Equivalents
IR oxycodone 60 mg	60 mg (i.e., 90 mg − 30 mg)
SR morphine 120 mg	120 mg
Total	180 mg oral morphine

- Calculate the IV morphine drip rate.

Oral Morphine	Parenteral Dose	IV Drip Rate
180 mg	60 mg (180 mg/3)	2.5 mg/hr (60 mg/24 hr)

Another patient who needed to switch from oral to intravenous opioids was taking 180 mg of SR oxycodone a day and hydromorphone for rescue. He took 24 mg of oral hydromorphone on the day before admission. Intravenous hydromorphone could be used, but for this example, assume that you wish to prescribe morphine.

CONVERTING FROM ORAL SR OXYCODONE PLUS HYDROMORPHONE TO AN EQUIVALENT PARENTERAL MORPHINE DOSE

- Calculate oral morphine equivalents taken in the past 24 hours and decrease doses of other opioids by one-third to adjust for incomplete cross-tolerance.

Current Medications	Oral Morphine Equivalents
SR oxycodone 180 mg	180 mg (i.e., 270 mg − 90 mg)
Hydromorphone 24 mg oral	64 mg ([{24 mg/7.5} × 30] − 32)
Total	244 mg oral morphine

- Calculate the IV morphine drip rate.

Oral Morphine	Parenteral Dose	IV Drip Rate
244 mg	81 mg (244 mg/3)	3.4 mg/hr (81 mg/24 hr)

Some patients are admitted with pain despite taking oral opioids. I give them the exact equivalent in morphine, which, in effect, is a 33 percent increase in dose. For example, you might want to start an intravenous morphine drip for a patient whose average pain intensity is 6 despite taking two Percodan every 4 hours (i.e., 10 mg oxycodone × 6 doses = 60 mg IR oxycodone) and 60 mg of SR oxycodone every 12 hours.

If the patient has not received intravenous opioids before, it is important to explain to him why you are using this route. I learned this from a young patient with testicular cancer who was admitted with severe retroperitoneal pain resulting from metastases.

Dire Implications of a "Morphine Drip"

Joe was an 18-year-old student referred to me by his family physician, who had discovered a testicular mass. Joe had decided to finish the school year before com-

---

CONVERTING FROM ORAL IR AND SR OXYCODONE TO A PARENTERAL MORPHINE DOSE FOR A PATIENT IN MODERATE PAIN

- Calculate oral morphine equivalents taken in the past 24 hours.

Current Medications	Oral Morphine Equivalents
IR oxycodone 60 mg	90 mg
SR oxycodone 120 mg	180 mg
Total 270 mg oral morphine	

- Calculate the IV morphine drip rate.

Oral Morphine	Parenteral Dose	IV Drip Rate
270 mg	90 mg (270 mg/3)	3.75 mg/hr (90 mg/24 hr)

---

ing to see me, and by the time he arrived, he had extensive painful retroperitoneal adenopathy.

To relieve his pain I ordered a morphine drip. When I next went to see Joe he was in tears. I asked what was the matter, and he replied, "I knew from Dr. Porter that I was sick, but he never told me I was about to die!" I was taken aback and told him that, on the contrary, he had every chance of being cured by the chemotherapy. When I asked what had made him think he was terminally ill, he said, "Well, you started a morphine drip. And the only time I saw that used before was with my Aunt Jane; they started one on her just a few days before she died."

Since this experience, I have been careful to explain to a patient why I am choosing intravenous opioids. I say something like,

> *I know you are having very severe pain and I want to lower the level of the pain as fast as I can. To do this, I need to give you opioid medications, and I need to give them intravenously. This doesn't mean you're about to die; it's just that this is the fastest way I can bring your pain under control. As soon as I know what dose of opioids you need, I'll switch you to oral medications at the equivalent dose.*

I have frightened many fewer patients since I adopted this technique.

Changing from Pills to a Transdermal Fentanyl Patch and Vice Versa.   The technique for changing patients from oral medications to a transdermal fentanyl patch includes not only determining the equianalgesic dose (Table 5.5) but also providing pain relief during the time it takes for the patch to begin providing adequate analgesia. This is very easy to do if the patient is taking an SR morphine or oxycodone preparation. Avinza relieves pain for 24 hours, Kadian relieves pain for 12 to 24 hours and the other SR preparations relieve pain for about 12 hours, which is almost the same amount of time it takes for the patch to begin providing adequate pain relief. Therefore, instruct the patient to take the last dose of the SR opioid pills (or 50% of the Avinza dose) at the time he applies the first patch and to use the rescue doses if needed.

If pain control is inadequate, the dose of fentanyl is usually titrated upward at 72 hours. If, 72 hours after the patch is placed, the patient's pain control is not satisfactory or her rescue doses of morphine exceed 25 percent of the total daily opioid dose, increase the fentanyl dose. Further dose titrations may be needed over the ensuing weeks.

To convert from a fentanyl patch to oral medications, you must take into consideration the significant amount of fentanyl that remains in the skin reservoir after the patient has removed the patch. Therefore, ask the patient to refrain from taking the usual scheduled opioid for the first 12 hours after the patch is removed, and instead to take rescue medication if pain recurs. At 12 hours after patch removal, since the skin reservoir is still half full, the patient should take half the equianalgesic dose of the

---

CONVERTING FROM ORAL OPIOIDS TO TRANSDERMAL FENTANYL

Example. A patient taking SR morphine 150 mg p.o. every 12 hours would like to switch to transdermal fentanyl.

- Refer to Table 5.5 for the fentanyl dose that should be prescribed for each oral morphine dose. A further one-third decrease is not required.

Current Medications	*Transdermal Fentanyl Equivalents*
SR morphine 300 mg	150 μg/hr
Rescue dose: 30 mg IR morphine	

INCREASING THE DOSE OF TRANSDERMAL FENTANYL

Example. A patient who had been maintaining excellent pain relief using a 75 µg/hr fentanyl patch (equivalent to 150 mg of morphine) had for the past three days required six 15-mg doses daily (total 90 mg) of IR morphine (i.e., about 33 percent of the total daily opioid dose) for increased pain.

- Refer to Table 5.5 for the fentanyl dose equivalent to the oral morphine dose.

Current Medications	Transdermal Fentanyl Equivalents
Fentanyl 75 µg/hr	75 µg/hr
IR morphine 90 mg	45 µg/hr
New patch strength	125 µg/hr

- Calculate new rescue dose.

Fentanyl Dose	Morphine Equivalent
125 µg/hr	250 mg
Rescue dose	10 percent of 250 mg ≈ 30 mg IR morphine

---

oral opioid agent. Twenty-four hours after the patch is removed, the patient may resume taking the full equianalgesic dose of oral opioid.

RAPIDLY RELIEVING EXCRUCIATING PAIN

Rarely, you will admit a patient who has a pain "emergency": the pain has been severe (≥7 on a scale of 0 to 10) for at least six hours and has escalated over the past several days. The patient is in agony, and you want to relieve the pain as soon as possible. You can do this most expeditiously using morphine or hydromorphone intravenous bolus doses or a patient-controlled analgesia (PCA) with or without a basal rate. To do this safely, however, the patient must be monitored very closely. After the PCA is started or while the bolus doses are being given, the patient should be under continuous observation, with recordings at least every 15 minutes of vital signs, verbal pain scores, mental status changes, and other adverse events, until the pain level has fallen to <5. This process may take a number of hours.

CONVERTING FROM A TRANSDERMAL FENTANYL PATCH TO ORAL OPIOID

Example. A patient using a 100 μg/hr transdermal fentanyl patch is to be switched to the equivalent SR morphine dose.

• Referring to Table 5.5, select the equianalgesic dose.

Current Fentanyl Dose	Morphine Equivalent
100 μg/hr	200 mg morphine/24 hr

Rescue dose: 20 mg IR morphine
(e.g., 1 ml of a 20 mg/ml elixir)

• Patient removes the patch; takes IR morphine every 2 hours p.r.n. for the next 12 hours.
• Twelve hours later, the patient takes 45 mg of SR morphine (~50 percent of 100-mg dose).
• Twelve additional hours later, 24 hours after removing the patch, the patient begins 100 mg of SR morphine every 12 hours.

TREATING SEVERE PAIN (GREATER THAN 7/10) IN AN OPIOID-NAIVE PATIENT

• Begin a bowel regimen; monitor the patient for nausea/sedation due to opioids.
• PCA option.
  —Begin with loading dose, basal rate, and bolus dosing.
    Hydromorphone for patients with renal failure:
      0.2 to 0.5 mg loading dose + 0.01 mg/kg basal rate + 0.2 to 0.4 mg boluses every 7 minutes p.r.n.
      Sample calculation. For a 70-kg man, hydromorphone basal rate = 0.7 mg/hr. For very elderly patients or patients with CO_2 retention, begin at 0.35 mg/hr.
    Morphine for other patients:
      2 to 5 mg loading dose + 0.05 mg/kg basal rate + 2 to 4 mg boluses every 7 minutes p.r.n.
      Sample calculation. For a 70-kg man, morphine basal rate = 3.5 mg/hr.

(continued)

For very elderly patients or patients with CO_2 retention: begin at 0.25 mg/hr.

—Check vital signs including level of sedation every 15 minutes.

—Reevaluate pain hourly.

—Double bolus doses every hour until pain level falls below 5 or becomes tolerable.

—Increase the basal rate every 12 hours as needed, adjusting rate by the p.r.n. opioids received.

Example. A patient receiving 3 mg/hr IV morphine received 24 mg IV morphine over the past 12 hours.

New IV morphine basal rate: 3 mg/hr + 24 mg/12 hr = 5 mg/hr

- IV bolus option.

—Give 5 to 10 mg of IV morphine over 15 minutes; evaluate vital signs and pain relief 15 minutes after the infusion is complete.

—If pain level is unchanged, double the bolus dose; check vital signs; reevaluate pain 15 minutes after this bolus fusion is complete. If still unchanged, repeat.

—When pain level decreases but is still ≥5, repeat the *same* bolus dose; check vital signs; reevaluate pain level 15 min after this bolus infusion is complete. If still ≥5, repeat.

—When pain level <5, give the effective bolus dose q2h as needed for next 12 hours.

—When pain control is adequate, begin continuous infusion or oral or transdermal opioid based on the opioid used in the past 12 hours.

Example.

Morphine to reduce pain level to <5: 35 mg over 2 hours (5 mg + 10 mg + 20 mg).

Three additional 20-mg boluses required in the next 12 hours.

Total morphine taken in 12 hours: 95 mg IV.

Options: morphine drip at 8 mg/hr or oral or transdermal opioid equivalent to 95 mg/12 hr parenteral morphine with 20 mg IV morphine q2h p.r.n. rescue.

Rapid dose escalation is usually needed to overcome severe pain in both opioid-naive patients and patients who are already taking opioids. In both situations, prescribing a bowel regimen and insuring close monitoring for opioid-induced nausea and sedation are required. With careful patient observation, opioid doses can be increased substantially without excessive toxicity. Suggestions for dosing via PCA or IV boluses and recommended monitoring parameters for both types of patients are given in the boxes describing the treatment of severe pain.

TREATING SEVERE PAIN IN A PATIENT ALREADY TAKING OPIOIDS

- Continue the bowel regimen; monitor the patient for nausea or sedation caused by the increased opioid dose.
- Continue the previous oral SR or transdermal opioid; add additional opioid by PCA or IV bolus.

Example.
Oral morphine: 100 mg every 12 hours.
Current rescue dose: 15 mg every 2 hours p.o. = 5 mg every 2 hours IV.

- PCA option.
  —Start IV morphine PCA with basal rate at twice the current rescue dose.
  Basal rate: 10 mg/hr IV morphine, with boluses of 5 mg morphine IV every 7 minutes p.r.n.
  —Reevaluate vital signs including sedation every 15 minutes, pain hourly.
  —Double bolus doses every hour until pain level falls below 5 or becomes tolerable. Continue the effective bolus dose.
  —Increase the basal rate every 12 hours p.r.n., adjusting for bolus doses taken.
  Example. A patient receiving 10 mg/hr IV morphine required 12 boluses of IV morphine in the past 12 hours (5 mg + 10 mg + [20 mg × 10]).
  New basal rate: 10 mg/hr + 215 mg/12 hr = 28 mg/hr.
- IV bolus option.
  —Give 10 to 20 mg IV morphine over 15 minutes; evaluate pain relief.
  —If pain level ≥7 and unchanged, double the bolus dose; check vital signs every 15 minutes; reevaluate pain in 30 minutes. If still ≥5, repeat the same dose. If pain level is unchanged, double the bolus dose.
  —When pain level <5, give effective bolus doses q2h as needed for next 24 hours.

(continued)

- When pain control is adequate, convert to new, higher dose of oral or transdermal opioid.
  Example. The IV bolus option is used in a patient taking 100 mg of SR morphine every 12 hours.
  Morphine to reduce pain level to <5: 70 mg over 2 hours (10 mg + 20 mg + 40 mg). Three additional 40-mg boluses required in the next 22 hours.
  Total morphine taken in 24 hours: 190 mg IV (= 570 mg p.o.) + 200 mg p.o. = 770 mg p.o.
  Resume oral or transdermal opioid at a dose equivalent to 770 mg oral morphine/24 hr with 80 mg MSIR p.o. q4h p.r.n.

A more rapid titration of morphine (2 mg IV every 2 minutes) has been found effective in decreasing the excruciating pain of both opioid-naive and opioid-tolerant patients to a tolerable level (<4) within 15 minutes (Mercadante et al. 2002). The majority of patients (30 of 45) were not receiving morphine prior to the onset of the excruciating pain. Doses required to achieve pain levels of <4 were modest (mean dose of 8.5 mg, Confidence Interval 6.5 to 10.5 mg IV morphine). Doses of up to 40 mg IV were given, and no significant adverse events noted.

Another report demonstrated that a rapid titration of intravenous fentanyl could control severe pain in as little as 10 minutes (Soares et al. 2003). The patients did not have neuropathic pain, and all had been taking morphine for at least 2 weeks before the pain emergency occurred. The fentanyl dose was calculated from the previous morphine dose, using 10 percent of the previous 24-hour opioid dose and a ratio of 1 mg morphine to 10 μg fentanyl. For example, if a patient was taking 150 mg/day of oral morphine, the IV equivalent is 50 mg/day; 10 percent of that is 5 mg IV morphine. The equivalent fentanyl dose is 50 μg. The patient would receive a 50 μg fentanyl bolus. If the pain remained at ≥4 after 5 minutes, a second 50 μg bolus was given; if the pain remained at ≥4 after an additional 5 minutes, the fentanyl dose was increased by 50 percent. The last dose (i.e., 75 μg) could be given again 5 minutes later if necessary. All 18 patients treated were carefully monitored in the emergency department, and all had relief of pain, with an average time to control of 11 minutes, and without adverse effects.

When satisfactory pain relief is finally achieved, the patient usually falls asleep. This is not a signal to decrease the opioid drip rate. The patient is not overdosed; he is simply exhausted by loss of sleep due to the excruciating pain. I do lower the drip rate for patients who are difficult to arouse or who have depressed respirations (<10/min), but otherwise I let the patient sleep as long as necessary. When he awakens, continue careful evaluations of pain intensity and side effects. Once the pain has been controlled for a day or two, the patient is likely to require less opioid to maintain the same level of pain relief.

SUMMARY

As clinicians, we strive to help even our sickest patients accomplish the goals they have set for themselves. To succeed, we must relieve uncontrolled pain. The pharmacologic agents and other treatment modalities discussed in this chapter, along with the nonpharmacologic techniques reviewed in Chapter 6, enable us to control the pain of 90 percent or more of our patients with cancer and minimize the associated side effects. Our patients will not ask us to relieve their suffering by helping them to kill themselves; instead, when they have accomplished their final tasks, they will—despite the urgings of the poet Dylan Thomas to the contrary—"go gentle into that good night."

TABLES

Tables 5.1 to 5.14 follow on pages 254–263.

Table 5.1 Nonsteroidal Anti-inflammatory Drugs (NSAIDs)

Chemical Class	Generic Name	Interval	Initial Dose (mg)[1]	Max. 24-hr Dose (mg)
p-Aminophenol salicylates	Acetaminophen[2]	q4–6h	650	4000
	Aspirin[2,3]	q4–6h	650	4000
	Salsalate	q8–12h	750–1000	3000
	Diflunisol	q12h	500	1500
Propionic acid derivatives	Ibuprofen	q4–6h	400	2400
	Fenoprofen	q4–6h	200	2400
	Ketoprofen[2]	q6–8h	25	225
	Naproxen[2,3]	q6–8h	250	1000
	Oxaprozin	q12–24h	600	1200
Acetic acid derivatives	Indomethacin[2,3]	q8–12h	25	150
	Tolmetin	q8h	400	1800
	Diclofenac[2]	q8h	50	150
	Sulindac	q12h	150	400
	Ketorolac	q6h	30–60 IV load, 15–30 IV q6h (p.o. 10 mg q6h)	150 mg day 1, 120 mg days 2–7 (p.o. 40 mg)
COX-2 "selective"[4]	Etodolac	q8–12h	200–400	1200
	Nabumetone	q12–24h	1000/24 hr	1500
	Celecoxib	q12–24h	100–200	400
	Valdecoxib	q12–24h	10	40

Source: Modified with permission from N. Coyle, N. Cherny, and R. K. Portenoy, Pharmacologic management in cancer pain, in *Cancer Pain Management*, 2nd ed, D. B. McGuire, C. H. Yarbro, B. R. Ferell (eds), Boston: Jones and Bartlett, 1995; Miaskowski C, Cleary J, Burney R, et al. *Guideline for the Management of Cancer Pain in Adults and Children*, APS Clinical Practice Guidelines Series, No. 3. Glenview, Ill.: American Pain Society, 2005. www.ampainsoc.org.

[1] In the elderly and in patients with renal insufficiency, start at one-half to two-thirds of these doses.

[2] Bioavailable p.r. via custom-made suppository or microenema (Davis et al. 2002).

[3] Available in suppository form.

[4] Rofecoxib (Vioxx), withdrawn in September 2004, may again be available. Use with caution in patients with increased cardiac risk factors. Dosing is 25 mg q12–24h,

Table 5.2   Cost Comparison for Equianalgesic Doses of Opioids

Drug	Dose	Comparative Cost, One-Month Supply[1]
MSIR®	45 mg q4h	++
MS Contin®	150 mg q12h	+++
Oramorph®	150 mg q12h	+++
Kadian®	150 mg q12h	++++
Avinza®	300 mg q24h	+++
Oxycodone IR	30 mg q4h	++
OxyContin®	100 mg q12h	++++
Hydromorphone	12 mg q4h	+++
Duragesic®	150 µg/hr	++++
Methadone	10 mg q8h	+

Source: Average wholesale price from *Red Book®,* Montvale, N.J.: Medical Economics Company, 2004.
[1]Cost: + = less than $50; ++ = $51 to $250; +++ = $251 to $600; ++++ greater than $600.

Table 5.3   Commonly Used Step 2 Opioids: Preparations Available

Name	Initial Dose (mg), Oral[1]	Dose Interval (hr)	Dose Adjustments Needed	Preparations Available[2]
Hydrocodone	10	3–4	None	IR, comb
Codeine	60	3–4	Severe hepatic or renal failure	IR, comb, IM, SQ, p.r.
Oxycodone[3]	5–10	3–4	Severe hepatic or renal failure	Comb, p.r.
Tramadol	50	6	Cirrhosis or renal failure	IR, p.r. comb

Source: Miaskowski C, Cleary J, Burney R, et al. *Guideline for the Management of Cancer Pain in Adults and Children,* APS Clinical Practice Guidelines Series, No. 3. Glenview Ill.: American Pain Society, 2005. www.ampainsoc.org.
[1]For patients weighing over 110 pounds who have moderate to severe pain.
[2]Preparations: IR = oral, immediate-release; comb = oral combination preparation with an NSAID (acetaminophen, aspirin, ibuprofen, etc.); IM = parenteral—suitable for intramuscular use; SQ = subcutaneous; p.r. = per rectum via commercial or custom-made suppository or microenema (Davis et al. 2002).
[3]See also Table 5.4 for oxycodone not in a combination preparation; that is, IR, sustained-release (SR), liquid (liq), or liquid concentrate (liq conc) oxycodone.

Table 5.4   Commonly Used Step 3 Opioids: Preparations Available

Name	Initial Dose (mg)[1] Oral	Initial Dose (mg)[1] IM/IV	Dose Interval (hr)	Dose Adjustments Needed	Preparations Available[2]
Morphine	15–30	10	3–4	Renal failure	IV/SQ, IR, p.r., liq, liq conc
Morphine, SR	15–30	n/a	8–12	Renal/hepatic failure	SR, p.r.
Morphine, SR	30	n/a	24	Renal/hepatic failure	SR
Hydromorphone	4–8	1.5	4	Hepatic failure	IV/SQ, IR, p.r.
Hydromorphone, SR[3]	12	n/a	24	Hepatic failure	SR
Oxycodone	10	n/a	3–4	Renal failure	IR, liq, liq conc, p.r.
Oxycodone, SR	10	n/a	12	Renal/hepatic failure	SR
Fentanyl[3]	n/a	25 µg/hr	72	Hepatic failure	Transdermal
Fentanyl	200 µg	n/a	2		Transmucosal
Methadone	5	2.5	6–8	Renal/hepatic failure	IV/SQ, IR, liq, p.r.
Oxymorphone	n/a	1	3–4	Renal failure	IV/SQ, p.r.
Demerol®[4]	N/R	N/R	N/R	Renal failure	IV, IR

Source: Miaskowski C, Cleary J, Burney R, et al. *Guideline for the Management of Cancer Pain in Adults and Children,* APS Clinical Practice Guidelines Series, No. 3. Glenview, Ill.: American Pain Society, 2005. www.ampainsoc.org

[1] For patients weighing over 110 pounds who have moderate to severe pain.

[2] Preparations: p.r. = per rectum via commercial or custom-made suppository or microenema (Davis et al. 2002); IV = parenteral—suitable for intravenous use; SQ = subcutaneous; IR = oral, immediate-release; SR = oral, sustained-release; liq = liquid; liq conc = concentrated liquid solution; N/R = not recommended.

[3] Only use as an initial dose if the patient is already taking the equivalent of oral morphine.

[4] Not recommended for use other than for a limited time (see text).

Table 5.5   Commonly Used Opioids: Equianalgesic Doses

Drug	Oral/Rectal Dose (mg)	Parenteral Dose (mg)
Morphine	30	10
Hydromorphone	7.5	1.5
Oxycodone	20	n/a
Methadone[1]	10	5
Levorphanol	4	2
Oxymorphone	n/a	1
Meperidine[2]	300	75

Conversion from fentanyl transdermal patch
to parenteral or oral morphine

Fentanyl	Morphine (mg/24 hr)	
(μg/hr)	p.o.	IM/IV
25	50	17
50	100	33
75	150	50
100	200	67
125	250	83
150	300	100

Source: American Pain Society, *Principles of Analgesic Use in the Treatment of Acute Pain and Cancer Pain,* 5th ed., Glenview, Ill.: American Pain Society, 2003.
[1]For dosing of methadone, see discussion in text.
[2]Not recommended for cancer patients (see text).

Table 5.6   Laxatives to Prevent and Treat Opioid-Induced Constipation Syndromes

Drug	Mechanism	Initial Dosage
GENERAL		
Senna	Myenteric plexus stimulant	2 p.o. b.i.d.
Senokot-S®	Senna + stool hydrating agent	2 p.o. b.i.d.
Bisacodyl (Dulcolax®)	Myenteric plexus stimulant	2 p.o. h.s.
Milk of Magnesia (MOM®)	Osmotic	30–60 ml p.o. t.i.d.
Lactulose	Osmotic	15–30 ml p.o. h.s.
Polyethylene glycol	Osmotic	17 g in 4 oz water p.o. daily
MOM® + mineral oil	Osmotic	30–60 ml MOM + 15–30 ml mineral oil q.d. or b.i.d.
OPIOID BOWEL SYNDROME		
Metoclopramide (Reglan®)	Vagal stimulant	5–10 mg p.o. q.i.d. to 20 mg p.o. q.i.d.; or 1–3 mg/hr IV
Clonidine	Prevents withdrawal	0.1–0.3 mg transdermal patch
Naloxone	Antagonizes opioid binding to gut opiate receptors	4 mg p.o. b.i.d. to t.i.d.

Table 5.7   Antiemetics

Etiology of Nausea	Drug	Dose
Initiation of opioid therapy	Prochlorperazine (Compazine®)	10 mg p.o. t.i.d. to q.i.d.or 25 mg p.r. b.i.d.
Stimulation of chemoreceptor trigger zone	Haloperidol (Haldol®)	1–2 mg p.o. b.i.d. to q.i.d., 0.5–1 mg IV b.i.d. to q.i.d.
	Prochlorperazine (Compazine®)	10 mg p.o. t.i.d. to q.i.d. or 25 mg p.r. b.i.d.
Delayed gastric emptying	Metoclopramide (Reglan®)	10–20 mg b.i.d. to q.i.d. or 1–3 mg/hr IV
Vertigo	Scopolamine (Transderm Scōp®)	1 patch q72h
	Meclizine (Bonine®, Antivert®)	25 mg t.i.d. p.o.
Unclear	Ondansetron (Zofran®)	4–8 mg p.o. b.i.d. to t.i.d.
	Olanzapine (Zyprexa®, Zydis®)	2.5–5 mg p.o./SL qhs to b.i.d.
	Lorazepam (Ativan®)	0.5–1 mg p.o./SL/IV q4h

Note: For nausea, initial steps should be (1) treat cause, if identified; (2) consider changing to a different opioid agent (see text); and (3) use adjuvants to decrease opioid dose (see Table 5.6, opioid bowel syndrome). SL = sublingual dissolving tablets/wafers.

Table 5.8   Psychostimulants

Drug	Dose
Methylphenidate (Ritalin®)	2.5–5 mg p.o. every morning; may repeat at noon if needed
Dextroamphetamine (Dexedrine®)	2.5–5 mg p.o. every morning; may repeat at noon if needed
Modafinil (Provigil®)	200 mg p.o. every morning; can increase to 400 mg/day

Note: For sedation, initial steps should be (1) treat cause, if identified; (2) use SR and IR preparations effectively; (3) discontinue other sedating agents (see text); and (4) use adjuvants to decrease opioid dose (see Table 5.6, opioid bowel syndrome).

Table 5.9   Treatment of Delirium

Drug	Dose	Comments
Haloperidol (Haldol®)	0.5–5 mg p.o., IV, SQ. Repeat q2–12h as needed.	Do not exceed 20 mg in 24 hr. Maintain the patient on the effective dose (divided into a b.i.d. dose) for 3–4 days, then taper over 1 week, as tolerated.
Olanzapine (Zyprexa®, Zydis®)	2.5–5 mg p.o./SL h.s. to b.i.d.	Can add 2.5 mg q4h p.r.n.
Chlorpromazine (Thorazine®)	25–100 mg p.o., IV or p.r., b.i.d. to q.i.d.	May cause significant hypotension.
Lorazepam[1] (Ativan®)	0.5–1 mg p.o./SL q1–2h	Add to haloperidol for patients with an agitated delirium. Tablets can be used p.r. for terminal delirium.
Diazepam[1] (Valium®)	5–10 mg p.o. b.i.d.	Useful p.r. for patients unable to take oral medication.
Clonazepam[1] (Klonopin®)	0.5–5 mg p.o./SL t.i.d.	Tablets have been used p.r. for terminal delirium. Do not exceed 20 mg/24 hr.
Midazolam[1] (Versed®)	30–100 mg IV/SQ over 24 hr	IV drip or SQ infusion for terminal delirium.

Note: In delirious patients, attempt first to identify the underlying cause and begin to correct it as you give the agents listed. Make the patient's surroundings as familiar as possible. Ask a family member or friend to sit with the patient. SL = sublingual dissolving tablets/wafers.

[1]*Caution:* Any benzodiazepine may exacerbate delirium, especially in older adults (>70).

Table 5.10 Adjuvants for Neuropathic Pain

Class/Drug	Dose	Comments
Corticosteroids		
Prednisone	20–40 mg in divided doses; taper to q.o.d. as tolerated	Add acylovir for acute herpes zoster (see text).
Dexamethasone	10–100 mg bolus; 6 mg p.o./IV q.i.d.; taper as tolerated	Spinal cord compression
	4–6 mg b.i.d. to q.i.d.	Other neuropathic pain
Anticonvulsants		
Gabapentin (Neurontin®)	900–3600 mg/day p.o.	Initial dose: 100 mg b.i.d. to t.i.d.; increase by 100 mg q3d.
Phenytoin (Dilantin®)	1000 mg load; 200–300 mg/day	Cannot be given IM.
Carbamazepine (Tegretol®)	200 mg p.o. h.s., increase q3d	Suspension available for rectal administration. Do not exceed 1200 mg/24 hr.
Clonazepam (Klonopin®)	0.5 mg p.o. t.i.d. SL; increase by 0.5 mg q3d	Rarely used for neuropathic pain. Do not exceed 20 mg/24 hr.
Lamotrigine (Lamictal®)	100–200 mg/day p.o.	Initial dose 25 mg/day p.o.; increase by 25 mg/day q. 2 weeks.
Topiramate (Topamax®)	200–400 mg/day p.o.	Initial dose 25–50 mg/day p.o.; increase 25–50 mg/day q. week.
Oxcarbazepine (Trileptal®)	2400 mg/day p.o.	Initial dose 300 mg p.o. b.i.d.; increase by 300 mg q3d.
Levetiracetam (Keppra®)	3000 mg/day p.o.	Initial dose 500 mg p.o. q12h; increase by 1000 mg/day q. 2 weeks.
GABA antagonist		
Baclofen (Lioresal®)	5 mg t.i.d.; increase by 5 mg q3d	Used for tic douloureux-like pain. Target dose: 40–80 mg/24 hr
Alpha-2 adrenergic agonist		
Clonidine	0.1–0.3 mg patch	
NMDA Antagonist		
Ketamine	0.1–0.2 mg/kg IV initial	Double dose q15min until pain is relieved; then begin drip at equivalent amount per hour. Scopolamine may be needed for increased salivation.
Anesthetic		
Lidocaine	1–3 mg/kg load IV over 20–30 min, followed by infusion of 0.5–2 mg/kg/hr	Close monitoring of vital signs and patient symptoms required.

Table 5.11   Antidepressants as Adjuvant Analgesics

Name	Dose	Comments

Tricyclic antidepressants
  Amitriptyline (Elavil®)
  Imipramine (Tofranil®)
  Doxepin (Sinequan®)
  Clomipramine
    (Anafranil®)
  Desipramine
    (Norpramin®)
  Nortriptyline
    (Pamelor®)
	Begin at 10–25 mg p.o. h.s.;
	  increase to therapeutic dose
	  (50–150 mg in divided doses)
		Side effects: anticholinergic,
		  sedation, cardiac arrhythmias,
		  orthostatic hypotension.
		Amitriptyline: most sedating.
		Desipramine: least sedating,
		  minimal cardiotoxicity; may
		  need 150–300 mg for
		  therapeutic effect.
		Nortriptyline: least orthostatic
		  hypotension; minimal
		  sedation.

Table 5.12   Adjuvants for Bone Pain

Drug	Dose	Comments
Bisphosphonates		Caution in renal insufficiency.

Zoledronic acid
    (Zometa®)
	4 mg IV over 15 min
	  q. month	

Pamidronate
    (Aredia®)
	60–90 mg IV over
	  2 hr, q. month	

Calcitonin	100–200 IU SQ b.i.d.	Often effective for weeks to a few
		  months; can cause symptomatic
		  hypocalcemia.

Strontium chloride 89		Induces significant cytopenias;
		  contraindicated in hypercalcemic
		  patients.

Samarium 153 lexidronam		Induces significant cytopenias.

Note: For NSAIDs and corticosteroids, see text and Tables 5.1 and 5.10.

Table 5.13   Topical and Oral Anesthetics

Drug	Preparation	Comments
ELA-Max	Cream (lidocaine 4%)	For procedure-related pain.
EMLA®	Cream (lidocaine 2.5% + prilocaine 2.5%)	For procedure-related pain; may help in post-herpetic neuralgia.
Lidocaine	Ointment (5%, 10%), gel (5%), patch (5%)	Post-herpetic neuralgia; peripheral sensory neuropathy.
Capsaicin	Cream (0.025%, 0.075%)	Bone pain; post-herpetic neuralgia. Avoid heat to areas where cream is used.
Mexiletine (Mexitil®)	Pill	Initial dose: 150 mg q.d.; do not exceed 300 mg t.i.d.

Table 5.14   Pain Behaviors in Elderly Patients Who Are Cognitively Impaired

Facial expressions
   Slight frown; sad, frightened face
   Grimacing, wrinkled forehead, closed
     or tightened eyes
   Any distorted expression
   Rapid blinking
Verbalizations, vocalizations
   Sighing, moaning, groaning
   Grunting, chanting, calling out
   Noisy breathing
   Asking for help
   Verbally abusive
Body movements
   Rigid, tense body posture, guarding
   Fidgeting
   Increased pacing, rocking
   Restricted movement
   Gait or mobility changes

Changes in interpersonal reactions
   Aggressive, combative, resisting care
   Decreased social interactions
   Socially inappropriate, disruptive
   Withdrawn
Changes in activity patterns or routines
   Refusing food, appetite changes
   Increase in rest periods
   Sleep, rest pattern changes
   Sudden cessation of common routines
   Increased wandering
Mental status changes
   Crying or tears
   Increased confusion
   Irritability or distress

Note: Some patients demonstrate little or no specific behavior associated with severe pain.

Source: Table 3 in AGS Panel on Persistent Pain in Older Persons, The management of persistent pain in older persons, *Journal of the American Geriatrics Society,* 50:S205–S224, 2002. Blackwell Publishers; reprinted with permission.

Bibliography

The references are grouped by subject, following the order of discussion in the chapter.

GENERAL REFERENCES
American Pain Society. 2003. *Principles of Analgesic Use in the Treatment of Acute Pain and Cancer Pain*, 5th ed. Glenview, Ill.: American Pain Society.

Coyle N, Cherny N, Portenoy RK. 1995. Pharmacologic management of cancer pain. In *Cancer Pain Management*, 2nd ed, McGuire DB, Yarbro CH, Ferrell BR (eds). Boston: Jones and Bartlett.

Foley KM. 2005. Management of cancer pain. In *Cancer: Principles and Practice of Oncology*, 7th ed, DeVita VT, Hellman S, Rosenberg SA (eds). Philadelphia: Lippincott-Raven.

Jacox A, Carr DB, Payne R. 1994. New clinical-practice guidelines for the management of pain in patients with cancer. *N Engl J Med* 330:651–655.

Levy MH. 1996. Pharmacologic treatment of cancer pain. *N Engl J Med* 335:1124–1132.

Mercadante S. 1999. Pain treatment and outcomes for patients with advanced cancer who receive follow-up care at home. *Cancer* 85:1849–1858.

Miaskowski C, Cleary J, Burney R, et al. 2005. *Guideline for the Management of Cancer Pain in Adults and Children*. APS Clinical Practice Guidelines Series, No. 3. Glenview, Ill.: American Pain Society. www. ampainsoc.org.

National Comprehensive Cancer Network (NCCN). 2004. NCCN Pain Guideline VI. www.nccn.org.

Schug SA, Zech D, Dorr U. 1990. Cancer pain management according to WHO analgesic guidelines. *J Pain Symptom Manage* 5:27–32.

World Health Organization. 1996. *Cancer Pain Relief: With a Guide to Opioid Availability*, 2nd ed. Geneva: World Health Organization.

Zech D, Grond S, Lynch J, et al. 1995. Validation of World Health Organization Guidelines for cancer pain relief: a 10-year prospective study. *Pain* 63:65–76.

DRUG USE IN RENAL FAILURE
Kurella M, Bennett WM, Chertow GM. 2003. Analgesia in patients with ESRD: a review of available evidence. *Am J Kidney Dis* 42:217–228.

NSAIDs
GENERAL DISCUSSION
McQuay HJ, Moore E. 2004. Non-opioid analgesics. In *Oxford Textbook of Palliative Medicine*, 3rd ed, Doyle D, Hanks G, Cherny N, Calman K (eds). Oxford: Oxford University Press.

Vane JR. 1971. Inhibition of prostaglandin synthesis as a mechanism of action for aspirin-like drugs. *Nature* 231:232–235.

EFFICACY
Buckley MM, Brogden RN. 1990. Ketorolac: a review of its pharmacodynamic and pharmacokinetic properties, and therapeutic potential. *Drugs* 39:86–109.

Eisenberg E, Berkey CS, Carr DB, et al. 1994. Efficacy and safety of non-steroidal anti-inflammatory drugs for cancer pain: a meta-analysis. *J Clin Oncol* 12:2756–2765.

Mercadante S, Sapio M, Caligara M, et al. 1997. Opioid-sparing effect of diclofenac in cancer pain. *J Pain Symptom Manage* 14:15–20.

Reynolds LW, Hoo RK, Brill RJ, et al. 2003. The COX-2 specific inhibitor, valdecoxib, is an effective, opioid-sparing analgesic in patients undergoing total knee arthroplasty. *J Pain Symptom Manage* 25:133–141.

Stuart MJ, Murphy SM, Oski FA, et al. 1972. Platelet function in recipients of platelets from donors ingesting aspirin. *N Engl J Med* 287:1105–1109.

Wallenstein SL. 1975. Analgesic studies of aspirin in cancer patients. In *Proceedings of the Aspirin Symposium*. London: Aspirin Foundation.

Warren DE. 1996. Practical use of rectal medications in palliative care. *J Pain Symptom Manage* 11:378–387.

SIDE EFFECTS AND COMPLICATIONS

Chan FFKL, Hung LCT, Suen BY, et al. 2002. Celecoxib versus diclofenac and omeprazole in reducing the risk of recurrent ulcer bleeding in patients with arthritis. *N Engl J Med* 347:2104–2110.

DeMaria AN, Weir MR. 2003. Coxibs—beyond the GI tract: renal and cardiovascular issues. *J Pain Symptom Manage* 25S:S41–49.

Gloth FM. 1996. Concerns with chronic analgesic therapy in elderly patients. *Am J Med 101* (suppl 1):9S–24S.

Hawkey CJ, Karrasch KA, Szczepanski L, et al. 1998. Omeprazole compared with misoprostol for ulcers associated with nonsteroidal antiinflammatory drugs. *N Engl J Med* 338:727–734.

Hollander D. 1994. Gastrointestinal complications of nonsteroidal anti-inflammatory drugs: prophylactic and therapeutic strategies. *Am J Med* 96:274–281.

Laine L. 2003. Gastrointestinal effects of NSAIDs and coxibs. *J Pain Symptom Manage* 25S:S32–40.

Roth SH. 1989. Merits and liabilities of NSAID therapy. *Rheum Dis Clin North Am* 15:479–498.

Scheiman JM. 1996. NSAIDs, gastrointestinal injury, and cytoprotection. *Gastroenterol Clin North Am* 25:279–298.

Schlondorff D. 1993. Renal complications of nonsteroidal anti-inflammatory drugs. *Kidney Int* 44:643–653.

Strom BL. 1994. Adverse reactions to over-the-counter analgesics taken for therapeutic purposes. *JAMA* 272:1866–1867.

Whitcomb DC, Block GD. 1994. Association of acetaminophen hepatotoxicity with fasting and ethanol use. *JAMA* 272:1845–1850.

Yeomans ND, Tulassay Z, Juhasz L, et al. 1998. A comparison of omeprazole with ranitidine for ulcers associated with nonsteroidal antiinflammatory drugs. *N Engl J Med* 338:719–726.

OPIOIDS

GENERAL GUIDELINES

Goldfrank L, Weisman RS, Errick JK, Lo MW. 1996. A nomogram for continuous intravenous naloxone. *Ann Emerg Med* 15:566.

Hanks GWC, Cherny N, Fallon M. 2004. Opioid analgesic therapy. In *Oxford Textbook of Palliative Medicine*, 3rd ed, Doyle D, Hanks G, Cherny N, Colman K (eds). Oxford: Oxford University Press.

Levy MH. 1996. Pharmacologic treatment of cancer pain. *N Engl J Med* 335:1124–1132.

Medical Board of California. *Action Report*, vol 87, pp 1, 4–6. Sacramento Medical Board of California, October 2003.

Medical Economics Company. 2004. *Red Book®*. Montvale, N.J.: Medical Economics Company.

Mercadante S. 1999. Pain treatment and outcomes for patients with advanced cancer who receive follow-up care at home. *Cancer* 85:1849–1858.

Thomas SH, Silen W, Cheema F, et al. 2003. Effects of morphine analgesia on diagnostic accuracy in emergency department patients with abdominal pain: a prospective, randomized trial. *J Am Coll Surg* 196:18–31.

Weinberg BBBA, Inturissi CE, Reidenberg B, et al. 1988. Sublingual absorption of selected opioid analgesics. *Clin Pharmacol Ther* 44:335–342.

ORAL ROUTE

The opioids commonly taken orally are listed alphabetically.

Avinza 24-Hour Efficacy

Caldwell JR, Rapoport RJ, Davis JC, et al., for the Avinza™ TR G004-04 Study Group. 2002. Efficacy and safety of a once-daily morphine formulation in chronic, moderate-to-severe osteoarthritis pain: results from a randomized, placebo-controlled, double-blind trial and an open-label extension trial. *J Pain Symptom Manage* 23:278–291.

Portenoy RK, Sciberras A, Eliot L, et al. 2002. Steady-state pharmacokinetic comparison of a new extended release, once-daily morphine formulation, Avinza™, and a twice-daily controlled release morphine formulation in patients with chronic moderate-to-severe pain. *J Pain Symptom Manage* 23:292–300.

Codeine

Desmeules J, Gascon M-P, Dayer P, Magistris M. 1991. Impact of environmental and genetic factors on codeine analgesia. *Eur J Clin Pharmacol* 41:23–26.

Sindrup SH, Arendt-Nielson L, Rosen K, et al. 1992. The effect of quinidine on the analgesic effect of codeine. *Eur J Clin Pharmacol* 42:587–591.

Meperidine

Kaiko RF, Foley KM, Grabinski PY, et al. 1983. Central nervous system excitatory effects of meperidine in cancer patients. *Ann Intern Med* 13:180–185.

Methadone

Bruera E, Sweeney C. 2002. Methadone use in cancer patients with pain: a review. *J Palliat Med* 5:127–138.

Fainsinger R, Schoeller T, Bruera E. 1993. Methadone in the management of cancer pain: a review. *Pain* 52:137–147.

Foley KM. 2003. Opioids and chronic neuropathic pain. *N Engl J Med* 348:1279–1281.

Foley KM, Houde RW. 1998. Methadone in cancer pain management: individualize dose and titrate to effect (editorial). *J Clin Oncol* 16:3213–3215.

Mercadante S, Casuccio A, Agnello A, et al. 1998. Morphine versus methadone in the pain treatment of advanced cancer patients followed at home. *J Clin Oncol* 16:3656–3661.

Ripamonti C, Groff L, Brunelli C, et al. 1998. Switching from morphine to oral methadone in treating cancer pain: what is the equianalgesic dose ratio? *J Clin Oncol* 16:3216–3221.

Tarumi Y, Pereira J, Watanabe S. 2002. Methadone and fluconazole: respiratory depression by drug interaction. *J Pain Symptom Manage* 23:148–153.

Morphine (Sustained-Release Kadian [also marketed as Kapanol])

Broomhead A, Kerr R, Tester W, et al. 1997. Comparison of a once-a-day sustained-release morphine formulation with standard oral morphine treatment for cancer pain. *J Pain Symptom Manage* 14:63–73.

Gourlay GK, Cherry DA, Onley MM, et al. 1997. Pharmacokinetics and pharmacodynamics of twenty-four-hourly Kapanol compared to twelve-hourly MS Contin in the treatment of severe cancer pain. *Pain* 69:295–302.

Jones R, Hale E, Talosim L, Phillips R. 1996. Kapanol™ capsules: pellet formulation provides alternative methods of administration of sustained-release morphine sulfate. *Clin Drug Invest* 12:88–93.

Maccarone C, West RJ, Broomhead AF, Hudson GP. 1994. Single dose pharmacokinetics of Kapanol™, a new oral sustained-release morphine formulation. *Clin Drug Invest* 7:262–274.

Oxycodone (Sustained-Release)

Bruera E, Belzile M, Pituskin E, et al. 1998. Randomized, double-blind, cross-over trial comparing safety and efficacy of oral controlled-release oxycodone with controlled-release morphine in patients with cancer pain. *J Clin Oncol* 16:3222–3229.

Kaiko RF, Benziger DP, Fitzmartin RD, et al. 1996a. Pharmacokinetic-pharmacodynamic relationships of controlled-release oxycodone. *Clin Pharmacol Ther* 59:52–61.

Kaiko R, Lacouture P, Hopf K, et al. 1996b. Analgesic onset and potency of oral controlled-release (CR) oxycodone and CR morphine. *Clin Pharmacol Ther* 59:130.

Kaplan R, Parris WC-V, Citron ML, et al. 1998. Comparison of controlled-release and immediate-release oxycodone tablets in patients with cancer pain. *J Clin Oncol* 16:3230–3237.

Tramadol

Bodalia B, Mcdonald CJ, Smith KJ, et al. 2003. A comparison of the pharmacokinetics, clinical effects and tolerability of once-daily tramadol tablets with normal release tramadol capsules. *J Pain Symptom Manage* 25:142–149.

Gobel H, Stadler T. 1995. Treatment of pain due to postherpetic neuralgia with tramadol—results of an open, parallel pilot study vs clomipramine with or without levomepromazine. *Clin Drug Invest* 10:208–214.

Tramadol—a new oral analgesic. 1995. *Med Lett* 37:59–60.

Wilder-Smith CH, Schimke J, Osterwalder B, Senn HJ. 1994. Oral tramadol, a mu-opioid agonist and monoamine reuptake-blocker, and morphine for strong cancer-related pain. *Ann Oncol* 5:141–146.

ORAL TRANSMUCOSAL FENTANYL

Christie JM, Simmonds M, Patt R, et al. 1998. Dose-titration, multicenter study of oral transmucosal fentanyl citrate for the treatment of breakthrough pain in cancer patients using transdermal fentanyl for persistent pain. *J Clin Oncol* 16:3238–3245.

Fine PG, Marcus M, Just De Boer A, Van der Oord B. 1991. An open label study of oral transmucosal fentanyl citrate (OTFC) for the treatment of breakthrough cancer pain. *Pain* 45:149–153.

Payne R, Caluzzi P, Hart L, et al. 2001. Long-term safety of oral transmucosal fentanyl citrate (OTFC) for breakthrough cancer pain. *J Pain Symptom Manage* 22: 579–583.

Rees E. 2002. The role of oral transmucosal fentanyl citrate in the management of breakthrough cancer pain. *Int J Palliat Nurs* 8:304–308.

Zhang H, Zhang J, Streisand JB. 2002. Oral mucosal drug delivery: clinical pharmacokinetic and therapeutic applications. *Clin Pharmacokinet* 41:661–680.

TOPICAL OPIOIDS

Flock P. 2003. Pilot study to determine the effectiveness of diamorphine gel to control pressure ulcer pain. *J Pain Symptom Manage* 25:547–554.

Krajnik M, Zylicz Z, Finlay I, et al. 1999. Potential uses of topical opioids in palliative care—report of 6 cases. *Pain* 80:121–125.

Stein C. 1995. The control of pain in peripheral tissue by opioids. *N Engl J Med* 332: 1685–1690.

Zeppetella G, Paul J, Ribeiro MDC. 2003. Analgesic efficacy of morphine applied topically to painful ulcers. *J Pain Symptom Manage* 25:555–558.

TRANSDERMAL FENTANYL

Ahmedzai S, Brooks D, on behalf of the TTS-Fentanyl Comparative Trial Group. 1997. Transdermal fentanyl versus sustained-release oral morphine in cancer pain: preference, efficacy, and quality of life. *J Pain Symptom Manage* 13:254–261.

Donner B, Zena M, Tryba M, Strumpf M. 1996. Direct conversion from oral morphine to transdermal fentanyl: a multicenter study in patients with cancer pain. *Pain* 64:527–534.

Hough SW, Bajwa ZH, Warfield CA. 2003. Pharmacological therapy of cancer pain. www.uptodate.com.

Payne R, Mathias SD, Pasta DJ, et al. 1998. Quality of life and cancer pain: satisfaction and side effects with transdermal fentanyl versus oral morphine. *J Clin Oncol* 16:1588–1593.

Portenoy RK, Southam MA, Gupta SK, et al. 1993. Transdermal fentanyl for cancer pain: repeated dose pharmacokinetics. *Anesthesiology* 78:36–43.

Varvel JR, Shafer SL, Hwang SS, et al. 1989. Absorption characteristics of transdermally administered fentanyl. *Anesthesiology* 70:928–934.

RECTAL ROUTE

Bruera E, Fainsinger R, Spachynski K, et al. 1995. Clinical efficacy and safety of a novel controlled release morphine suppository and subcutaneous morphine in cancer pain: a randomized evaluation. *J Clin Oncol* 13.1520–1527.

Davis MP, Walsh D, LeGrand SB, Naughton M. 2002. Symptom control in cancer patients: the clinical pharmacology and therapeutic role of suppositories and rectal suspensions. *Support Care Cancer* 10:117–138.

De Conno F, Ripamonti C, Saiti L, et al. 1995. Role of rectal route in treating cancer pain: a randomized crossover clinical trial of oral versus rectal morphine administration in opioid-naive cancer patients with pain. *J Clin Oncol* 13:1004–1008.

Watanabe S, Belzile M, Kuehn N, et al. 1996. Capsules and suppositories of methadone for patients on high-dose opioids for cancer pain: clinical and economic considerations. *Cancer Treat Rev* 22:131–136.

Westerling D, Lindahl S, Anderson KE, Anderson A. 1982. Absorption and bioavailability of rectally administered morphine in women. *Eur J Clin Pharmacol* 23:59.

INTRAVENOUS ROUTE

Citron ML, Kaira J-M, Seltzer VL, et al. 1992. Patient-controlled analgesia for cancer pain: a long-term study of inpatient and outpatient use. *Cancer Invest* 10:335–341.

Coyle N, Adelhardt J, Foley KM, Portenoy RK. 1990. Character of terminal illness in the advanced cancer patient: pain and other symptoms during the last four weeks of life. *J Pain Symptom Manage* 5:83–93.

Hagen NA, Elwood T, Ernst S. 1997. Cancer pain emergencies: a protocol for management. *J Pain Symptom Manage* 14:45–50.

Lichter I. 1994. Accelerated titration of morphine for rapid relief of cancer pain. *N Z Med J* 107:488–490.

Portenoy RK, Moulin DE, Rogers A, et al. 1986. IV infusion of opioids for cancer pain: clinical review and guidelines for use. *Cancer Treat Rep* 70:575–581.

SUBCUTANEOUS ROUTE

Bruera E, Fainsinger R, Moore M, et al. 1991. Local toxicity with subcutaneous methadone: experience of two centers. *Pain* 45:141–145.

Coyle N, Cherny NI, Portenoy RK. 1994. Subcutaneous opioid infusions in the home. *Oncology* 8:21–27.

Storey P, Hill H, St. Louis R, Tarver E. 1990. Subcutaneous infusions for control of cancer symptoms. *J Pain Symptom Manage* 5:33–46.

SPINAL OPIOIDS/ANESTHETICS

Cousins MJ, Walker SM, Goudas LC, Carr DB. 2002. Spinal opioid and non-opioid drugs. IARS 2002 Review Course Lectures. *Anesth Analg* 95(suppl):S38–44.

Du Pen SL, Kharasch ED, Williams A, et al. 1992. Chronic epidural bupivacaine-opioid infusion in intractable cancer pain. *Pain* 49:293–300.

Du Pen S, Williams A. 1994. The clinical dilemma of systemic to epidural morphine conversion: development of a conversion tool for cancer pain patients. *Pain* 56:113–118.

Eisenach JC, Du Pen S, Dubois M, et al., the Epidural Clonidine Study Group. 1995. Epidural clonidine analgesia for intractable cancer pain. *Pain* 61:391–398.

Johnson SM, Duggan AW. 1981. Evidence that opiate receptors at the substantia gelatinosa contribute to the depression by intravenous morphine of the spinal transmission of impulses in the unmyelinated primary afferents. *Brain Res* 207:223–228.

Kitahata LM, Collins JG. 1981. Spinal action of narcotic analgesics. *Anesthesiology* 54:153–163.

Krames ES. 1996. Intraspinal opioid therapy for chronic nonmalignant pain: current practice and clinical guidelines. *J Pain Symptom Manage* 11:333–352.

Marlowe S, Engstrom R, White PF. 1989. Epidural patient-controlled analgesia (PCA): an alternative to continuous epidural infusions. *Pain* 37:97–101.

Paice JA, Magolan JM. 1991. Intraspinal drug therapy. *Nurs Clin North Am* 26:477–498.

Paice JA, Williams AR. 1995. Intraspinal drugs for pain. In *Cancer Pain Management*, 2nd ed, McGuire DB, Yarbro CH, Ferrell BR (eds). Boston: Jones and Bartlett.

Smith TJ, Coyne P, Staats PS, et al. 2003. Implantable drug delivery system (IDDA) provides sustained pain control, less drug toxicity, and better survival compared to medical management (CMM) (abstr #2967). *Proc Am Soc Clin Oncol* 22:738.

Smith TJ, Staats PS, Deer T, et al. 2002. Randomized clinical trial of an implantable drug delivery system compared with comprehensive medical management for refractory pain: impact on pain, drug related toxicity, and survival. *J Clin Oncol* 20:4040–4049.

Swarm RA, Karanikolas M, Cousins MJ. 2004. Anesthetic techniques for pain control. In *Oxford Textbook of Palliative Medicine,* 3rd ed, Doyle D, Hanks G, Cherny N, Calman K (eds). Oxford: Oxford University Press.

Waldman SD, Coombs DW. 1989. Selection of implantable narcotic delivery systems. *Anesth Analg* 68:377–384.

Walker SM, Goudas LC, Cousins MJ, Carr DB. 2002. Combination spinal analgesic chemotherapy: a systematic review. *Anesth Analg* 95:674–715.

OPIOID-INDUCED SIDE EFFECTS

CONSTIPATION

Bruera E, Suarez-Almazor M, Velasco A, et al. 1994. The assessment of constipation in terminal cancer patients admitted to a palliative care unit: a retrospective review. *J Pain Symptom Manage* 9:515–519.

Canty SL. 1994. Constipation as a side effect of opioids. *Oncol Nurs Forum* 21:739–745.

Cleveland MJB, Flavin DP, Ruben RA, et al. 2001. New polyethylene glycol laxative for treatment of constipation in adults: a randomized, double-blind, placebo-controlled study. *South Med J* 94:478–481.

Currow DC, Coughlan M, Fardell B, Cooney NJ. 1997. Use of ondansetron in palliative medicine. *J Pain Symptom Manage* 13:302–307.

Curtis E, Krech R, Walsh T. 1991. Common symptoms in patients with advanced cancer. *J Palliat Care* 7:25–29.

Dalal S, Melzack R. 1998. Potentiation of opioid analgesia by psychostimulant drugs: a review. *J Pain Symptom Manage* 16:245–253.

Kosten TR, O'Connor PG. 2003. Management of drug and alcohol withdrawal. *N Engl J Med* 348:1786–1795.

Levy MH. 1991. Constipation and diarrhea in cancer patients. *Cancer Bull* 43:412–422.

Lublin M, Schwartzentruber BJ. 2002. Bowel obstruction. In *Principles and Practice of Supportive Oncology,* Berger AM, Portenoy RK, Weissman DE (eds). Philadelphia: Lippincott-Raven.

Portenoy RK. 1987. Constipation in the cancer patient: causes and management. *Med Clin North Am* 71:303–311.

Thomas J, Portenoy R, Moehl M, et al. 2003. A phase II randomized dose finding trial of methylnaltrexone for the relief of opioid-induced constipation in hospice patients. *Proc ASCO* 22:729.

Twycross R. 1994. *Pain Relief in Advanced Cancer.* London: Churchill Livingstone.

Twycross RG, Harcourt JMV. 1991. The use of laxatives at a palliative care center. *Palliat Med* 5:27.

NAUSEA

Baines M. 1988. Nausea and vomiting in the patient with advanced cancer. *J Pain Symptom Manage* 3:81–85.

Currow DC, Coughlan M, Fardell B, Cooney NJ. 1997. Use of ondansetron in palliative medicine. *J Pain Symptom Manage* 13:302–307.

Ferris FD, Kerr IG, Sone M, Parcuzzi M. 1991. Transdermal scopolamine use in the control of narcotic-induced nausea. *J Pain Symptom Manage* 6:389–393.

SEDATION

Breitbart W, Passik SD. 1993. Psychiatric approaches to cancer pain management. In *Psychiatric Aspects of Symptom Management in Cancer Patients*, Breitbart W, Holland JC (eds). Washington, D.C.: American Psychiatric Press.

Bruera E, Watanabe S. 1994. Psychostimulants as adjuvant analgesics. *J Pain Symptom Manage* 9:412–415.

Cox JM, Pappagallo M. 2001. Modafinil: a gift to portmanteau. *Am J Hospice Palliat Care* 18:408–410.

Fishbain DA, Cutler RB, Rosomoff HL, Rosomoff RS. 2003. Are opioid-dependent/tolerant patients impaired in driving-related skills? A structured evidence-based review. *J Pain Symptom Manage* 25:559–577.

Kreeger L, Duncan A, Cowap J. 1996. Psychostimulants used for opioid-induced drowsiness. *J Pain Symptom Manage* 11:1–2.

Rozans M, Dreisbach A, Lertora JJL, Kahn M. 2002. Palliative uses of methylphenidate in patients with cancer: a review. *J Clin Oncol* 20:335–339.

Vainio A, Ollila J, Matikainen E, et al. 1995. Driving ability in cancer patients receiving long-term morphine analgesia. *Lancet* 346:667–670.

Wilwerding MB, Loprinzi CL, Mailliard JA, et al. 1995. A randomized crossover evaluation of methylphenidate in cancer patients receiving strong narcotics. *Support Care Cancer* 3:135–138.

DELIRIUM

Breitbart W, Chochinov HM, Passik SD. 2004. Psychiatric symptoms in palliative medicine. In *Oxford Textbook of Palliative Medicine*, 3rd ed, Doyle D, Hanks G, Cherny N, Calman K (eds). Oxford: Oxford University Press.

de Stoutz ND, Bruera E, Suarez-Almazor M. 1995. Opioid rotation for toxicity reduction in terminal cancer patients. *J Pain Symptom Manage* 10:378–384.

de Stoutz ND, Tapper M, Fainsinger R. 1995. Reversible delirium in terminally ill patients. *J Pain Symptom Manage* 10:249–253.

Fürst CJ, Doyle D. 2004. The terminal phase. In *Oxford Textbook of Palliative Medicine*, 3rd ed, Doyle D, Hanks G, Cherny N, Calman K (eds). Oxford: Oxford University Press.

Ingham JM, Caraceni AT. 2002. Delirium. In *Principles and Practice of Supportive Oncology*, 2nd ed, Berger AM, Portenoy RK, Weissman DE (eds). Philadelphia: Lippincott-Raven.

Lawlor PG, Gagnon B, Mancini IL, Pereira JL, et al. 2000. Occurrence, causes, and outcome of delirium in patients with advanced cancer: a prospective study. *Arch Intern Med* 160:786–794.

Stiefel F, Fainsinger R, Bruera E. 1992. Acute confusional state in patients with advanced cancer. *J Pain Symptom Manage* 7:94–98.

Warren DE. 1996. Practical use of rectal medications in palliative care. *J Pain Symptom Manage* 11:378–387.

RESPIRATORY DEPRESSION

Citron ML, Jonston-Earley A, Fossieck BE, et al. 1984. Safety and efficacy of continuous intravenous morphine for severe cancer pain. *Am J Med* 77:199–204.

Goldfrank L, Weisman RS, Errick JK, Lo MW. 1986. A dosing nomogram for continuous infusion intravenous naloxone. *Ann Emerg Med* 15:566–570.

Legrand SB, Estfan B, Walsh D, et al. 2004. Parenteral opioid dose titration and ventilatory function. *J Clin Oncol* 22(14S):8005.

MYOCLONUS

Hagen N, Swanson R. 1997. Strychnine-like multifocal myoclonus and seizures in extremely high dose opioid administration: treatment strategies. *J Pain Symptom Manage* 14:51–58.

PRURITUS

Hough SW, Bajwa ZH, Warfield CA. 2003. Pharmacological therapy of cancer pain. www.uptodate.com.

McNicol E, Horowicz-Mehler N, Fisk RA, et al. 2003. Management of opioid side-effects in cancer-related and chronic noncancer pain: a systematic review. *J Pain* 4:231–256.

Zylicz Z, Smits C, Prajnik M. 1998. Paroxetine for pruritus in advanced cancer. *J Pain Symptom Manage* 16:121.

ADJUVANT ANALGESICS

ANTIDEPRESSANTS

Max MB, Culnane M, Schafer SC, et al. 1987. Amitriptyline relieves diabetic neuropathy pain in patients with normal or depressed mood. *Neurology* 37:589–596.

NEUROPATHIC ADJUVANTS

General Discussions

Beydoun A, Backonja M-M. 2003. Mechanistic stratification of antineuralgia agents. *J Pain Symptom Manage* 25:S18–30.

Kost RG, Straus SE. 1996. Postherpetic neuralgia—pathogenesis, treatment, and prevention. *N Engl J Med* 335:32–42.

Lussier D, Portenoy RK. 2004. Adjuvant analgesics in pain management. In *Oxford Textbook of Palliative Medicine,* 3rd ed, Doyle D, Hanks G, Cherny N, Calman K (eds). Oxford: Oxford University Press.

Rowbotham MC, Twilling L, Davies PS, et al. 2003. Oral opioid therapy for chronic peripheral and central neuropathic pain. *N Engl J Med* 348:1223–1232.

Warren DE. 1996. Practical use of rectal medications in palliative care. *J Pain Symptom Manage* 11:378–387.

Corticosteroids

Abrahm JL. 2004. Assessment and treatment of patients with malignant spinal cord compression. *J Support Oncol* 2:377–391.

Bruera E, Roca E, Cedaro L, et al. 1985. Action of oral methylprednisolone in terminal cancer patients: a prospective randomized double-blind study. *Cancer Treat Rep* 69:751–754.

Heimdal K, Hirschberg H, Slettebo H, et al. 1992. High incidence of serious side-effects of high-dose dexamethasone treatment in patients with epidural spinal cord compression. *J Neurooncol* 12:141–144.

Loblaw DA, Lapierre NJ. 1998. Emergency treatment of malignant extradural spinal cord compression: an evidence-based guideline. *J Clin Oncol* 16:1613–1624.

Loblaw DA, Laperriere N, Perry J, Chambers A, and Members of the Neuro-Oncology Disease Site Group. Malignant extradural spinal cord compression: diagnosis and management. Evidence summary report #9-9. Cancer Care Ontario. www.cancercare.on.ca/pdf/pebc9-9esf.pdf.

Maranzano E, Latini P, Beneventi S, et al. 1996. Radiotherapy without steroids in selected metastatic spinal cord compression patients: a phase II trial. *J Clin Oncol* 19:179–183.

Patchell R, Tibbs PA, Regine WF, et al. 2003. A randomized trial of direct decompressive surgical resection in the treatment of spinal cord compression caused by metastasis (abstr #2). *Proc Am Soc Clin Oncol* 22:1.

Robertson CL, Marques CB, Gralla RJ, Rittenberg CN. 1997. Documenting the rapidity of pain relief and palliation of other lung cancer symptoms with the use of dexamethasone. *Proc Am Soc Clin Oncol* 16:80a.

Schiff D. 2003. Spinal cord compression. Neurol Clin 21:67–86.

Sorensen S, Helweg-Larsen S, Mouridsen H, et al. 1994. Effect of high dose dexamethasone in carcinomatous metastatic spinal cord compression treated with radiotherapy: a randomised trial. *Eur J Cancer* 1:22–27.

Watanabe S, Bruera E. 1994. Corticosteroids as adjuvant analgesics. *J Pain Symptom Manage* 9:442–445.

Whitley RJ, Weiss H, Gnann JW, et al., and the National Institute of Allergy and Infectious Diseases Collaborative Antiviral Study Group. 1996. Acyclovir with and without prednisone for the treatment of herpes zoster. *Ann Intern Med* 125:376–383.

Wood MJ, Johnson RW, McKendrick MW, et al. 1994. A randomized trial of acyclovir for 7 days or 21 days with and without prednisone for treatment of acute herpes zoster. *N Engl J Med* 330:896–900.

Anticonvulsants

Backonja M, Glanzman RL. 2003. Gabapentin dosing for neuropathic pain: evidence from randomized, placebo-controlled clinical trials. *Clin Ther* 25:81–104.

Berde CB. 1997. New and old anticonvulsants for management of pain. *IASP Newsletter* Jan–Feb.

Farrar JT, Portenoy RK. 2001. Neuropathic cancer pain: the role of adjuvant analgesics. *Oncology* 15:1435–1442, 1445.

Rowbotham M, Harden N, Stacey B, et al. 1998. Gabapentin for the treatment of postherpetic neuralgia: a randomized, controlled trial. *JAMA* 280:1837–1842.

Benzodiazepines

Fernandez F, Adams F, Holmes VF. 1987. Analgesic effect of alprazolam in patients with chronic, organic pain of malignant origin. *J Clin Psychopharmacol* 3:167–169.

Scavone JM, Greenblatt DJ, Goddard JE, et al. 1992. The pharmacokinetics and pharmacodynamics of sublingual and oral alprazolam in the post-prandial state. *Eur J Clin Pharm* 42:439–443.

Baclofen

Fromm GH, Terrence CF, Chattha AS. 1984. Baclofen in the treatment of trigeminal neuralgia: double-blind study and long-term follow-up. *Ann Neurol* 15:240–244.

Ketamine

Bell RF, Eccleston C, Kalso E. 2003. Ketamine as adjuvant to opioids for cancer pain: a qualitative systematic review. *J Pain Symptom Manage* 26:867–875.

Fine PG. 1999. Low-dose ketamine in the management of opioid resistant terminal cancer pain. *J Pain Symptom Manage* 17:296–300.

Fine PG. 2003. Ketamine: from anesthesia to palliative care. *AAHPM Bull* 3:1, 6.

Fitzgibbon EJ, Hall P, Schroder C, et al. 2002. Low dose ketamine as an analgesic adjuvant in difficult pain syndromes: a strategy of conversion from parenteral to oral ketamine. *J Pain Symptom Manage* 23:165–170.

Mercadante S, Arouri E, Tirelli W, Casuccio A. 2000. Analgesic effect of intravenous ketamine in cancer patients on morphine therapy: a randomized, controlled, double-blind, crossover, double dose study. *J Pain Symptom Manage* 4:246–251.

Yang C-Y, Wong C-S, Chang J-Y. 1996. Intrathecal ketamine reduces morphine requirements in patients with terminal cancer pain. *Can J Anaesth* 43:379–383.

ADJUVANTS FOR BONE PAIN

External Beam Radiation and Radiopharmaceuticals

Janjan NA. 2001. Bone metastases: approaches to management. *Semin Oncol* 28(suppl 11):28–34.

Kan MK. 1995. Bone pain palliation in metastatic cancer with Sr-89. *Cancer Nurs* 18:286–291.

McCready VR, O'Sullivan JM. 2002. Future directions for unsealed source radionuclide therapy for bone metastases. *Eur J Nucl Med Mol Imaging* 29:1271–1275.

McEwan AJB. 1997. Unsealed source therapy of painful bone metastases: an update. *Semin Nucl Med* 27:165–182.

Palmedo H, Guhlke S, Bender H, et al. 2000. Dose escalation study with rhenium-188 HEDP in prostate cancer patients with osseous metastases. *Eur J Nucl Med* 27:123–130.

Palmedo H, Manka-Waluch A, Albers P, et al. 2003. Repeated bone-targeted therapy for hormone-refractory prostate carcinoma: randomized phase II trial with the new, high-energy radiopharmaceutical rhenium-188 hydroxyethylidenediphosphonate. *J Clin Oncol* 21:2869–2875.

Porter AT, McEwan AJB, Powe JE, et al. 1993. Results of a randomized phase III trial to evaluate the efficacy of strontium-89 adjuvant to local field external beam irradiation in the management of endocrine resistant metastatic prostatic cancer. *Int J Radiat Oncol Biol Phys* 25:805–813.

Resche I, Chatal J-F, Pecking A, et al. 1997. A dose-controlled study of 153Sm-ethylenediaminetetramethylene phosphonate (EDTMP) in the treatment of patients with painful bone metastases. *Eur J Cancer* 133:1583–1591.

Serafini AN, Houston SJ, Resche I, et al. 1998. Palliation of pain associated with metastatic bone cancer using samarium-153 lexidronam: a double-blind placebo-controlled trial. *J Clin Oncol* 16:1574–1581.

Biphosphonates

Berenson JR, Lichtenstein A, Porter L, et al. 1998. Long-term pamidronate treatment of advanced multiple myeloma patients reduces skeletal events. *J Clin Oncol* 16:593–602.

Hortobagyi GN, Theriault RL, Lipton A, et al. 1998. Efficacy of longterm prevention of skeletal complications of metastatic breast cancer with pamidronate. *J Clin Oncol* 16:2038–2044.

Johnson KB, Gable P, Kaime EM, et al. 2003. Significant deterioration in renal function with the new bisphosphonate, zoledronic acid. *Proc ASCO* 22:738.

Kloth DD, McDermott RS, Rogatko A, Langer CJ. 2003. Impact of zolendronic acid on renal function in patients with cancer: is constant monitoring necessary? *Proc ASCO* 22:755a.

Rosen LS, Gordon O, Tchekmedyian WS, et al. 2004. Long-term efficacy and safety of zoledronic acid in the treatment of skeletal matastases in patients with non-small cell lung carcinoma and other solid tumors: a randomized, Phase II double-blind placebo-controlled trial. *Cancer* 100:2613–2621.

Reitsma DJ. 1998. Efficacy of longterm prevention of skeletal complications of metastatic breast cancer with pamidronate. *J Clin Oncol* 16:2038–2044.

Saad F, Gleason DM, Murray R, et al. 2002. A randomized, placebo-controlled trial of zoledronic acid in patients with hormone-refractory metastatic prostate carcinoma. *J Natl Cancer Inst* 94:58–68.

Kyphoplasty/Vertebroplasty

Jensen ME, Kallmes DK. 2002. Percutaneous vertebroplasty in the treatment of malignant spinal disease. *Cancer J* 8:194–206.

Papaioannou A, Watts NB, Kendler DL, et al. 2002. Diagnosis and management of vertebral fractures in elderly adults. *Am J Med* 113:220–228.

Watts NB, Harris ST, Genant HK. 2001. Treatment of painful osteoporotic vertebral fractures with percutaneous vertebroplasty or kyphoplasty. *Osteoporos Int* 12:429–437.

Zoarski GH, Snow P, Olan WJ, et al. 2002. Percutaneous vertebroplasty for osteoporotic compression fractures: quantitative prospective evaluation of long-term outcomes. *J Vasc Interv Radiol* 13:139–148.

Radiofrequency Ablation

Goetz MP, Callstrom MR, Charboneau JW, et al. 2004. Percutaneous image-guided radiofrequency ablation of painful metastases involving bone: a multicenter study. *J Clin Oncol* 122:300–306.

Patti JW, Neeman Z, Wood BJ. 2002. Radiofrequency ablation for cancer-associated pain. *J Pain* 3:471–473.

NEUROLEPTICS

Beaver WT, et al. 1966. A comparison of the analgesic effect of methotrimeprazine and morphine in patients with cancer. *Clin Pharm Ther* 7:436.

ANESTHETIC METHODS

TOPICAL AGENTS

Argoff CE. 2003. Targeted topical peripheral analgesics in the management of pain. *Curr Pain Headache Rep* 7:34–38.

EMLA

Rice LJ, Cravero J. 1994. Relieving the pain and anxiety of needle injections—experience with EMLA® cream (lidocaine 2.5 percent and prilocaine 2.5 percent) dermal anesthetic. *Today's Ther Trends* 11:175–185.

Stow PJ, Glynn CJ, Minor B. 1989. EMLA cream in the treatment of post-herpetic neuralgia: efficacy and pharmacokinetic profile. *Pain* 39:301–305.

Lidocaine

Galer BS, Jensen MP, Ma T, et al. 2002. The lidocaine patch 5% effectively treats all neuropathic pain qualities: results of a randomized, double-blind, vehicle-controlled, 3-week efficacy study with use of the neuropathic pain scale. *Clin J Pain* 18:297–301.

Gammaitoni AR, Davis MW. 2002. Pharmacokinetics and tolerability of lidocaine 5% patch with extended dosing. *Ann Pharmacother* 36:236–240.

Katz NP, Gammaitoni AR, Davis MW, et al. 2002. Lidocaine patch 5% reduces pain intensity and interference with quality of life in patients with postherpetic neuralgia: an effectiveness trial. *Pain Med* 3:1–10.

Rowbotham MC, Davies PS, Fields HL. 1995. Topical lidocaine gel relieves postherpetic neuralgia. *Ann Neurol* 37:246–253.

Capsaicin

Ellison N, Loprinzi CL, Kugler J, et al. 1997. Phase III placebo-controlled trial of capsaicin cream in the management of surgical neuropathic pain in cancer patients. *J Clin Oncol* 15:2974–2980.

Watson CPN, Evans RJ, Watt VR. 1988. Postherpetic neuralgia and topical capsaicin. *Pain* 33:333–340.

Watson CPN, Evans RJ, Watt VR. 1989. The post-mastectomy pain syndrome and the effect of topical capsaicin. *Pain* 38:177–186.

Watson CPN, Tyler KL, Bickers DR, et al. 1993. A randomized vehicle-controlled trial of topical capsaicin in the treatment of post-herpetic neuralgia. *Clin Ther* 15:510–526.

ORAL ANESTHETICS

Glazer S, Portenoy RK. 1991. Systemic local anesthetics in pain control. *J Pain Symptom Manage* 6:30–39.

PARENTERAL ANESTHETICS

Ferrini R. 2000. Parenteral lidocaine for severe intractable pain in six hospice patients continued at home. *J Palliat Med* 3:193–200.

Mao J, Chen LL. 2000. Systemic lidocaine for neuropathic pain relief. *Pain* 87:7–17.

Rowbotham MC, Reisner-Keller LA, Fields HL. 1991. Both intravenous lidocaine and morphine reduce the pain of postherpetic neuralgia. *Neurology* 41:1024–1028.

NEURAL BLOCKADE AND NEUROABLATION

Backonja M-M. 1994. Local anesthetics as adjuvant analgesics. *J Pain Symptom Manage* 9:491–499.

Ferrante FM, Bedder M, Caplan RA, et al. 1996. Practice Guidelines for Cancer Pain Management: a report by the American Society of Anesthesiologists' Task Force on Pain Management, Cancer Pain Section. *Anesthesiology* 84:1243–1257.

Slatkin NE, Rhiner M. 2003. Phenol saddle blocks for intractable pain at the end of life: report of four cases and literature review. *Am J Hospice Palliat Care* 20:62–66.

Swarm RA, Karanikolas M, Cousins MJ. 2004. Anaesthetic techniques for pain control. In *Oxford Textbook of Palliative Medicine*, 3rd ed, Doyle D, Hanks G, Cherny N, Calman K (eds). Oxford: Oxford University Press.

Postherpetic Neuralgia
Alper B, Lewis PR. 2002. Treatment of postherpetic neuralgia: a systemic review of the literature. *J Fam Pract* 51:121–128.
Rowbotham M, Harden N, Stacey B, et al. 1998. Gabapentin for the treatment of postherpetic neuralgia: a randomized controlled trial. *JAMA* 280:1837–1842.

RELIEVING PAIN IN OLDER PERSONS
AGS Panel on Persistent Pain in Older Persons. 2002. The management of persistent pain in older persons. *J Am Geriatr Soc* 50:S205–224.
Barsky AJ, Hochstrasser B, Coles NA, et al. 1990. Silent myocardial ischemia: is the person or the event silent? *JAMA* 264:1132–1135.
Bernabei R, Gambassi G, Lapane K, et al., for the SAGE Study Group. 1998. Management of pain in elderly patients with cancer. *JAMA* 279:1877–1882.
Ferrell BA, Ferrell BR, Rivera L. 1995. Pain in cognitively impaired nursing home patients. *J Pain Symptom Manage* 10:591–598.
Ferrell BR, Ferrell BA (eds). 1996. *Pain in the Elderly.* Seattle: International Association for the Study of Pain Press.
Forman WB. 1996. Opioid analgesic drugs in the elderly. *Clin Geriatr Med* 12:489–500.
Gloth FM. 2001. Pain management in older adults: prevention and treatment. *J Am Geriatr Soc* 49:188–199.
Kerr KA, Mobily PR. 1993. Comparison of selected pain assessment tools for use with the elderly. *Appl Nurs Res* 6:39–46.
Popp B, Portenoy RK. 1996. Management of chronic pain in the elderly: pharmacology of opioids and other analgesic drugs. In *Pain in the Elderly,* Ferrell BR, Ferrell BA (eds). Seattle: International Association for the Study of Pain Press.
Stein WM. 1996. Cancer pain in the elderly. In *Pain in the Elderly,* Ferrell BR, Ferrell BA (eds). Seattle: International Association for the Study of Pain Press.
Stein WM, Miech RP. 1993. Cancer pain in the elderly hospice patient. *J Pain Symptom Manage* 8:474–482.
Von Strauss EM, Viitanen D, De Ronchi D, et al. 1999. Aging and the occurrence of dementia. *Arch Neurol* 56:587–592.
Warden V, Hurley AC, Volicer L. 2003. Development and psychometric evaluation of the pain assessment in advanced dementia (PAINAD) scale. *J Am Med Dir Assoc* 4:9–15.

RELIEVING PAIN IN SUBSTANCE ABUSERS
Gonzales GR, Coyle N. 1992. Treatment of cancer pain in a former opioid abuser: fears of the patient and staff and their influence on care. *J Pain Symptom Manage* 7:246–249.
Wesson DR, Ling W, Smith DE. 1993. Prescription of opioids for treatment of pain in patients with addictive disease. *J Pain Symptom Manage* 8:289–296.

COMMON CLINICAL SITUATIONS: RAPIDLY RELIEVING EXCRUCIATING PAIN
Hagen NA, Elwood T, Ernst S. 1997. Cancer pain emergencies: a protocol for management. *J Pain Symptom Manage* 14:45–50.

Lichter I. 1994. Accelerated titration of morphine for rapid relief of cancer pain. *N Z Med J* 107:488–490.

Mercadante S, Villari P, Ferrera P, et al. 2002. Rapid titration with intravenous morphines for severe cancer pain and immediate oral conversion. *Cancer* 95:203–208.

Soares LGL, Martins M, Uchoa R. 2003. Intravenous fentanyl for cancer pain: a "fast titration" protocol for the emergency room. *J Pain Symptom Manage* 26:876–881.

Nonpharmacologic Strategies for Pain and Symptom Management

Although they do not replace drug therapies, nonpharmacologic techniques are valuable adjuncts and should be incorporated into pain and symptom management strategies. These techniques, though generally "low-tech," involve skilled practitioners: acupuncturists; yoga teachers;

therapists skilled in massage or physical, occupational, speech, music, and art therapies; social workers, psychiatrists, and psychologists skilled in the other cognitive therapies; and spiritual counselors. Because many of the techniques can be performed by properly trained laypersons, the practitioner often serves both as therapist and as teacher, instructing patients or family members in how they can perform techniques by themselves.

Oncologists often are unaware of the utility of nonpharmacologic therapies for cancer patients and rarely prescribe them. One study, for example, found that fewer than 2 percent of cancer patients were receiving any form of nonpharmacologic therapy (Ferrell et al. 1991). Many primary care physicians and their patients, however, are aware of these techniques. In one survey, patients reported that 50 percent of referrals to physicians who were alternative medicine practitioners were either given or approved by their primary care physicians. In a telephone survey, 34 percent of Americans said they had visited such a practitioner (Eisenberg et al. 1993). Cancer patients, however, may be reluctant to volunteer that they have adopted these unorthodox practices for fear that their physician will ridicule either the practices or them.

Clinicians who select appropriate nonpharmacologic therapies as adjuncts can open an important line of communication with patients who either are using or are considering using these treatments. At a minimum, patients will be much more likely to tell us which of these unorthodox agents or practices they have adopted.

The National Center for Complementary and Alternative Medicine has defined five domains of these therapies. The domains are (1) alternative medical systems, (2) manipulative and body-based methods, (3) mind-body interventions, (4) biologically based therapies, and (5) energy therapies. Alternative medical systems include philosophies and practices that are completely independent of the usual medical approach. Homeopathic, naturopathic, Ayurvedic, and Native American medicine are examples of alternative medical systems. Manipulative and body-based methods include chiropractic, osteopathy, and massage. Among the mind-body interventions are education, cognitive and behavioral interventions, and art and music therapy. Biologically based treatments include special diets, such as the Atkins or Ornish diets; herbal treatments; megadose vitamin therapy; or use of particular substances not proven effective by conventional medical studies, such as laetrile. Energy therapies focus on energy fields within the body (biofield therapies) or outside the body (electromagnetic fields). Qi gong, Therapeutic Touch, Reiki, and healing touch are examples of these therapies.

In this chapter, I review the nonpharmacologic techniques that I consider have the most evidence supporting their effectiveness in relieving pain and other sources of distress in cancer patients: selected alternative medical systems (acupuncture/acupressure and yoga), selected manipulative and body-based methods, and mind-body interventions. Readers interested in a more comprehensive discussion of the domains not reviewed here can refer to the work of Dr. Barrie Cassileth (1998; Cassileth and Chapman 1996).

ALTERNATIVE MEDICAL SYSTEMS

Alternative medical systems embrace a theory of what promotes health of the mind, body, and spirit, what causes illness, and how health and balance can be regained, which differs from that of standard medical practice.

ACUPUNCTURE/ACUPRESSURE/AURICULOTHERAPY

Acupuncture is part of classic Chinese medicine in which, as described by Helms,*

> The language . . . reflects nature and agrarian village metaphors and describes a philosophy of man functioning harmoniously within an orderly universe. The models of health, disease, and treatment are presented in terms of patients' harmony or disharmony within this larger order, and involve their responses to external extremes of wind, heat, damp, dryness, and cold, as well as to internal extremes of anger, excitement, worry, sadness, and fear. Illnesses likewise are described and defined poetically, by divisions of the yin and yang polar opposites (interior or exterior, cold or hot, deficient or excessive), by descriptors attached to elemental qualities (wood, fire, earth, metal,

---

*From Joseph M. Helms, An overview of medical acupuncture, www.medicalacupuncture.org, modified from a chapter in *Essentials of Complementary and Alternative Medicine*, Jonas WB, Levin JS (eds), Baltimore: Lippincott Williams & Wilkins, in press; used with permission from Dr. Helms.

and water), and by the functional influences traditionally associated with each of the internal organs.

Acupuncture anatomy is a multilayered, interconnecting network of channels that establishes an interface between an individual's internal and external environments, permitting energy to move through the muscles and the various organs.

In acupuncture, needles are inserted beneath the skin to stimulate peripheral nerves to provide pain relief. The practitioner uses his or her knowledge of acupuncture meridian points, extra-meridian odd points, and new points to choose the appropriate areas of the skin to stimulate, either mechanically or electrically. Acupuncture alters the pain experiences of healthy volunteers tested in a variety of pain-inducing experiments (e.g., tooth pain). In general, from fifteen to forty minutes after stimulation, pain relief becomes apparent and often lasts for up to several days. Unfortunately, less information is available about its use in cancer patients.

It is known that pain relief through acupuncture requires peripheral nerve stimulation, because anesthetizing the skin into which the acupuncture needle is inserted abolishes the effect. The spinal cord is also involved in a segmental, bilateral fashion, as was demonstrated by experiments with patients who were hemiplegic or paraplegic.

The delay in the onset of pain relief after stimulation suggests that inhibitory signals descending from the central nervous system are mediating the pain relief. The patient's hypnotic susceptibility may also be a factor—those who are not at all susceptible to hypnosis do not get pain relief from acupuncture. Endogenous endorphin release may contribute as well (Thompson and Filshie 1997).

It is difficult to comment on the efficacy of *real* versus *sham* acupuncture (in which the needles do not pierce the skin), because of the nature of the currently available studies. The existence of extra-meridian and new points makes choosing placebo sites difficult. In addition, these studies did not enroll a sufficient number of patients to determine whether there was a real difference in pain response between the two procedures. This does not mean that acupuncture is ineffective, just that its efficacy has not yet been satisfactorily demonstrated. I would not discourage a patient with musculoskeletal or nerve pain from trying acupuncture.

Dr. Weiger and her colleagues reviewed the evidence from one or more small, randomized, controlled trials that looked at the use of acupuncture (Weiger et al. 2002). The evidence supports the use of acupuncture for chemotherapy-related nausea and vomiting, and for dyspnea due to bronchospasm or chronic obstructive pulmonary disease (Cassileth and Shulman 2004). Acupuncture for pain is less well studied, but Weiger believes it can be recommended. According to the American Association of Medical Acupuncture, the World Health Organization, in its listing of disorders for which acupuncture is effective, includes spasm of the esophagus and cardia, hiccups, constipation, and paralytic ileus.

Acupressure involves stimulating the same acupuncture points, but pressure is used instead of needles to relieve pain (e.g., headache, backache). Acupressure may have a role in reducing nausea associated with pregnancy, motion sickness, or surgery, but the data are conflicting and there are no reliable studies in cancer patients with chronic nausea.

Auriculotherapy (electrical stimulation of the outer ear), however, has not been shown in rigorously controlled trials to relieve chronic pain either from nerve injury or from low back or musculoskeletal pain syndromes. I cannot recommend its use to relieve pain in cancer patients.

Yoga

Yoga is "a discipline that nurtures the union of body, mind and spirit and emphasizes that as human beings, we are part of a larger whole and not just isolated individuals. One of the underlying beliefs of yoga is that there is more right with us than wrong with us, and that despite experiences of illness or disease, we are more than our illness or disease" (Ott 2002). Of the eight major branches of yoga, hatha yoga is the most often used in the medical context. The practice of hatha yoga has been shown to have significant effects in increasing strength and flexibility, normalizing heart rate and blood pressure and depth and pace of breathing, and increasing metabolic rate. It has been shown to improve the pain of patients with osteoarthritis and carpal tunnel syndrome. Breathing using yoga techniques substantially reduces the chemoreflex response to hypoxia so that patients with congestive heart failure can improve their exercise tolerance (Raub 2002).

The practice of hatha yoga usually "includes a combination of asanas (physical postures), pranayama (breathing), chanting (working with sound), shavasana (relaxation), and meditation" (Ott 2002). Patients who are bedridden can practice yoga using specially modified asanas. In fact, the effects on anxiety, strength, flexibility, and breathing can help bedridden patients become sufficiently reconditioned to graduate to more vigorous physical therapy. Patients who are anxious about their medical procedures or the limitations, losses, and other changes induced by their disease or its treatment can benefit greatly from yoga training and practice. They can be taught how to regain control of situations that seem out of their control, and to increase their self-esteem and their endurance.

Yoga practice for practitioners and families has similar benefits. Being present to suffering is one of the hardest things I have ever had to do. While I do not yet practice yoga daily, the techniques taught to me by Mary Jane Ott, M.N., M.A., R.N.C.S., a member of our pain and palliative care team, have made it possible for me to find the equanimity I need. She teaches our team many ways to use the breath to steady ourselves before or during clinical encounters, and to deal with suffering by breathing in the suffering and breathing out compassion. She has also taught us yoga postures we can do at our desks, or while waiting for elevators, that help decrease stress and increase our energy.

MANIPULATIVE AND BODY-BASED METHODS

Manipulative and body-based methods for relief of pain and other causes of distress include a variety of cutaneous interventions, massage and vibration, transcutaneous nerve stimulation, and positioning and exercise. All these therapies can be given in the patient's home by family members or by therapists. They can add significantly to any pharmacology-based regimen.

CUTANEOUS INTERVENTIONS
Cutaneous interventions are of particular value when the pain is localized, when muscle tension or guarding is apparent, or when the pa-

---

MANIPULATIVE AND BODY-BASED METHODS
- Cutaneous interventions
- Massage and vibration
- Transcutaneous electrical nerve stimulation (TENS)
- Positioning and exercise

tient is waiting for a diagnostic procedure, for treatment, or for a pain medicine to take effect. Cold and warmth are routinely used in benign orthopedic and arthritic conditions. They are also very effective for cancer pain, especially that caused by bony metastases or nerve involvement.

Cold has been noted to be particularly helpful for patients suffering from skeletal muscle spasm induced by nerve injury. It interrupts the cycle of nerve ischemia caused by muscle spasms and decreases itching and hyperesthesia. Cold also seems to help patients with inflamed joints, possibly by creating numbness, but it may also decrease the release of chemical mediators of pain.

Cold wraps, gel packs, ice bags, and menthol are common ways of delivering cold. Cold massage can be done by filling a small paper cup with water, freezing it, and then massaging the painful area with the ice that forms in the cup. The mechanism of the pain relief induced by the ice massage is thought to be "hyperstimulation analgesia" or "counter-irritation." According to this theory, a mildly painful stimulus paradoxically relieves severe pain by bombarding the spinal relay system with inconsequential messages that block the transmission of the more severe pain signal. You may have experienced the effect of counter-irritation if, after getting an insect bite, rather than scratch the bite itself you've slapped or scratched the skin an inch or so away from the bite. In most cases, the itch disappears.

Patients usually tolerate cold well, but rarely they may develop a hypersensitivity syndrome that clinically resembles cold urticaria. Cold should not be used for analgesia in patients with peripheral vascular disease or for the rare patient with cryoglobulinemia or cold agglutinin disease.

Dry or moist heat can be delivered using a heating pad, a tub full of water, a hot water bottle, plastic wrap, or a commercial hot wrap, which maximizes patient mobility. To avoid burning the skin, sessions should not last more than twenty minutes. Patients should be cautioned against using a menthol product with heat because this, too, may cause the skin to burn.

Heat is contraindicated in areas where the patient is anesthetic and in areas with inadequate vascular supply, such as an extremity in a patient with atherosclerotic or diabetic vascular insufficiency. Tissue necrosis can result from the increased metabolic demands in the heated area. Heat is also contraindicated for patients with bleeding disorders, which can be exacerbated by the increase in blood flow. Short-wave diathermy cannot be used near a metal implant, including metal-containing intrauterine devices and cardiac pacemakers, or near contact lenses, because serious burns may result.

Cold and heat can be used to prevent the incident type of breakthrough pain. Some patients find alternating the two treatments to be soothing, while others find it most helpful to combine them with any of the imaging and relaxation techniques or the other cutaneous techniques summarized below.

MASSAGE AND VIBRATION

Massage, like the relaxation techniques described below, also slows heart and respiratory rates, lowers blood pressure, and even lessens pain and anxiety. And it can deliver a nonverbal message of affection and support.

Massage is specifically helpful for patients with muscle spasm resulting from tension or nerve injury. It is also generally useful for anxious patients, those who are limited in their ability to communicate, or those who can benefit from the closeness such touch can offer. Some patients, however, find it too personal or see it as an invitation to more intimacy than the person giving the massage intends.

Massage can include stroking, compression, percussion, or vibration and can be done with the hands, with ice, or with vibration, with or without added heat (see below). Massage should not be offered to patients with coagulation abnormalities or thrombophlebitis, whom it might harm. Nurses, physical therapists, and massage therapists can all do massage and teach caregivers of bed-bound patients the basic techniques.

Vibration, either from the hands or from an electrically powered device, is also useful for pain relief. It facilitates muscle relaxation and, possibly by counter-irritation (i.e., stimulating large-diameter fibers), may also decrease sensation in the painful area. It is indicated for the same patients who can benefit from massage, but can also help patients with neuropathic or phantom limb pain or can substitute for the TENS machine (see below). A variety of devices are available, offering a number of settings and additional heat. The patient should work with the therapist to determine the optimal setting and duration of treatment.

Dr. Weiger and her colleagues have reviewed the evidence supporting the use of massage techniques to relieve pain or other symptoms (Weiger et al. 2002). Massage, in the absence of specific contraindications, can be recommended for anxiety, pain, lymphedema, and nausea related to autologous bone marrow transplantation. Evidence for its efficacy in each of these areas comes from one or more small, randomized controlled trials.

Transcutaneous Electrical Nerve Stimulation (TENS)

TENS has documented utility in several nonmalignant pain syndromes, but its effectiveness has not been demonstrated in patients with cancer pain. The TENS machines are portable battery-operated stimulators that activate the large-diameter fibers of peripheral nerves, thereby diminishing transmission of the pain signal.

The machines are attached to small electrodes that are placed on the skin over the nerve that is thought to be sending the pain signal, and a special current is then applied. When low-intensity, low-frequency current is applied, the patient's original pain is replaced by a feeling of numbness or of "pins and needles." If higher-intensity, low-frequency (acupuncture-like) current is applied, muscle contraction may occur.

TENS machines are especially helpful for patients with *dermatomal* pain such as that of post-herpetic neuralgia, fractured ribs, diabetic neuropathy, or radiculopathy due to disk disease or spinal cord compression. There have also been reports of its utility in post-mastectomy pain and phantom limb pain. It may take as long as a week of use for the maximal pain relief to be achieved, and the relief provided by the TENS machine usually lasts no more than two or three months.

TENS units cannot be used for patients who have demand pacemakers, and electrodes cannot be placed over the eye, near the carotid sinus, or over metal implants (doing so may cause short circuits). TENS should be used with caution in emotionally disturbed, mentally handicapped, or senile patients, or for patients with lymphedema, which has been reported to worsen with the use of TENS. In routine use, the most common complication, occurring in 10 percent of patients, is allergic dermatitis from the tape used to secure the electrodes. If the conducting gel is used improperly, electrical skin burns can also occur.

Properly trained and experienced physiatrists and physical therapists are key to the successful use of TENS machines. They choose the appropriate stimulator and electrodes, place the electrodes on the skin, and pick the correct electrical wave form and intensity. They also educate the patient and the family about the procedures required, as well as the potential usefulness and limitations of the machines.

POSITIONING AND EXERCISE

Physiatrists and occupational therapists should be consulted for planning the care of patients who would benefit from proper positioning and exercise. They are familiar with the proper equipment (beds, wheelchairs, shower/bath assisting devices, toilets), and they can teach positioning, range-of-motion exercises, energy conservation techniques, and safe techniques for transferring patients from beds to chairs. For those with only one arm, the therapist can demonstrate how to dress, undress, and use assisting devices with only one hand.

POSITIONING.   Cancer patients with pain may lose the spontaneous pain-relieving movements that healthy people use to minimize tissue ischemia. To relieve their pain and minimize complications such as frozen joints, decubitus ulcers, or contractures, nurses, aides, therapists, or family members need to help patients change their position. The goal is to achieve a "loose-packed" position that minimizes stress on joints. Recommended joint flexion angles are 45° at the elbow and 30° at the hip, and the hip should also be abducted 20°. This does not need to be exact, however; patients can be helped into any position that is comfortable for them.

Custom-made cushions or pillows for beds or chairs, as well as cradles to keep bedclothes off the legs, can be very helpful. Electric beds with specially designed mattresses that distribute the patient's weight uniformly are also important. For selected patients, the physical or occupational therapist may also recommend splints, orthotics, or support devices.

Dyspnea and discomfort in the chest due to excessive secretions can be ameliorated by a combination of chest physical therapy, teaching correct coughing techniques, correctly positioning the patient, and teaching techniques that relax the head, neck, shoulder girdle, and thorax (see below).

EXERCISE.   Carefully constructed exercise plans can maximize patient mobility, minimize pain, and help patients function independently for as long as possible. Exercise is especially important for patients with limited joint motion due to pain, paraparesis, or paraplegia to prevent even more loss of function. The exercise can be done with or without assistance from a therapist, aide, or trained family member. Range-of-motion exercises can be done *for* the patient by one of these caregivers.

Contractures, deformities, and pressure sores are painful conditions that can often be prevented by such exercise regimens. Canes, walkers, manual or electric wheelchairs, chairs in which the seat lifts the patient to a standing position, and other assistance devices should be used as needed to maintain as much mobility as possible.

Severe lymphedema often responds to an aggressive daily regimen of massage, compression bandages, and exercise, after which the now smaller limb can be fitted with an elastic compression stocking or glove.

MIND-BODY INTERVENTIONS

Pain and psychological distress are, ultimately, cognitive experiences. The neospinothalamic and paleospinothalamic pathways carry pain stimuli from the periphery to the thalamus, and from there the pain signal is transmitted to numerous cortical projections. When the cortex has been severely damaged (e.g., by prolonged hypoxia), there are reflex reactions to noxious stimuli but no experience of pain.

The cortex is also intimately involved in modifying the transmission of those ascending pain signals. It has extensive input into descending neural pathways that carry inhibitory messages via the dorsolateral funiculus to the dorsal horn entry zones in the spinal cord, where they in-

---

MIND-BODY INTERVENTIONS
- Education and reassurance
- Diversion of attention
- Relaxation and breathing
- Mindfulness meditation
- Hypnosis
- Biofeedback
- Music therapy
- Art therapy
- Counseling

hibit transmission of an ascending pain stimulus. Thus, if we can change the way a patient views his disease or his pain, we may be able to lessen his suffering without eliminating the noxious stimulus. Similarly, we can use cognitive techniques to modify nausea, dyspnea, and insomnia.

Something as simple as a room with a view, for example, has been shown to diminish postoperative suffering and decrease the number of days spent in the hospital (Ulrich 1984). This was demonstrated some years ago in a study that compared the experiences of cholecystectomy patients housed in rooms with two different types of views: a view of a brick wall or of a stand of trees. The rooms were otherwise identical.

Those with the wall view did much worse than those with the tree view. They went home one day later, and nurses recorded four times as many negative comments about these patients (e.g., "upset and crying," "needs much encouragement"). In addition, during the second to fifth postoperative days, those with the wall view asked for significantly more analgesic doses, and the type of analgesic they took was most often an opioid. Those with the tree view most often took aspirin or acetaminophen.

What patients were looking at significantly affected their recovery. A tree view led to less pain and an earlier discharge. To produce the mental equivalent of a tree view for my cancer patients, I use the variety of mind-body interventions described below. With these adjunctive techniques, I can eliminate a number of sources of distress not amenable to opioids. And, in addition, I can diminish the pain intensity of those who do require opioids, lessen their need for pain medication, and thereby minimize the side effects they experience.

EDUCATION AND REASSURANCE

A diagnosis of cancer carries the risk of transforming a *person* into a *patient*. Physicians who are patients are at least at home in the hospital setting and are aware of the procedures they will have to undergo during their cancer staging and treatment. Therefore, though they retain their anxiety about their prognosis and the effects of the treatment, they will at least be in familiar surroundings.

People who are not physicians or health care workers enter an alien environment when they become patients, and they have no idea what to expect. They do not know what tests will be ordered, or why, or what those tests will entail. Education and reassurance can be very helpful in ameliorating their anxiety.

> **PRACTICE POINTS: PREPARING PATIENTS FOR PROCEDURES**
> - Explain which tests are planned and why they are important.
> - Describe what the procedure will be like, including elements from as many senses as possible (sight, smell, sound, feeling, taste).
> - If surgery is planned, rehearse the major events the patient will experience while awake.
> - Anticipate and correct common misunderstandings about test results.

When, for example, you send patients for their first CT scan, MRI, echocardiogram, or intravenous pyelogram (IVP), you might take a few minutes to explain the procedure to them. It is important to include as many senses as possible in the description: what the room will look and smell like, what temperature it will be, what noises the machines will make, who will be there, and what will happen during the procedure.

To describe an IVP, you might say something like,

> *You'll be in a hospital gown on a gurney, waiting outside in a cold hall, and then you'll be wheeled into an even colder room. You'll lie on a table under the x-ray machine, and you'll have a small needle connected to plastic tubing in a vein in your arm. When they put the dye in the tubing to look at the kidneys, it will go into your bloodstream and you're likely to feel very warm and maybe even flushed. Don't worry, that's normal and will pass. There will be plenty of people there to help you, so let them know if you have any questions. You'll be awake the whole time.*

As the patient listens to this thorough description, you are giving him a chance to rehearse the procedure in his mind and raise any questions that occur to him. Later, as he actually goes through the procedure, he will become calmer and calmer as your predictions come true. Confident in his knowledge of what is coming next, he can relax.

Similarly, a rehearsal of a planned surgery is very helpful. In one study, two groups of patients who were to have the same surgery were given either just the usual pre-anesthesia evaluation or a rehearsal of what was planned for the next day, including how much pain they should expect and how they could deal with it (Egbert et al. 1964). The patients in the group that received the rehearsal needed less anesthesia and less pain medicine after the operation, and went home almost three days earlier than the patients in the other group.

In addition to rehearsing planned procedures, it is often useful to anticipate the possible findings and explain these to the patient, as well. If you don't, they are sure to come to their own, often incorrect, conclusions. Take, for example, a woman with a newly diagnosed breast cancer who has to undergo staging tests.

The Importance of Dispelling Misconceptions

Except for extensive osteoarthritis, my aunt Ruth had been very healthy all her life and rarely saw a physician outside the family setting (her brother, niece, and nephew were all doctors). When she was 75, she noticed a small breast lump and it proved to be cancerous. When I called, she told me she was scheduled for bone and CT scans to help plan her therapy. She was understandably apprehensive, but I was able to reassure her that this was all routine and that, at her age, it was likely that the cancer was still localized.

Luckily, as we were talking, I remembered her osteoarthritis, and I imagined what that would look like on a bone scan. So I said to her,

> Now Auntie Ruth, I need to explain about your bone scan. The scan can't tell the difference between cancer and arthritis in a bone. It will be abnormal wherever you have a bone that is arthritic, and, because you have so much arthritis, the scan is likely to light up like a Christmas tree. They will want to take an x-ray of everywhere that lights up. When that happens, remember what I told you and don't worry—it's not the cancer; it's your arthritis.

When I next called to see how she was doing, she said,

> You know, it went just as you said it would. After the scan, they came in and told me I would have to have several x-rays. I was very upset because I was sure the cancer had spread everywhere. Then I remembered what you told me—that everywhere I have arthritis would be abnormal on the scan. So I calmed down right away and felt much better.

As it turned out, all the abnormalities were due to her arthritis; her other test results were also negative and she has been in remission for ten years since her local therapy. I was able to prevent her distress by anticipating both the results of the bone scan and her reaction to them and then educating and reassuring her. She, in turn, was able to use what she had learned to deal with her initial fears.

Education can also lessen the intensity of pain, especially when a patient is misinterpreting its source. A patient of mine with lung cancer and liver metastases developed acute cholecystitis. He was usually rather stoic, but seemed extremely distressed, even between bouts of colicky pain. It seems that he had decided that the jaundice he had developed meant that his disease had progressed and that he was dying. Not only was he relieved when I told him that he had gallbladder disease, but his pain intensity dropped by a third and his distress by over a half, and he regained his usual coping skills.

Dr. Henry Beecher, an army surgeon in World War II, found that the degree of pain reported and the amount of analgesia required to alleviate pain correlated more with the setting and significance of the wound than with the extent of the injury. As an army surgeon, Dr. Beecher treated extensively wounded soldiers who had survived the assault on Anzio. He found that they requested minimal or no analgesia for their wounds (Beecher 1946). Later, in his civilian practice, he found that with injuries comparable to those sustained by the soldiers, his civilian patients required much more analgesia. For these civilians, the injuries meant disruption of their usual lives and routines, loss of income, and impaired functioning. For the soldiers, however, the injury had guaranteed a ticket home. The meaning of the pain had altered the intensity of the pain experience and changed the analgesic requirements (Beecher 1956).

Whenever possible educate patients, even if they don't directly ask, to diminish their fear and thereby decrease the intensity of the distressing stimulus.

Diversion of Attention

Distraction is a technique that can be used to decrease the pain and distress of cancer patients undergoing diagnostic procedures. If, for example, a patient is scheduled to have a breast biopsy under local anesthesia, you might suggest that she take along a tape player with headphones and listen to music or a book on tape during the procedure. The surgeon and anesthetist usually don't mind (the anesthetist will often be happy to change the tapes!), and the patient will be spared having to listen to the operating room chatter. Distraction techniques, including a head-mounted virtual reality device, can also help patients receiving chemotherapy (Schneider et al. 2004).

Similarly, patients should be encouraged to find activities at home or in their community that engage their attention and so distract them from their pain. Music (either listening to or playing an instrument), television, movies, card-playing, visitors, crafts, or interesting scenery can all be useful distractions.

RELAXATION AND BREATHING

Sometimes, however, the pain is too insistent for distraction to be effective, and a technique directed specifically at lowering the pain intensity is required. Relaxation and breathing techniques are designed to do just that. They can free muscles from tension so that they hurt less. Stress decreases and patients become more relaxed; they experience less pain and are better able to cope with any residual pain.

For patients with low levels of pain or stress, relaxation alone may be effective. For those with more intense pain, who usually require pharmacologic therapy, relaxation therapies can be very effective adjuvants. The best studied of these techniques are breathing modification and progressive muscle relaxation.

You probably are most familiar with the use of breathing techniques to control the pain of childbirth (e.g., the Lamaze method), but they are also very effective for patients experiencing other types of pain (see Sample Relaxation Exercise, below). Progressive muscle relaxation can be used by the vast majority of patients, but because of the need to tense certain muscles before they are relaxed, it should be avoided in the minority whose lesions make the muscle-tensing maneuvers too painful. It is often a component of a hypnotic trance induction (see below), but can also be helpful in itself. The therapist (e.g., a trained nurse or psychologist) or a trained family member helps the patient learn a sequence of muscle relaxation exercises, or a sequence of muscle tensing that is followed by muscle relaxing. There is a variety of regimens, each prescribing a different number of sessions each day. Each session can last from five to twenty minutes and can be repeated up to three times a day.

When the sequence is complete, the muscle tension has usually diminished markedly and the patient is usually much more comfortable. The patient's blood pressure, pulse, and respiratory rate decrease; peripheral vasodilatation increases; and concentration and susceptibility to suggestions made by the therapist increase. During the exercise, the patients are very still, remaining in the same position unless given permission to move "if needed" by the therapist; they are silent and seem oblivious to external surroundings (this is also what a person in a hypnotic trance looks like).

In short, they look relaxed, and their vital signs confirm that they are. And in this relaxed state, patients are more susceptible to suggestions made by the therapist about how to control their symptoms and how to feel better about themselves. The patients themselves report that, indeed, they feel much better in a number of ways: they feel more "in control," sleep better, are less nauseated, eat and drink more, and experience less pain and less anxiety. Comparable patients receiving the same psychological supportive therapy but not taught these techniques do not experience these benefits.

SAMPLE RELAXATION EXERCISE.   For each patient interested in learning progressive relaxation, I improvise a custom-made "script." Each script includes breathing modification, progressive relaxation, imagery, and suggestions that build self-esteem. If I have taught the patient to use images to decrease pain (see Hypnosis, below), I incorporate these into the script as well.

To create the most evocative imagery, I try to determine whether the patient has an aural, visual, or kinesthetic imagination. I also take a thorough travel history, noting which sites she liked and which she would rather avoid, and I record any allergies, fears, and phobias. I would not want to ask someone who can't swim to imagine she is sailing, or suggest to someone who is allergic to ragweed that she's walking in a field. That would hardly be conducive to relaxation!

Before I begin the relaxation exercise, I make sure the patient is comfortably positioned, in a quiet room with subdued lighting, if possible. Then I begin talking. Here is a sample script for a patient named Susan Harrison. In the script, the number of dots in each ellipsis indicates how long I pause before saying the next word. For example, . . . is a short pause, ... a longer one. I begin by directing her breathing, and then I time my words to her inhalations and exhalations:

> Susan . . I'd like you to close your eyes . . . that's right . . . Now take a deep
> breath in. . . . . . and out. . . . . . in . . . . . and out. . . . . . [I am breathing at the
> same rate, to model the behavior for her, taking longer with the exhalations.] And with each breath in . . . that's right . . . and out. . . . . [talking
> more slowly now] you can begin to feel more. . . . . . and more. . . . . . comfortable . . If at any time you need to move . . . to make yourself EVEN . .

MORE . . COMFORTABLE . . . you can do that. . . . The only voice . . you need to pay attention to . . is mine. . . . . No other sounds . . need disturb us. . . . And with each breath in . . . and out . . . . . . you're able to LET GO . . of more . . . and more [said on the inhale]. *. . . . . . tension* [said on the exhale] *. . . more . . . and more . . . of anything . . that might be on your mind . . . letting it* [said on the inhale] *. . . all out* [said on the exhale, in a lower-pitched voice].

Now I begin the progressive muscle relaxation, using imagery.

Maybe . . you'll find yourself . . on a beach in the mid-morning. . . . . or by a stream. . . . . or a small lake. . . . . You are walking along . . . at a comfortable pace . . . or lying on a soft patch of ground. . . . . The sun . . is gently warming . . the back of your neck. . . . . your shoulders. . . . . all the way down . . your arms. . . . . to the tips of your fingers. . . . . feeling warm . . . and COMFORTABLE. . . . . . . and the warmth . . is now spreading. . . . from the back of your neck. . . . ALL THE WAY DOWN [said in a lower voice] *your back. . . . . . to the bottom of your spine . . . down the back of your legs . . . and the front . . . to the tips of your toes. . . . . . the muscles of your neck . . shoulders . . arms . . back . . and legs. . . . unwinding. . . . . . . like a braid unwinds in the water. . . . . . more and more comfortable. . . . . . more and more loose . . . like a rag doll. . . . . . free. . . . . . . and loose. . . . . and. . . . FINE. . . . . Notice the feel of the soft . . warm . . breeze against your skin. . . . . . the smell of the air. . . . . . the light . . as it comes through the trees . . or glints off the water . . . the feel of the ground under you. . . . . and the wonderfully safe. . . . comfortable. . . . . free . . feeling of this place. . . . . . YOU'RE DOING VERY, VERY WELL.*

If I'm doing hypnosis work to diminish her pain, I begin that here; at the end of the work, I bring her back from this special place, gently.

And each time. . . . you sit . . or lie down comfortably at home. . . . in a quiet . . dark . . private . . space. . . . . and practice. . . . . closing your eyes. . . . . breathing in. . . . . and out. . . . . and then feeling the sun gently warm your muscles . . . ALL THE WAY DOWN. . . . . . . unwinding them . . . like a braid unwinds . . . in the water. . . . . it will be easier . . and easier . . for you to get back here . . . to your special place . . . to this wonderful . . peaceful . . . very relaxed. . . . . . feeling . . . This is something you can do for yourself . . . YOU ARE VERY GOOD AT IT . . . and it is very good for you. . . . . . . It is important that you take this time out of time for yourself . . . whenever you need it . . . And you can bring that feeling back with you . . . as you gently return . . . feeling very pleased . . with how VERY well . . . you have done today . . . and you will do again . . . gently . . . safely . . . comfortably . . . back [with the pitch and volume of my voice rising to the end of the sentence, as the signal for her to come back].

Both my patients and I feel relaxed and refreshed after these sessions. Given the time it takes to describe the technique, take the history, and conduct the first relaxation experience, I usually reserve thirty minutes for this initial session. Subsequent sessions usually take only fifteen minutes.

And it is easy for patients to practice at home. Each session can take as little as five to ten minutes, or can last thirty minutes or more—whatever the patient prefers. Many people ask for a tape of the session to play at home to help them practice the exercise. I ask them to be sure to let me know, after they use the tape, how I can improve it for them. They might, for example, have specific suggestions for a different "special place" they'd like me to describe during the session.

A note on referring patients to specialists in relaxation techniques is included at the end of the discussion of hypnosis.

I very much enjoy using relaxation therapy with my patients. I find it creates a special bond that improves communication between us, a bond that is very helpful if the illness progresses.

MINDFULNESS MEDITATION

The three general types of meditation are concentrative, contemplative, and mindfulness. Transcendental meditation, and meditation in which the practitioner focuses on a word, mantra, or image, are concentrative. Prayer is a type of contemplative meditation. Classic examples of mindfulness meditation are the vipassana and Soto Zen traditions. The mindfulness practitioner is paying attention to everything that is going on "right here, right now," even if this includes painful or frightening physical sensations or emotions. The patient is encouraged to "observe" these feelings and thoughts as they arise during the meditation and to separate the sensations from the emotions that are occurring. Such observation can often help the patient later reframe the meanings of the sensations so that they are less frightening or less able to provoke anxiety. During a mindfulness meditation, if memories of past events and emotions, or visions of future events, arise, they are dismissed in favor of the focus on the present. Through the concentration on present sensations and emotions, patients with cancer can learn to be still, to allow time to pass. Medications have time to take effect; patients achieve emotional distance from a troubling turn of events, regain control of themselves, and are able to make decisions more easily.

Dr. Jon Kabat-Zinn, who integrated mindfulness into his stress reduction practice, has demonstrated in seven randomized clinical trials significant health benefits for persons who maintain a routine practice of mindfulness. Medical and premedical students can reduce their stress with routine mindfulness practice (Shapiro et al. 1998). People who participate in mindfulness meditation classes learn three types of meditation: (1) a body scan meditation, which they do lying down; (2) sitting meditation, done on a chair or the floor; and (3) mindful hatha yoga, in which asanas are performed mindfully (Kabat-Zinn et al. 1998). Patients are given audiotapes and asked to practice these meditations in 45-minute sessions, six days a week. They also practice different informal meditations each week, which involve being mindful during normal daily activities.

Patients who practice mindfulness meditation generally have less pain, anxiety, depression, and fatigue. In a recent pilot study at the Dana-Farber Cancer Institute and Brigham and Women's Hospital, patients undergoing stem cell or bone marrow transplantation who practiced mindful meditation showed an immediate decrease in heart rate and pain, lowered anxiety, and an increase in feelings of control (Bauer-Wu 2004, personal communication). Some patients who have attended silent mindfulness meditation retreats, however, have reported increased anxiety, depression, or confusion, which in rare cases necessitated emergency psychiatric intervention. There are not enough data to identify which patients are at risk for such an event. Research in this area and in the benefits of mindfulness meditation is growing, and results of new studies may help define the role of mindfulness meditation for patients with cancer and their families.

Mary Jane Ott, whom I mentioned in the discussion of yoga, is also a trained teacher of mindfulness meditation (she is also a Reiki master and a trained family therapist). She starts our pain and palliative care team meetings with a meditation, which she often begins by bringing our attention to the fact that "we have arrived." She helps us focus on the present so that we can attend to the tasks before us, and as she ends, we often hear her urge us to be "right here, right now." For each of us, those two to five minutes bring our scattered minds to the room in which we are gathered, and when we are done, we are often refreshed and focused in a way that greatly enhances the work we need to do.

HYPNOSIS

While relaxation therapy is helpful in itself, it is also used by practitioners of hypnosis as an induction into the trance state. Hypnosis is an ancient and powerful technique that has a number of medical, dental, obstetric, dermatologic, and psychiatric uses. Hypnosis is particularly effective in relief of pain and other symptoms in cancer patients. It is even effective in decreasing bleeding (as Rasputin knew well).

Aesculapius and his followers used hypnosis-like techniques, as did Franz Anton Mesmer. John Elliotson and James Esdaile, British surgeons familiar with Mesmer's work, also believed that the power of the mind could be used to fight pain. Esdaile (1850) performed thousands of operations in India with hypnosis as the only analgesia, with convincing results, though when he returned to England he was ridiculed. James Braid, a Scottish contemporary of Esdaile, mislabeled the phenomenon "hypnosis" meaning a sleep-like state, only to discover later that patients under hypnosis are not asleep.

In the second half of the nineteenth century, the French physicians Ambrose August Liebeault and Hippolyte-Marie Bernheim promoted hypnosis and introduced the concepts of suggestion and suggestibility. They considered hypnosis to be a function of normal behavior. Freud studied with Bernheim, who was a noted neurologist, but when Freud found he did not need trance for the work he was doing with his patients, he abandoned it.

As long ago as the 1950s, hypnosis was accredited as a safe, effective procedure in both the United States and England. And during the last fifteen years, experienced practitioners have noted an increase in its use for habit control and for relief of pain of malignant and nonmalignant origin.

Hypnosis is a set of techniques through which patients can be taught to regain control over situations from which much control has been lost. They can minimize their suffering while waiting for pain or antiemetic medications to take effect and can minimize the amount of medication they need, along with the associated side effects. Appetite may be enhanced and insomnia reduced. Patients often experience newly gained independence and power, which can help even bedridden patients achieve appreciation of their own capabilities and gain a heightened sense of self-control and self-respect.

If you are interested in being trained in hypnotic techniques, I recommend that you attend one of the monthly four-day training sessions held by the American Society for Clinical Hypnosis (140 N. Bloomingdale Road, Bloomingdale, IL 60108-1017; telephone: 630-980-4740; fax: 630-351-8490; e-mail: info@asch.net; website: www.asch.net). The society holds classes for beginning, intermediate, and advanced practitioners, and you will be able to use hypnosis as soon as you finish the initial training.

DEFINITIONS.   There are a number of terms that have special meaning in the context of a discussion of hypnosis. These include *trance, induction, self-hypnosis, heterohypnosis, suggestion, distraction, dissociation,* and *negative* and *positive hallucinations*. A hypnotic *trance* is a state of altered awareness in which communication between the patient and the hypnotist is facilitated. *Induction* is the method used to help attain the hypnotic state. The hypnotist does not induce a trance, but rather assists the patient to experience one. If the trance is induced by the patient himself, it is called *self-hypnosis*. Trance induced by the hypnotist is called *heterohypnosis*. Frequently, a trance-like state is spontaneously induced by events of everyday life. An athlete who is "playing through the pain" can do so because he is in trance; trance can also occur at the theater, as when a play is so engrossing that you discover, only when the lights go on, that the seats that were empty on both sides of you are now occupied.

A *suggestion* is an idea that is presented to a patient in trance and is therefore accepted with a minimum of analysis, criticism, and resistance. *Distraction* is a diversion of attention. *Dissociation* means that the patient perceives that one part of the body or personality has been split from another, or that the body is in one location but, in some form, the person is elsewhere. A *negative hallucination* eliminates the perception of something that is objectively present. For example, if one is in a trance, a loudly flapping window shade will not be heard if the suggestion is made not to hear it. *Positive hallucinations* induce the perception of something that is not objectively present. They can be auditory, visual, or tactile. It is not hard, for example, to induce an injured child to watch a favorite program on an imaginary television while his wound is being treated. As I discuss below, any or all of these modes may be helpful in blocking pain perception.

MISCONCEPTIONS.   Despite its medical utility, there are numerous misconceptions about hypnosis. The prevalence of "hypnotists" in casino shows or on cruise ships, turning people into chickens, may account for some of these. Used for medical or dental purposes, however, hypnosis is not an entertainment but a therapeutic technique. Patients in trance are *not* asleep. Their eyes may be open and they may be sitting comfortably or walking while in trance. No one can be made to enter a trance unwillingly, and what occurs during the trance is entirely up to the subject. Nothing can be done that violates the individual's moral or ethical beliefs. People leave the trance state whenever they want to do so—the hypnotist cannot keep them there against their will.

PRACTICE POINTS: USING HYPNOSIS IN MANAGING THE SYMPTOMS OF CANCER PATIENTS

- Hypnosis itself is not therapy, but therapy can take place while the patient is in a trance.
- Almost everyone can experience a useful trance.
- The more motivated the patient, the more he or she will benefit from work in trance.
- Hypnosis helps patients suffering from insomnia, anxiety, feelings of helplessness, or feelings of loss of control.
- Patients modify the experience of distressing symptoms through imagery and metaphor.
- Patients with chronic, "meaningless" pain learn how to "put the pain away for now" and to experience only "today's" pain, not yesterday's or tomorrow's.

Hypnosis itself is not therapy, but therapy can take place while the patient is in trance. The hypnotist teaches the patient how to experience a state of trance and may give helpful suggestions while the patient is in trance. The hypnotic state itself facilitates the giving and receiving of suggestions relative to specific goals.

HYPNOTIC SUSCEPTIBILITY.   Almost everyone can experience a useful trance. Only 5 to 10 percent of the population cannot experience trance to any degree. About 10 percent of people are so adept that they can use suggestions made during trance as their only anesthetic when they undergo surgery. Differences in degrees of suggestibility, which can be assessed, may affect what can be accomplished by hypnosis. For pain relief, however, results of controlled studies differ; some have found a correlation between degree of hypnotizability and pain relief achieved, and others have found no such correlation.

Clinically, the ability to benefit from trance depends on the degree of the patient's motivation. The patient has to want to use trance to solve a problem, such as pain. In general, creative individuals with a good work history, many friends, good family relationships, and leisure activities, who are not severely depressed, tend to make the best subjects. However, even severely depressed people can benefit if they are well motivated.

UTILITY IN CANCER PATIENTS.   Hypnosis has many uses for cancer patients. It can help treat nausea, vomiting, anorexia, sleeplessness, anxiety, and feelings of helplessness and loss of control. The rehearsal technique described above is particularly vivid for a patient in trance and has special efficacy in helping patients deal with anticipated pain or discomfort prior to surgery, radiation, or chemotherapy.

In carefully controlled studies, hypnosis has also proved to be of significant benefit in relieving acute nonmalignant pain (e.g., dental), acute iatrogenic pain, and cancer pain. In these studies, patients using hypnosis had significantly less pain than those who did not. More controversial, it seems, is whether hypnosis is more beneficial than other cognitive techniques that reduce pain. Most studies have shown equivalency, though in some areas hypnosis was superior.

While in a hypnotic trance, patients can use images or metaphors to change the intensity of their pain or other symptom. For example, you can ask the patient to visualize a car speedometer with a 0 to 100 scale. Ask her to move the indicator to the number that reflects the cause of her distress. Next, suggest that she imagine the indicator to have moved to a higher number and ask if the symptom has also increased in intensity. It usually has. Then suggest that she move the indicator to a position lower than it was initially, and as she does so she will experience a lower intensity of the symptom. With appropriate suggestions, the diminished symptom intensity will persist when she comes out of trance.

It is important to determine which images are likely to be most compelling for a given patient. The speedometer image will be useful for people who are mechanically inclined or who just like to drive. But it may not be helpful for someone with different interests. For those who are musical, you can use the image of the volume control on a radio. For very visual people, you can suggest they use a rheostat to change the symptom intensity just as they do the intensity of light in a room. Visual people also find they can change the "color" of their symptom, from a hot, painful color such as red to a cooler, more comfortable one such as blue.

If a patient has chronic pain that is not serving as a danger signal, you can help him find an old trunk in the attic in which he can "put the pain" and "check on it" whenever he feels the need. He will still react to new pains or to changes in the existing pain, which he can report to you for evaluation. Children like to go to the deck of a spaceship and search for the colored wire and matching light switch that correspond to their pain. When they find them, they turn the switch—and the pain that came with it—to "off." You can create any number of metaphors and images once you know the patient's personality and his likes and dislikes.

You can also alter time subjectively, as you know if you've ever been to a boring lecture or an exciting sports event. Using hypnosis, you can prolong patients' pain-free periods and shorten the painful ones. And you can use patients' memories of other episodes of anesthesia, such as spinal anesthesia, to teach them to bring back that numbness to relieve their pain. They can also be taught to develop anesthesia in a glove-like distribution and to use that "anesthetized" hand to spread a feeling of numbness to painful body parts.

DISTRACTION.   Montaigne once wrote, "We feel one cut from the surgeon's scalpel more than ten blows of the sword in the heat of battle." Our peacetime warriors, the weekend football and basketball players, experience the same phenomenon—it is not until after the distraction of the game is gone that the bruises or even broken bones become apparent. Distraction, then, is a powerful modifier of the pain experience.

Without even realizing it, most of us use distraction when we need to do something that may make a patient uncomfortable. Performing a pelvic or rectal exam, for example, we engage our patient's attention by talking about something interesting. I have seen hematologists extract sternal bone marrow samples with no other anesthesia than the fascinating story they were telling—they were out of the door before the patient even realized a needle had been stuck in his chest, marrow extracted, and a Band-Aid placed on the wound.

Distraction is much more powerful, however, when the patient is in a hypnotic trance. Trance is especially likely to be effective in the emergency room, when it is spontaneously induced by both the injury and the setting. You might have a patient with a serious limb laceration, for example. Using your voice and nonverbal cues such as a hand on the shoulder to help induce or simply deepen the trance, you can suggest that the patient imagine that the injured limb is covered with newly fallen snow, which is lightweight and cold. You can then suggest that the coolness and comfort are spreading throughout the injured limb. This image is likely to lessen the bleeding as well. While the wound is being closed, you can ask the patient to concentrate on guessing how many stitches it will take. Engrossed in that discussion, and in trance, she will often be distracted from the associated pain. This technique is especially effective with children.

DISSOCIATION.   Bedridden patients can often use dissociation during trance to escape from their pain. They can "go" to their favorite vacation spot and retrieve enjoyable experiences while in trance, through self-hypnosis or heterohypnosis. You don't even have to be there to help them; you can make them tapes filled with suggestions that enhance their ability to dissociate.

Patients can also be taught during trance to dissociate a painful part of their body; they will then experience that body part as "not there" or "not theirs." The former is a negative hallucination; the latter is dissociation. A patient might, for example, dissociate the body part in anticipation of a painful procedure. Putting in an IV, for example, can be less painful if you make the suggestion that the arm is not really part of the body and what happens to it doesn't need to affect how the patient feels.

You can further enhance patients' comfort during this procedure by helping them induce anesthesia in the arm. When they are in trance, you might suggest that they use the cool sensation created by the alcohol swab to help them recall any previous feelings of numbness they've had, and extend the feeling of coolness in the arm to that numb feeling; then, when the needle enters the skin, they will feel it, but it won't hurt. When the procedure is completed, you must suggest that the sensation will return to normal, otherwise the arm might stay numb for some time and not respond normally to a painful stimulus (e.g., extreme heat).

MAKING A REFERRAL FOR RELAXATION THERAPY OR HYPNOSIS.   While you can do a great deal with the techniques outlined above, some patients will benefit from more intensive work with someone fully trained in the use of hypnosis and relaxation techniques to relieve pain. You may find, however, that patients resist such referrals. They may misinterpret your suggestion as implying that you don't really believe they are having pain. Or they may just be afraid of the techniques themselves. I therefore preface the referral by saying something along the following lines:

> *The pain syndrome you are experiencing is a very complex one, but there are a number of effective treatments for it. Remember when you were first diagnosed with cancer and your oncologist felt that you would benefit from both surgery and radiation treatments? That probably seemed reasonable to you, since the side effects of each treatment would be minimized, and yet you would obtain the best possible result. Well, I think we also need to use a number of different treatments to relieve your pain.*
>
> *In addition to taking the medications I will prescribe, I want you to learn some other techniques to lessen your pain. Two of these are hypnosis and relaxation therapy. People with the kind of pain you have can benefit a lot from these techniques. And since you won't need as much pain medicine, you'll have fewer side effects from it. Unfortunately, I am not really an expert in teaching relaxation techniques, but* [the psychologist, psychiatrist, social worker, nurse] *is and would be happy to teach them to you.*
>
> [She] *may, in fact, offer to teach you a number of techniques that can help you relieve your pain. When you first meet* [the practitioner, she] *will assess your pain, as I did, so that* [she] *can choose the most effective techniques to use or to teach you to use at home.* [The practitioner] *would also be happy to teach these skills to anyone in your family who is interested. Your work with* [her] *will be confidential, just like yours is with me.*
>
> *You, your family,* [the practitioner], *and I will continue to work together to be sure you achieve a degree of pain relief that is satisfactory to you. So I'd very much like to hear which treatments you are using and how each of them is helpful.*

Implicit in such an introduction is my belief that the patient is really in pain. I have also communicated my faith in the colleague I've recommended and in the techniques he or she will suggest to ameliorate the pain.

BIOFEEDBACK

Biofeedback, in its narrowest sense, is an electronic teaching aid that helps patients monitor certain physiological functions, such as muscle tension or skin temperature, and modify them. It has been found to be efficacious for patients with a number of nonmalignant conditions, in-

cluding spasmodic torticollis, spasticity, or paresis resulting from cere-
brovascular accidents, urinary or fecal incontinence, and for the elderly.
It is also effective in mild hypertension and in some patients with mi-
graine or tension headaches, but is no more effective than other methods of relaxation for these conditions. However, there are no controlled
studies of its efficacy for patients with pain of other etiologies, including
cancer pain.

Music Therapy

Introduced into palliative care in the United States and in Canada in
the 1970s by Lucanne Magill, Susan Munro, and Balfour Mount, music
therapy is "the creative and professionally informed use of music in a
therapeutic relationship with people identified as needing physical,
psychosocial, or spiritual help, or with people aspiring to experience
further self-awareness, enabling increased life satisfaction" (O'Callaghan
2004). Music therapy can be done with individuals or groups in the outpatient, home, or hospital setting.

Music therapy offers diversion, distraction, and enhanced relaxation.
It may benefit some patients with complex pain problems, though few
studies documenting its impact are available. Music therapists are specially trained individuals who involve patients in active music making,
song writing, and selecting the recorded music that is meaningful to
them. Therapists trained in the Bonny method of guided imagery and
music incorporate music into a program of guided imagery and relaxation aimed at helping patients gain more self-awareness and individual
development. Therapists or volunteers can also assist patients in selecting tapes designed for relaxation or can make personal tapes for them.

Music therapy is particularly useful in assisting patients with life review. It takes them back into memorable times of their life through the
music that was associated with those times. Patients can also work with
therapists to create music-related legacies. They can put music that has
been meaningful to them on a CD or on a portable digital music player
(such as iPod), rewrite the lyrics of familiar songs, or create new songs
that reflect what they need to say. Observational studies indicate that patients, families, and staff have positive responses to this therapy, so long
as they can choose the music or musical style. Not only were they able to
remember good times, but in many cases they felt "transported" to new,
pleasant experiences (O'Callaghan 2004).

Practitioners of music thanatology use music to alleviate the distress of dying patients (Horrigan 2001). Therese Schroeder-Sheker is a harpist, singer, composer, clinician, and educator who founded the field of music thanatology thirty years ago: the Chalice of Repose Project, and the School of Music Thanatology at St. Patrick's Hospital and Health Sciences Center in Missoula, Montana. Training in music thanatology requires five semesters plus a one-year internship.

Schroeder-Sheker recommends a polyphonic instrument to "deliver prescriptive music": a piano, organ, lute, guitar, or harp, or a keyboard that simulates these instruments. She considers the harp to be "particularly effective" in this work. Instrumentalists position themselves on either side of the patient's bed; Schroeder-Sheker always uses two harpists for the vigils she conducts. Vigils can last for an hour or more.

Before and after each session, music thanatologists assess the patient's pulse rate and strength, pattern of breathing, temperature, and any indications in the face or movements of the body that suggest distress. The music is synchronized to the dying patient's heartbeat and respirations, and can produce a profoundly calming, peaceful result. Breathing becomes deeper and easier, grimacing and muscle tremors resolve, and a deep sleep begins in patients who were unable to sleep before the session.

Schroeder-Sheker draws the parallel between childbirth and the dying process, both of which can be eased by the right partnering. Music thanatologists act as such partners. They help the patient, and they help the family and loved ones express their emotions and say good-bye (Hilliard 2001). They are "called to protect the sacredness of some events, and death is one such sacred mystery."

Art Therapy

Art therapy enables patients and families to use symbolic representations to express and explore their thoughts, hopes, and fears. Patients under active treatment, or bereaved family members (including children and adolescents), can participate (Pratt and Wood 1998). They create an art piece and then, with the help of the art therapist, reflect on its implications. Often the *process* is more important than the quality of the artwork. The making of the piece may enable the patient to express feelings that otherwise would be suppressed. Anger or frustration that cannot be directed at the physician or at God can manifest, for example, as pounding on clay; these emotions can be noted and then discussed with the art therapist. Hope, gratitude, and love can also be expressed in artistic creations when words do not come easily or do not suffice.

Art therapists are trained at a postgraduate level and certified. They can work in the outpatient setting or in homes, hospices, or hospitals. Art therapy is particularly helpful when patients or their families are having difficulty communicating verbally about their struggle with the illness and what it has meant for their lives, either because of language or cultural differences or because of a sense of unease in talking about such important issues. Physical, social, psychological, and spiritual struggles, concerns about body image, and lack of self-esteem are all areas that can be explored by art therapists. Studies supporting the benefits of art therapy suggest it can contribute to patients' sense of well-being (Reynolds 2000), but more research is needed (Wood 2003).

COUNSELING

Patients and their families often benefit from psychological and spiritual counseling. I discuss psychological counseling when I review the assessment and treatment of anxiety and depression in Chapter 7, so here the focus is on spiritual counseling.

Spiritual needs may be defined as the need to give and receive love, to have hope, to be able to express ourselves creatively, and to have meaning and purpose in our lives (Highfield and Cason 1983). We need to be reconciled with those from whom we have been estranged (Cosh 1995), and we need to resolve feelings of guilt and shame (Fitchett and Handzo 1998). Spiritual counseling addresses these needs, reestablishes hope and meaning, and, for the terminally ill, enables them to resolve issues that might otherwise prevent a peaceful death.

GOALS OF SPIRITUAL COUNSELING

- Enable patients to give and receive love, have hope, express themselves creatively, and have meaning and purpose in their lives.
- Help patients reconcile with those from whom they have been estranged.
- Eliminate feelings of guilt and shame.

A diagnosis of cancer is often an occasion to reflect on past events—achievements, failures, loves won and lost—and a time to put everything into perspective. It is also a time when we reexamine our relationship with God, with those we love, and with those who love us. We need to be reconciled to our failures and to bring closure to relationships left unsettled. And we look for hope, if not for a cure. We'd like to know we can accomplish those goals that remain to us and that we will die a dignified, pain-free death.

For some people, this will be a time of great creativity as they seek a way to communicate what their life has been or what they think is most important. Be it through an audiotape or videotape, a book, a scrapbook, or a painting, that work will express what they need to leave behind.

There are patients, however, who cannot find the meaning alone, who feel that they have been forsaken by God or those they love, or who see no reason to hope. They may feel isolated, changed by their illness into someone they don't recognize, someone whom their family and friends cannot understand or love. Their resulting emptiness, confusion, or despair may be very painful. Chaplains, social workers, psychotherapists, and psychiatrists are particularly skilled in aiding such patients.

But even though we are not professionals in this area, Dr. Roderick Cosh urges us to develop some basic skills that will be very helpful to those in spiritual pain: the ability to be with people and to listen to them. As he says, we are accustomed to "doing things for people" (Cosh 1995). We need to think about spending the time we would otherwise spend retrieving and analyzing test results, conferring with consultants, and writing orders in just being with our terminally ill patients, especially if they are in pain. We need to listen to their spiritual questions, understanding that they don't really expect answers from us. In some patients we may detect signs of spiritual health, as I should have in Miss Brown ("I'm all right, dear. Are you?"; see Chapter 1). In others, we may determine during the course of our listening that the patient has specific problems that could benefit from the extra time another team member could give, especially the hospice or hospital chaplain.

Paula Balber (1995), in her discussion of the "Hermes listener," suggests that if we choose to do the listening ourselves, we should ask questions that enable patients to develop their own myths—to go on their own hero's journey, as described by Joseph Campbell. This journey, as Campbell recounts it, begins with taking leave of the familiar after the arrival of the messenger with the bad news (that's us, giving them their diagnosis and prognosis). The hero acquires a guide and traveling companion who will take him to the second step of the journey, where he will encounter all the issues that keep him from being able to face death with a quiet mind and spirit.

Health care professionals, clergy, or family and friends can serve as this guide and protective figure (Balber 1995). And they can help as patients relate stories in which they recast moments of the past to give meaning and purpose to their lives, reconciling themselves to what has gone before, and creating their legacies.

Listening to such stories is hard work, though it may be very rewarding. In addition to standard questions such as "What was your childhood like? Tell me about your family. What did you do for a living? What do you think will happen next?" (Balber 1995), you might ask questions with a more personal focus (Betts 1988):

> Do you have any objects that you cannot throw away? What were your lucky breaks? Where were your life's turning points? What is your favorite memory? How was your life different from what you expected? In what family members do you recognize yourself? What would you like to have done instead of the work that you chose? How have you coped with the deaths of ones you've loved?

These questions are likely to lead to the kinds of stories that will help patients address the issues they need to address.

In the stories, you are likely to notice metaphors for the problems that the patient is currently facing. The patient may reveal her fears, how she overcame or dealt with them in the past, and how she regained control of the situation. You can share your admiration for how she overcame each of these problems before and in so doing, without actually mentioning current problems, you will be expressing your confidence that she will be able to deal just as well with them.

The stories may also be vehicles in which patients can release their anger, resentment, or disappointment. With the help of the listener, the patient may be able to understand the purpose of past painful events or reconcile with those he wants to see again before he dies. Individual stories become part of the whole tale of his life, helping the patient regain perspective and meaning.

SPEECH AND LANGUAGE THERAPY

Speech and language therapy can help patients regain the ability to communicate. This therapy also enables some patients with swallowing difficulties to eat again. Speech, language, and swallowing problems affect about a quarter of patients enrolled in hospice programs (Jackson et al. 1996). It is important to refer patients early whenever problems can be expected. Patients with brain metastases, for example, who may develop cognitive decline, or patients who may lose their ability to speak postoperatively or following prolonged intubation for respiratory compromise, can benefit from a therapist's training them in other communication techniques (e.g., using a communication board) well before they are actually impaired. After initial assessment, the therapist monitors changes, provides exercises to enhance audibility and clarity of speech, and teaches ways to compensate for loss of speech. The therapist can also provide clarification and education to family members, helping them cope with the changes, anticipate what is ahead, and learn how to maximize their ability to connect with the patient.

Speech and language therapists are also called in to assess and provide therapeutic suggestions for patients with difficulty swallowing due to oral and pharyngeal dysfunction. They can assess aspiration risk and suggest safer postures or positions for eating or how the food consistency can be modified to diminish the chance of aspiration. Referrals are indicated as soon as the patient or family notices frequent choking or coughing after eating, or difficulty handling normal oral secretions.

SUMMARY

The nonpharmacologic strategies for managing pain and other sources of suffering in cancer patients add an important dimension to the treatment plan. Acupuncture can be a significant adjunct to symptom management. Yoga practice brings together mind, body, and spirit, strengthening, refreshing, and energizing them all. Patients, their families, and the treatment team can benefit from yoga practice. Many of the manipulative and body-based methods for providing relief to patients can be performed by friends and family, and can be a significant source of satisfaction for these caregivers. The practice of relaxation, mindfulness meditation, or hypnosis, and work with a spiritual counselor, can offer a sense of control and hope, meaningfulness, and self-worth throughout the course of illness. Working with a speech and language therapist, patients can enhance both their ability to communicate and their ability to eat. These approaches, along with art and music therapy, enhance the lives of patients with cancer. The meditative techniques similarly can enhance the lives of their families and of the doctors and nurses who care for them.

Bibliography

GENERAL NONPHARMACOLOGIC STRATEGIES

Alternative Medicine: Implications for Clinical Practice. 1996. Videotape series (14 tapes with a 370-page syllabus), David Eisenberg, MD, Course Director. Harvard MED CME, PO Box 825, Boston, MA 02117-0825.

Cassileth BR. 1998. *The Alternative Medicine Handbook: The Complete Reference Guide to Alternative and Complementary Therapies.* New York: WW Norton.

Cassileth BR, Chapman CC. 1996. Alternative cancer medicine: a ten-year update. *Cancer Invest* 14:396–404.

Eisenberg DM, Kessler RC, Foster C, et al. 1993. Unconventional medicine in the United States. *N Engl J Med* 328:246–252.

Ferrell BR, Wisdom C, Rhiner M, Alletto J. 1991. Pain management as a quality assurance outcome. *J Nurs Quality Assurance* 5(2):50–58.

Lerner IJ, Kennedy BJ. 1992. The prevalence of questionable methods of cancer treatments in the United States. *CA Cancer J Clin* 42:181–191.

The physician and unorthodox cancer therapies. 1997. *J Clin Oncol* 15:401–406.

Weiger WA, Smith M, Boon H, et al. 2002. Advising patients who seek complementary and alternative medical therapies for cancer. *Ann Intern Med* 137:889–903.

ALTERNATIVE MEDICAL SYSTEMS

ACUPUNCTURE

American Academy of Medical Acupuncture. www.medicalacupuncture.org.

Cassileth BR, Shulman G. 2004. Complementary therapies in palliative medicine. In *Oxford Textbook of Palliative Medicine,* 3rd ed, Doyle D, Hanks G, Cherny N, Calman K (eds). Oxford: Oxford University Press.

Helms JM. 2004. An overview of medical acupuncture. In *Essentials of Complementary and Alternative Medicine,* Jonas WB, Levin JS (eds). Baltimore: Lippincott Williams & Wilkins (in press).

Mayer DJ. 2000. Acupuncture: an evidence-based review of the clinical literature. *Annu Rev Med* 51:49–63.

National Institutes of Health. 1998. National Institutes of Health Consensus Conference: acupuncture. *JAMA* 280:1518–1524.

Thompson JW, Filshie J. 1997. Transcutaneous electrical nerve stimulation (TENS) and acupuncture. In *Oxford Textbook of Palliative Medicine,* 2nd ed, Doyle D, Hanks GWC, MacDonald N (eds). Oxford: Oxford University Press.

YOGA

Coulter AH. 1998. Yoga and cancer: a move toward relaxation. *Altern Complement Ther* 4:150–158.

Feuerstein G. 1998. *The Yoga Tradition: Its History, Literature, Philosophy, and Practice.* Prescott, Ariz.: Hohm Press.

International Association of Yoga Therapists. www.iayt.org.

Khalsa SK. 1998. *Fly Like a Butterfly: Yoga for Children.* Portland, Ore.: Rudra Press.

Ott MJ. 2002. Yoga as a clinical intervention. *Advance for Nurse Practitioners* Jan:81–83, 90.

Raub JA. 2002. Psychophysiologic effects of hatha yoga on musculoskeletal and cardiopulmonary function: a literature review. *J Altern Complement Medicine* 8:797–812.

Salt of the Soul. 2000. Yoga Break: Yoga Exercises Designed for You at Your Desk or Workspace. Interactive CD-ROM. Salt of the Soul, Inc. www.yogabreak.com.

MANIPULATIVE AND BODY-BASED METHODS

Bowsher D. 1988. Modulation of nociceptive input. In *Pain Management in Physical Therapy,* Wells PE, Frampton V, Bowsher D (eds). Norwalk, Conn.: Appleton and Lange.

Ferrell BR, Rhiner M, Ferrell BA, Grant M. 1993. *Managing Cancer Pain at Home,* part of a Patient Education Kit, which includes two audiocassettes and a self-care log. City of Hope, Mayday Pain Resource Center, 1500 East Duarte Road, Duarte, CA 91010.

Ferrell-Torry A, Glick O. 1993. The use of therapeutic massage as a nursing intervention to modify anxiety and the perception of cancer pain. *Cancer Nurs* 16:93–101.

Houts PS (ed). 1994. *American College of Physicians Home Care Guide for Cancer.* Philadelphia: American College of Physicians.

Lehmann JF, de Lateur BJ. 1994. Ultrasound, shortwave, microwave, laser, superficial heat and cold in treatment of pain. In *Textbook of Pain,* 3rd ed, Wall PD, Melzack R (eds). New York: Churchill Livingstone.

McCaffery M, Wolff M. 1992. Pain relief using cutaneous modalities, positioning, and movement. *Hospice J* 8:121–154.

Melzack R. 1994. Folk medicine and the sensory modification of pain. In *Textbook of Pain,* 3rd ed, Wall PD, Melzack R (eds). New York: Churchill Livingstone.

O'Gorman B. 1995. Physiotherapy in terminal care. In *A Challenge for Living: Dying, Death and Bereavement,* Corless IB, Germino BB, Pittman MA (eds). Boston: Jones and Bartlett.

Rhiner M, Ferrell BR, Ferrell BA, Grant MM. 1993. A structured nondrug intervention program for cancer pain. *Cancer Pract* 1:137–143.

Sluka KA, Walsh D. 2003. Transcutaneous electrical nerve stimulation: basic science mechanisms and clinical effectiveness. *J Pain* 4:109–121.

Spross JA, Wolff Burke M. 1995. Nonpharmacological management of cancer pain. In *Cancer Pain Management,* 2nd ed, McGuire DB, Yarbro CH, Ferrell BR (eds). Boston: Jones and Bartlett.

Woolf CJ, Thompson JW. 1994. Stimulation-induced analgesia: transcutaneous electrical nerve stimulation (TENS) and vibration. In *Textbook of Pain,* 3rd ed, Wall PD, Melzack R (eds). New York: Churchill Livingstone.

MIND-BODY INTERVENTIONS

Barkwell DP. 1991. Ascribed meaning: a critical factor in coping and pain attenuation in patients with cancer-related pain. *J Palliat Care* 7(3):5–14.

Beecher HK. 1946. Pain in men wounded in battle. *Ann Surg* 123:96–105.

Beecher HK. 1956. Relationship of significance of wound to the pain experienced. *JAMA* 161:1609–1613.

Benson H, Beary JF, Carol MP. 1974. The relaxation response. *Psychiatry* 37:37–46.

Egbert LD, Battit GE, Welch CE, Bartlett MK. 1964. Reduction of postoperative pain by encouragement and instruction of patients. *N Engl J Med* 270:825–827.

Fields HL, Basbaum AI. 1989. Endogenous pain control mechanisms. In *Textbook of Pain*, 2nd ed, Wall PD, Melzack R (eds). New York: Churchill Livingstone.

Loscalzo M. 1996. Psychological approaches to the management of pain in patients with advanced cancer. *Hematol Oncol Clin North Am* 10:139–155.

Markenson JA. 1996. Mechanisms of pain. *Am J Med* 101(suppl 1A):6S–18S.

National Institutes of Health. 1995. *Integration of Behavioral and Relaxation Approaches into the Treatment of Chronic Pain and Insomnia*. NIH Technology Assessment Conference Statement. Bethesda, Md.: National Institutes of Health, US Department of Health and Human Services, Public Health Service.

Schneider SM, Prince-Paul M, Allen MJ, et al. 2004. Virtual reality as a distraction for women receiving chemotherapy. *Oncol Nurs Forum* 31:81–88.

Syrjala KL, Donaldson GW, Davis MW, et al. 1995. Relaxation and imagery and cognitive-behavioral training reduce pain during cancer treatment: a controlled clinical trial. *Pain* 63:189–198.

Talbot JD, Marrett S, Evans AC, et al. 1991. Multiple representations of pain in human cerebral cortex. *Science* 251:1355–1358.

Turk DC, Meichenbaum D. 1994. A cognitive-behavioral approach to pain management. In *Textbook of Pain*, 3rd ed, Wall PD, Melzack R (eds). New York: Churchill Livingstone.

Ulrich RS. 1984. View through a window may influence recovery from surgery. *Science* 224:420–421.

Wolsko PM, Eisenberg DM, Davis RB, Phillips RS. 2004. Use of mind-body medical therapies. *J Gen Intern Med* 19:43–50.

MINDFULNESS MEDITATION

Carlson LE, Ursuliak Z, Goodey E, et al. 2001. The effect of a mindfulness meditation–based stress reduction program on mood and symptoms of stress in cancer outpatients: 6-month follow-up. *Support Care Cancer* 9:112–123.

Center for Mindfulness in Medicine, Health Care, and Society. www.umassmed.edu/cfm.

Kabat-Zinn J. 1990. *Full Catastrophe Living: Using the Wisdom of Your Body and Mind to Face Stress, Pain, and Illness*. New York: Dell.

Kabat-Zinn J, Massion AO, Hebert JR, Rosenbaum E. 1998. Meditation. In *Psycho-Oncology*, Holland JC (ed). New York: Oxford University Press.

Shapiro SL, Schwartz GE, Bonner G. 1998. Effects of mindfulness-based stress reduction on medical and pre-medical students. *J Behav Med* 21:581–599.

Speca M, Carlson LE, Goodey E, Angen M. 2000. A randomized, wait-list controlled clinical trial: the effect of a mindfulness meditation-based stress reduction program on mood and symptoms of stress in cancer outpatients. *Psychosom Med* 62:613–622.

HYPNOSIS

Barber J (ed). 1996. *Hypnosis and Suggestion in the Treatment of Pain: A Clinical Guide.* New York: WW Norton.

Esdaile J. 1850. *Mesmerism in India and Its Practical Application in Surgery and Medicine.* Hartford, England: Silus Andrus and Son.

Genuis ML. 1995. The use of hypnosis in helping cancer patients control anxiety, pain and emesis: a review of recent empirical studies. *Am J Clin Hypn* 37:316–325.

Spanos NP, Carmanico SJ, Ellis JA. 1994. Hypnotic analgesia. In *Textbook of Pain,* 3rd ed, Wall PD, Melzack R (eds). New York: Churchill Livingstone.

Spiegel D, Moore R. 1997. Imagery and hypnosis in the treatment of cancer patients. *Oncology* 11:1179–1195.

Syrjala KL, Cummings C, Donaldson G. 1992. Hypnosis or cognitive-behavioral training for the reduction of pain and nausea during cancer treatment: a controlled clinical trial. *Pain* 48:137–146.

Syrjala KL, Roth-Roemer SL. 1996. Hypnosis and suggestion for managing cancer pain. In *Hypnosis and Suggestion in the Treatment of Pain,* Barber J (ed). New York: WW Norton.

Waxman D (ed). 1989. *Hartland's Medical and Dental Hypnosis,* 3rd ed. London: Balliere Tindall.

BIOFEEDBACK

Jessup BA, Gallegos X. 1994. Relaxation and biofeedback. In *Textbook of Pain,* 3rd ed, Wall PD, Melzack R (eds). New York: Churchill Livingstone.

MUSIC THERAPY

Aldridge D (ed). 1999. *Music Therapy in Palliative Care: New Voices.* London: Jessica Kingsley.

Hilliard RE. 2001. The use of music therapy in meeting the multidimensional needs of hospice and families. *J Palliat Care* 17:161–166.

Horrigan B. 2001. Interview with Therese Schroeder-Sheker: music thanatology and spiritual care for the dying. *Altern Ther* 7:69–77.

Music Therapy in Palliative Care. 2001. *J Palliat Care* 17(3).

O'Callaghan C. 2004. The contribution of music therapy to palliative medicine. In *Oxford Textbook of Palliative Medicine,* 3rd ed, Doyle D, Hanks G, Cherny N, Calman K (eds). Oxford: Oxford University Press.

Spross JA, Wolff Burke M. 1995. Nonpharmacological management of cancer pain. In *Cancer Pain Management,* 2nd ed, McGuire DB, Yarbro CH, Ferrell BR (eds). Boston: Jones and Bartlett.

ART THERAPY

Luzzatto P, Gabriel B. 1998. Art psychotherapy. In *Psycho-Oncology,* Holland JC (ed). New York: Oxford University Press.

Pratt M, Wood MJM. 1998. *Art Therapy in Palliative Care: The Creative Response.* London: Routledge.

Reynolds MW, Nabors L, Quinlan A. 2000. The effectiveness of art therapy: does it work? *Art Therapy: J Am Art Ther Assoc* 17:207–213.

Wood M. 2003. *The Contribution of Art Therapy to Palliative Medicine.* New York: Oxford University Press.

SPIRITUAL COUNSELING

Bailey SS. 1998. Comprehensive spiritual care. In *Principles and Practice of Supportive Oncology,* Berger AM, Portenoy RK, Weissman DE (eds). Philadelphia: Lippincott-Raven.

Balber PG. 1995. Stories of the living-dying: the Hermes listener. In *A Challenge for Living: Dying, Death and Bereavement,* Corless IB, Germino BB, Pittman MA (eds). Boston: Jones and Bartlett.

Betts D. 1988. Paper presented at the conference Telling Times: Stories of the Living-Dying. Chapel Hill, N.C.

Cosh R. 1995. Spiritual care of the dying. In *A Challenge for Living: Dying, Death and Bereavement,* Corless IB, Germino BB, Pittman MA (eds). Boston: Jones and Bartlett.

Fitchett G, Handzo G. 1998. Spiritual assessment, screening, and intervention. In *Psycho-Oncology,* Holland JC (ed). New York: Oxford University Press.

Highfield MF, Cason C. 1983. Spiritual needs of patients: are they recognized? *Cancer Nurs* June 6.

Lo B, Ruston D, Kates LW, et al. 2002. Discussing religious and spiritual issues at the end of life: a practical guide for physicians. *JAMA* 287:749–754.

Puchalski C, Romer AL. 2000. Taking a spiritual history allows clinicians to understand patients more fully. *J Palliat Med* 3:129–137.

Welch T. 1985. Existential and spiritual concerns. In *Outpatient Management of Advanced Cancer: Symptom Management, Support, and Hospice-in-the-Home,* Billings JA. Philadelphia: JB Lippincott.

SPEECH AND LANGUAGE THERAPY

Jackson P, Robbins M, Frankel S. 1996. Communication impediments in a group of hospice patients. *Palliat Med* 9:1–26.

Salt N, Davies S, Wilkinson S. 1999. The contribution of speech and language therapy to palliative care. *Eur J Palliat Care* 6:126–129.

7

Managing Other Distressing Problems

Patients with cancer suffer from a number of disorders that cause distress without causing pain. In this chapter I focus on the most common and the most distressing of these nonpain problems and their treatment. Palliative care and hospice teams (introduced in Chapter 3) are often involved in implementing these treatment plans. Their role is described further at the end of this chapter. Readers interested in a comprehensive discussion of palliative care may refer to the *Handbook of Palliative Care in Cancer* (1996), the *Oxford Textbook of Palliative Medicine,* third edition (2004), and *Principles and Practice of Supportive Care in Oncology,* second edition (2002) (see General References in the bibliography at the end of the chapter).

In the first section of the chapter, I address psychological distress. In 2003, the National Comprehensive Cancer Network (NCCN) recognized the magnitude of the problem of psychological distress by issuing guidelines for the evaluation and treatment of cancer-related distress. The panel who prepared this Clinical Practice Guideline (version 1.2003) documented a prevalence of 20 to 40 percent of cancer-related distress, but noted that fewer than 10 percent of patients were referred for help (NCCN 2003). Panel members included "representatives from all the disciplines involved in the delivery of supportive psychosocial services and counseling in NCCN institutions: social work, nursing, psychiatry, psychology, and clergy," along with two oncologists and a patient advocate. The guidelines offer proposed standards of care, screening tools (including a distress "thermometer" and checklist of practical, family, emotional, spiritual/religious, and physical problems), and assessment and treatment algorithms for patients suffering from psychological distress (dementia, delirium, mood disorder, adjustment disorder, anxiety disorder, substance abuse, personality disorder). The guidelines, updated in 2005, also include indications for referral to psychiatric, social work, and pastoral services. In this section I review anxiety, adjustment disorders, major depression, and counseling.

PSYCHOLOGICAL PROBLEMS

Cancer patients often experience anxiety or depression or both together. Following a diagnosis of cancer, almost 50 percent of patients will have an adjustment disorder, 10 to 20 percent an anxiety disorder, and 5 to 10 percent a major depression. Patients at high risk for anxiety include younger patients, women, patients with a history of substance abuse, and patients from lower socioeconomic strata (Stark et al. 2002). Anxiety often peaks during the initial cancer therapy, but it can persist for as much as a year, even when the patient has had a curative procedure. Anxiety lessens during adjuvant chemotherapy but peaks again at the cessation of the therapy, falling gradually as the remission lengthens. If the cancer recurs, as the disease advances the incidence of anxiety increases, and the incidence of major depression rises to between 23 and 58 percent. Anxiety and depression decrease the quality of life (Stark et al. 2002), but patients often can be treated effectively, even patients with very advanced disease.

ANXIETY

Patients may experience anxiety in different degrees and patterns. Some present with panic disorders, general anxiety disorders, and/or phobias (Stark et al. 2002). Anxiety may manifest, for example, as uncontrolled worry, a sense of impending doom, motor tension, restlessness, autonomic hyperactivity (e.g., palpitations, sweating, dry mouth, tightness in the chest), nausea/vomiting/diarrhea, feeling on edge, difficulty concentrating or relaxing, insomnia, or irritability. Anxious people often feel out of control and helpless.

Some patients may experience anxiety only before each chemotherapy treatment or before hearing results of follow-up scans. Others are chronically anxious. Their anxiety may exacerbate, but they are never anxiety-free. Some patients with severe anxiety are actually suffering from a delirium. If, in addition to being anxious, the patient has hallucinations or extreme psychomotor agitation, or is disoriented or paranoid, the anxiety is likely to be part of a delirium and should be treated with the therapies described in Chapter 5.

Assessment of the *intermittently* anxious patient includes exploring what the patient thinks might be contributing to the anxiety, what makes it better, what makes it worse. Ask whether he uses alcohol or other drugs to ameliorate it. Don't stop the questioning until you feel fairly confident that you know what this patient is afraid of, or you know that you've gone as far as he'll allow in the questioning. Your inquiry may reveal, for example, painful memories of the suffering of a close family member or friend who had cancer many years ago, fears of disfigurement, needle phobias, or claustrophobia, all of which may respond to directed interventions.

Finding a physiological cause for a patient's anxiety should not stop you from listening for additional psychological or spiritual problems that also cause anxiety. Mrs. Hanrahan was such a patient.

Curiosity, Not Certainty

Mrs. Hanrahan was a 59-year-old woman with extensive metastatic lung cancer that had been increasingly resistant to therapy. She worked for years as a superintendent of schools in a moderate-sized town, and was married, with four children. We were asked to see her for shortness of breath and for the recent onset of episodes of rapid heartbeat that had occurred in the night during her summer vacation in Maine. She had practiced relaxation and yoga in the past, but was unable to get her symptoms under control using these methods.

On initial questioning, we found that her dyspnea at rest was improved by increased oxygen, but was still problematic with exercise. She was waking up at night with a sensation that her heart was pounding, and when that occurred she increased the oxygen, to some effect. She also had these episodes during the daytime; they responded to lorazepam.

As I listened, I was thinking about how we could treat the dyspnea with more oxygen and the related anxiety with a different benzodiazepine, along with focused instruction to help her improve her use of yoga and relaxation techniques. But I suddenly realized that I really didn't know what had caused the anxiety. I had just assumed it was related to the pulmonary process. So I pursued the questioning a bit further.

Mrs. Hanrahan told me that during her vacation she had decided to retire from her position and not return to school in the fall. She also said tearfully that several of her children were having a great deal of difficulty coping with her increasing debility.

As she talked and cried, with her husband comforting her, I realized how close I had come to missing the most important part of the story. She was suffering from so many new losses—her position at work, her independence, her roles as mother and wife. Freed from the administrative burden of her job, she could focus considerable attention on her declining health and her powerlessness to help her family. Clearly these were important contributors to her anxiety, and I would need other solutions if I were to have any chance to make it better.

We explored together the potential causes of her anxiety, and how helpful a hospice program would be for her and her family (see Chapter 3). She and her husband were eager to enroll, with the understanding that if new promising therapies appeared, she could disenroll. She went home having made an appointment with her yoga instructor and with a promise of support from hospice.

Evaluation of a *chronically* anxious patient also includes a thorough psychiatric history, seeking evidence of generalized anxiety, depression, social phobia, panic disorders, obsessive compulsive disorder, or posttraumatic stress disorder. Also look for contributing medical causes, including cardiovascular, endocrine, metabolic, neurologic, and respiratory conditions.

ANXIETY: COMMON CONTRIBUTING MEDICAL CONDITIONS

- Cardiovascular: angina or infarction; arrhythmias; congestive heart failure; hypovolemia
- Endocrine: hypercalcemia or hypocalcemia; hypothyroidism or hyperthyroidism
- Metabolic: hyperkalemia; hypoglycemia; hypoxia; hyponatremia; fever
- Neurologic: akathisia; encephalopathy; partial complex seizure disorder
- Respiratory: asthma; chronic obstructive pulmonary disease (COPD); pneumothorax; pulmonary edema; pulmonary embolism
- Medications: glucocorticoids; antiemetics that cause akathisia (e.g., Compazine; Reglan); bronchodilators and beta-adrenergic agonists; stimulants (methylphenidate); antidepressants (e.g., fluoxetine, which also causes akathisia); caffeine; "rebound" from ultra-short-acting benzodiazepines (e.g., Xanax)
- Withdrawal syndromes: alcohol; benzodiazepines; opioids

(Adapted from Noyes et al. 1998, 555)

Patients with anxiety respond to both nonpharmacologic and pharmacologic therapies. Counseling is discussed later in this chapter. Relaxation, hypnosis, and behavioral training also benefit patients with anxiety, and these are discussed in detail in Chapter 6. Pharmacologic therapies for anxiety (other than that associated with delirium) include the benzodiazepines, selective serotonin reuptake inhibitors (SSRIs), and atypical antipsychotics (e.g., quetiapine [Seroquel] and mirtazapine [Remeron]). The benzodiazepines are used to treat patients with mild anxiety (Table 7.1). Lorazepam (Ativan) (0.5 mg to 1 mg p.o. or sublingual t.i.d.) is recommended for intermittent anxiety. Clonazepam (Klonopin) (0.25 to 0.5 mg p.o. b.i.d., with 0.5 to 1 mg at bedtime) can be added for patients with chronic anxiety that is mild to moderate. In some patients, however, anxiety may unpredictably worsen in response to lorazepam. Alprazolam (Xanax) (0.25 to 2.0 mg p.o. t.i.d. to q.i.d.) is rapidly effective but has a "rebound" effect that causes a return of the anxiety in a short period of time. Oxazepam (Serax) (15 to 30 mg p.o. at bedtime), temazepam (Restoril) (7.5 to 30 mg p.o. at bedtime), or zolpidem (Ambien) (5 to 10 mg p.o. at bedtime) are often used to treat insomnia due to anxiety. Clorazepate (Tranxene) (15 to 60 mg/day p.o.) is used for anxiety and acute alcohol withdrawal. Patients with more severe anxiety benefit from treatment with SSRIs (such as citalopram [Celexa] or escitalopram [Lexapro]) or with mirtazapine (Remeron) (see Table 7.1).

DEPRESSION

It can be difficult to discern which patients with advanced disease are depressed. Many of the usual somatic signs (e.g., anorexia, sleep disturbances, fatigue, or weight loss) are not helpful, because they may be due to the underlying illness. Depressed patients, however, will also feel sad, cry, be unable to get pleasure from any activity, or feel globally worthless, guilty, hopeless, or helpless.

PRACTICE POINTS: SIGNS OF DEPRESSION IN CANCER PATIENTS
- Appearing depressed or describing a feeling of depression
- Crying
- Inability to get pleasure from any activity
- Feeling of worthlessness, guilt, hopelessness, or helplessness

Note: Anorexia, sleep disturbances, weight loss, and fatigue occur in many patients with cancer; these signs do not identify those who are depressed.

Table 7.1 Pharmacologic Treatment of Anxiety and Depression

Class/Drug	Dose	Comments
Benzodiazepines		
Lorazepam (Ativan®)	0.5–2 mg q1–4h max 10 mg/24 h	Tablets, sublingual tabs, and liquid available; tablets can be used p.r.
Clonazepam (Klonopin®)	0.5–1 mg p.o.	Can be given h.s., or up to t.i.d.; tablets have been used p.r. Do not exceed 4 mg/24 hr.
Alprazolam (Xanax®)	0.25–2 mg p.o. t.i.d.	Severe "rebound" effect; not recommended for chronic use.
Diazepam (Valium®)	5–10 mg p.r. h.s.	Useful for patients unable to take oral medication.
Oxazepam (Serax®)	15–30 mg p.o. h.s.	Insomnia from anxiety.
Temazepam (Restoril®)	7.5–30 mg p.o. h.s.	Insomnia from anxiety.
Zolpidem (Ambien®)	5–10 mg p.o. h.s.	Insomnia from anxiety.
Selective serotonin reuptake inhibitors		
Citalopram (Celexa®)	20–40 mg p.o. h.s.	Minimal sexual dysfunction.
Escitalopram (Lexapro®)	10–20 mg p.o. h.s.	Minimal sexual dysfunction.
Sertraline (Zoloft®)	50–200 mg p.o.	
Venlafaxine (Effexor®)	75–225 mg p.o.	Used alone or added to initial SSRI.
Paroxetine (Paxil®)	20–60 mg p.o. h.s.	Sedation; can be difficult to discontinue.
Fluoxetine (Prozac®)	20–80 mg/day p.o.	Stimulating; causes anorexia.
Psychostimulants		
Methylphenidate (Ritalin®)	5–60 mg p.o.	Divided doses (8 a.m., noon).
Dextroamphetamine (Dexedrine®)	5–60 mg p.o.	Divided doses (8 a.m., noon).
Others		
Clorazepate (Tranxene®)	15–60 mg/day p.o.	For anxiety from alcohol withdrawal.
Mirtazapine (Remeron®)	15–45 mg p.o. h.s.	Also enhances appetite.
Trazodone (Desyrel®)	50–400 mg p.o. h.s.	Sedating.
Tricyclic antidepressants		
Amitriptyline, doxepin, clomipramine, desipramine, nortriptyline	10–25 mg/day p.o. h.s	Increase to therapeutic dose (50–150 mg in divided doses).

Terminally ill patients who respond "Yes" to the screening question "Are you depressed?" are very likely to be confirmed as depressed in a more comprehensive evaluation. Useful follow-up questions include: How do you see your future? What do you imagine is ahead for you with this illness? What aspects of your life do you feel most proud of? Most troubled by? Are you getting less enjoyment from your favorite things?

Depressive symptoms can be manifestations of a number of medical, social, spiritual, or psychiatric disorders. Common metabolic and medication-related causes of depression in cancer patients include hyponatremia, hypercalcemia, CNS tumor, high-dose interferon therapy, opioids, and corticosteroids. Stress from financial or family concerns or from simple sleep deprivation are also often contributory. If none of these is present, the patient may have either an adjustment disorder or, more rarely, a major depression.

Treatment of depression is often very effective. For cancer patients, as discussed in Chapter 4, care must be taken to optimize their pain control, because uncontrolled pain is a major risk factor both for depression and for suicide. Psychological strategies include psychopharmacology and psychotherapy.

There are a number of agents that are often effective in alleviating depression. The most rapidly acting antidepressants are the psychostimulants dextroamphetamine and methylphenidate (2.5 to 5 mg at 8 a.m. and noon, maximum 60 mg), which often act within a few days. The SSRIs are the first choice when immediate onset is not needed; they may take 4 to 6 weeks to show effect. Initial doses are usually small. They are given for 3 to 7 days and then increased every week or every other week until the patient notices a benefit or the maximum dose is reached. The SSRIs should not be stopped suddenly; they should be tapered if they are to be discontinued. If the patient is expected to live longer than weeks to a few months, a stimulant and an SSRI may be started simultaneously, and the stimulant can be titrated off 4 weeks later.

Suggested Initial and Maximal Doses for SSRIs
- Citalopram (Celexa) and paroxetine (Paxil), 10 mg/day orally for the first week. If no response, increase by 10 mg weekly to the maximum dose of 60 mg/day.
- Escitalopram (Lexapro), 10 mg/day orally for the first week, then increase to the maximum dose of 20 mg/day.
- Sertraline (Zoloft), 50 mg/day orally for the first week, then increase to

75 mg if needed for an additional week. Increase as needed by 25 mg to the maximum dose of 200 mg/day.

- Fluoxetine (Prozac), 5 to 10 mg/day orally for the first week; increase by 10 mg every 2 weeks to the maximum dose of 80 mg/day, as it has a long half-life.
- Venlafaxine (Effexor), 37.5 mg orally twice a day for the first week; increase by 75 mg per week to a maximum dose of 225 mg/day. Missing any dose of venlafaxine can cause symptoms similar to those experienced with opioid withdrawal, so the patient must be weaned off the drug carefully.

Major side effects of the SSRIs include hyponatremia, sexual dysfunction or loss of libido, and gastrointestinal complaints (e.g., nausea, diarrhea, and foul-smelling flatus).

The mechanism of action of the antidepressant mirtazapine (Remeron) (15 mg p.o. at bedtime, to a maximum of 45 mg/day p.o.) is unknown, but in addition to its antidepressant actions, it is useful for insomnia, as it is sedating, and it enhances appetite. Trazodone (Desyrel) is also sedating. Initial doses are 50 mg orally at bedtime, to a maximum of 400 mg/day. Tricyclic antidepressants (e.g., amitriptyline, nortriptyline, desipramine) are less useful for patients with advanced disease, because of their side-effect profile. But if the patient also has neuropathic pain, you can try to enhance tolerance of the drugs by starting at very low doses (10 mg at bedtime) and increasing by 10 to 20 mg weekly. If there is no effect, check blood levels to ensure that the therapeutic range has been reached. Checking ECGs to detect conduction disturbances may be necessary when giving higher doses.

If the patient does not respond to first-line agents, a psychiatrist should be consulted. Referral to a psychiatrist is also necessary in any of the following situations: the physician is unsure of the diagnosis; the patient is psychotic, confused, or delirious; the patient previously had a major psychiatric disorder; there are dysfunctional family dynamics; or the patient is suicidal or is requesting assisted suicide.

Factors that make cancer patients more likely to attempt suicide include advanced illness and poor prognosis; uncontrolled pain; depression and hopelessness; delirium and disinhibition; loss of control and helplessness; preexisting psychopathology; prior history of attempted suicide and family history of suicide; and exhaustion and fatigue. The psychiatrist will not necessarily advise hospitalization if the patient's physical condition makes that inadvisable; the psychiatrist will, however, help the home care agency and the family take appropriate precautions.

COUNSELING

PSYCHOLOGICAL THERAPY.   Social workers, psychologists, and psychiatrists are equipped with an array of cognitive techniques that can help the patient and family lessen the pain they are suffering. These clinicians can offer support and education and can help in developing coping skills, and they can diminish patients' anxiety, depression, or delirium that may exacerbate pain.

Psychiatric therapy can be offered to the patient (either individually or in a group) or to the family or significant friends. Groups can be particularly helpful for cancer patients because of the similarities of the psychological problems posed by the disease in its various stages. Those who have passed through one or another stage can share their successes with others now facing the same problems. By becoming teachers, patients and their families can increase their own sense of self-worth.

In addition to the strategies useful for clients who do not have or have never had cancer, there is now a large body of information on the specific psychological needs of cancer patients. Work has been done on the implications of a wide variety of cancer-related practices, from genetic testing and cancer screening to the psychological, social, and behavioral factors that influence the risk of cancer and survival from it. Information is available on the needs of cancer survivors, patients with specific cancers (e.g., lung cancer, breast cancer) and their families, and patients receiving specialized therapies (e.g., bone marrow transplants), and on the pharmacologic and nonpharmacologic interventions appropriate for them. Much is also known about the psychological stresses experienced by both the families and the professional caregivers of patients with cancer.

The new field of psycho-oncology is responsible for this wealth of information and research-based recommendations for care. A comprehensive overview of the breadth and depth of the field is found in the textbook *Psycho-Oncology,* edited by one of its pioneering practitioners and researchers, Dr. Jimmie Holland. As she states in the book's preface, "This present volume describes the many ways in which mental health professionals have indeed contributed to improving the lot of the cancer patient." A thorough discussion of psycho-oncology is beyond my expertise, but I refer those who are interested to this fascinating text. I discuss below the role of psychiatrists and counselors in the care of cancer patients.

PRACTICE POINTS: THE ROLE OF PSYCHIATRISTS AND COUNSELORS IN THE CARE OF CANCER PATIENTS

- Therapists provide psychological and emotional support and education about cancer and its treatment(s); they teach coping skills.
- Therapists facilitate communication of the patient's and family's concerns to and among health care providers.
- Therapists evaluate and address the psychological needs of the family.
- Therapists recognize and treat adjustment disorders, anxiety, depression, and delirium.

SUPPORT.   Using a crisis intervention model, therapists can support cancer patients by providing emotional support and by just "being there" for them throughout the disease process. Patients with cancer need continuity, but instead usually see a number of specialists during the process of diagnosis and treatment—the general internist, radiologist, and medical, surgical, or radiation oncologist. The therapist can provide the needed continuity and, when necessary, can be the spokesperson for the family and patient if they are unable to explain their needs to whichever oncologist is currently treating the patient.

EDUCATION.   The therapist can also provide information about the disease and help the patient gain useful self-knowledge. Therapists who work with cancer patients are usually very well informed about the disease and its treatment, and patients may find it easier to ask them the questions they are reluctant to "bother" their oncologist with. Therapists can also help dispel misconceptions such as those about taking pain medications, discussed in Chapter 2. They can clarify therapeutic goals and reinforce the legitimacy of reporting treatment-related side effects if they arise.

But therapists also anticipate the emotional and psychological stresses that patients are likely to face, and can help them prepare by rediscovering coping strategies that have served them well in the past. Cancer is rarely the first major crisis a person has faced. The first may have been something as simple as passing an important examination or as complex as being in a front-line unit in combat. Therapists can help patients recall a crisis that they managed successfully and then, along with the patient, analyze the strategies that worked and decide how to apply the same techniques to the current crisis: being a cancer patient.

SKILL DEVELOPMENT.   The task of helping patients develop new skills also puts therapists in the role of teacher as they instruct patients in the relaxation and other cognitive coping techniques described above. The therapist can also teach patients another skill that is crucial to obtaining the best care during their illness: how to explain their needs to health care professionals.

Patients are unaccustomed to being assertive with physicians or nurses; but they may need to assert themselves if they are to retain their rights as people, even as they are being forced to take on the role of patient. In hospital settings, common courtesy is often forgotten even when no medical emergency has supervened. There is no reason, for example, that a person has to stop eating breakfast because it is convenient for a house officer or a phlebotomist to draw a blood sample at that moment. If the timing is important, the patient is owed both an explanation and an apology for the inconvenience.

There is also no need for a patient to suffer because she is afraid to tell the physician that the pain regimen isn't working. Therapists can help patients feel comfortable relinquishing this Good Patient role. Not only will the patient then be able to retain her sense of control and self-esteem even in the hospital setting, but she is much more likely to share all her concerns with us and frankly inform us if our symptom-oriented therapies are not working.

TREATMENT OF RELATED PSYCHIATRIC DISORDERS: ANXIETY, DEPRESSION, AND DELIRIUM.   Psychotherapy for anxiety and depression is often as effective as pharmacologic therapies; it can be combined with them and, in selected patients, can substitute for them. And counseling can help unravel complicated relationships that are causing distress to patients and their families. It is often difficult for patients and their families to realize that they would benefit from psychiatric or psychological help (Breitbart et al. 2003). They might misinterpret your offer of a referral as indicating that you think they are "crazy." I often need to spend a little time to explain why I think patients and families need the referral and how, specifically, I expect the therapist to help them. The Abernathy family benefited significantly from the counseling they received.

The Benefits of Psychological Counseling

John and Mary Abernathy were the parents of my patient Patricia, a 26-year-old woman with extensive, refractory sarcoma. Patricia required large doses of opioids along with adjuvants for her pain, but she felt that the pain was well controlled, and she enjoyed going to movies and sports events with friends as her energy level allowed. Over several months, despite satisfactory pain control, the hospice nurses noted a gradual change in Patricia, which I confirmed on a visit to her parents' home, where she lived.

Patricia looked very sad, was eating less, and told me that even when she felt up to it, she had no desire to see friends or go out with them as before. Her mother brought in a tray with her lunch and after she left, Patricia dissolved in tears. She said she was feeling terribly guilty for being such a burden to her family, that she couldn't contribute a thing to the running of the household, and that she was just of no use to anyone. She did not want to end her life herself, but she didn't think it was really worth living anymore. She asked that I not tell her parents how she felt because that would just distress them further.

After I left her room, Patricia's parents also shared their concerns with me. They had noticed the change in their daughter, but ascribed it to "all the dope" I had prescribed for her pain. They didn't want to let Patricia know how upset they were about her changed condition, but wanted something done to alleviate her distress.

Before leaving that day, I spoke with Patricia and her parents about the differences in their perceptions and the communication difficulties they were having. I told everyone that I thought Patricia was depressed, that depression commonly affected patients whose cancer was as far advanced as Patricia's, but that I had every hope that the depression would respond to treatment. I suggested that in addition to individual therapy for Patricia, family therapy might help them understand each other's concerns and improve their ability to share them, and they agreed to try it.

The therapist later informed me that Patricia did improve considerably, as did communication within her family. The therapist continued to provide support and counseling until Patricia's death, and she helped Patricia's parents cope with their bereavement.

If you're able to convince your patients and their families to accept this type of help, you will have opened the door to a complementary therapeutic experience for them. In their relationship with the therapist, they can ventilate and explore their feelings toward the cancer without expressing any "unacceptable" doubts to you, to your staff, or to other family members.

With careful preparation, many patients will at least explore the possibility and accept the referral without feeling either betrayed or rejected by you. While you are focusing on the medical care, the social worker or other therapist can identify psychological or social problems that otherwise might never come to your attention and yet would be sources of distress for your patients and their families. And as part of a hospice team, therapists are often available 24 hours a day and can be very helpful in emergencies.

ORAL PROBLEMS

A number of simple measures can help patients maintain oral comfort. These include removing poorly fitting dentures; replacing vitamins and minerals that if deficient can result in mucositis (e.g., vitamins B, C; zinc); presenting food at moderate temperatures; avoiding dry, acidic, or highly spiced foods; and minimizing alcohol and tobacco use.

PRACTICE POINTS: MAINTAINING ORAL COMFORT
- Remove poorly fitting dentures.
- Correct vitamin and mineral deficiencies.
- Present foods at moderate temperatures.
- Avoid dry, acidic, or highly spiced foods.
- Minimize alcohol and tobacco use.
- Continue routine, prophylactic oral care, including brushing, flossing, and rinsing with an alcohol-free antibacterial mouthwash.

Oral comfort can also be maximized by continuing routine, prophylactic oral care, even for patients who are very debilitated (Table 7.2). Regular mouth care can be carried out by the patient or the family; it can help stimulate the patient's appetite and diminish discomfort from a variety of causes. Patients should be encouraged to continue brushing daily using a soft-bristle brush, flossing, and rinsing with an antibacterial mouthwash (that does not contain alcohol) or a solution of bicarbonate in water (e.g., 1 tsp. in a cup of water). More detailed oral care protocols are described in sources listed in the bibliography at the end of the chapter.

Table 7.2 Oral Care

Problem	Therapy
Routine maintenance	Multivitamins/minerals
	Brushing, flossing
	Antibacterial rinses (sans alcohol)
Candida	Troches (miconazole, clotrimazole) q.i.d.
	Ketoconazole (Nizoral®) 200 mg b.i.d. p.o.
	Fluconazole (Diflucan®) 200 mg p.o. day 1, then 100 mg/day p.o.
	Itraconazole (Sporanox®) (tablet or solution) 100–200 mg/day p.o.
	Amphotericin B solution (100 mg/ml) 1 ml t.i.d. to q.i.d., rinse and spit
Xerostomia	Sugar-free sour candies
	Moist gauze
	Pilocarpine (Salagen®) 5–10 mg t.i.d. p.o.
	Cevimeline (Evoxac®) 30 mg p.o. t.i.d.

Despite these preventive regimens, about half of cancer patients will develop oral discomfort, the most common causes of which are candida infections; treatment-induced mucositis; or xerostomia resulting from mouth breathing, previous radiation therapy, or medications for pain or other symptoms. Simple methods of treatment are often very effective.

CANDIDA

ETIOLOGY. As many as 90 percent of cancer patients have contracted an oral candida infection by the time they die. Oral and esophageal infection with candida can arise in patients who have recently been on a course of antibiotics, which alter the normal protective oral flora. Other patients are predisposed to developing yeast infections due to immunosuppression resulting from therapeutic steroid doses or malnutrition (albumin of <3 g/dl).

MANIFESTATIONS IN IMMUNOSUPPRESSED PATIENTS. Oral thrush presents most often as a burning tongue and pain when eating. Examination of the oral cavity may reveal only a beefy red tongue (in those who have just been taking antibiotics) or white plaques (which are easily wiped off, but with bleeding) along the sides of the tongue or cheeks, on the gums, or on the roof of the mouth. Patients who leave their dentures in place between meals are particularly prone to develop both angular cheilitis and candidal infections on the roof or floor of the mouth; these appear as red, edematous areas.

Candidal esophagitis can contribute to anorexia by causing dysphagia. The lower esophageal sphincter area is most commonly involved, but the pain or the sensation of food "sticking" can be present in the throat or chest as well as the upper abdomen. Topical antifungal medications that are effective for oral thrush unfortunately do not prevent esophageal candida infections.

THERAPY.   Ketoconazole (200 mg/day) provides very effective, inexpensive therapy for these patients. But ketoconazole is nauseating and it requires the presence of stomach acid to be adequately absorbed. Therefore, if a patient develops nausea or vomiting when taking ketoconazole, or is taking an antacid agent, I substitute the more expensive fluconazole (100 mg/day p.o.) or itraconazole (100 to 200 mg tablets or oral suspension daily). Miconazole and clotrimazole (Mycelex) troches are also effective, but patients must take four or five a day and allow the troches to dissolve in the mouth. This may be very inconvenient for a patient with advanced cancer and ineffective for those with concurrent xerostomia. Such patients may require an amphotericin B 100 mg/ml oral solution (1 ml t.i.d. to q.i.d.—swish and spit out).

TREATMENT-INDUCED MUCOSITIS

Treatment-induced mucositis is one of the most common and most distressing side effects from chemotherapy and radiotherapy and from bone marrow transplants. Patients generally treat this with an intensive regimen of oral cleansing with frequent saline and antiseptic rinses daily. The following have all been used: amifostine (a free-radical scavenger) and benzydamine hydrochloride; antimicrobials (which attenuate pro-inflammatory cytokines); l-glutamine (which replaces l-glutamine losses); granulocyte-monocyte colony stimulating factors; and superoxide dismutase inhibitors (Sonis 2004).

A novel therapy, recombinant human keratinocyte growth factor (rHu-KGF; palifermin from Amgen), improves soreness and ability to eat, drink, sleep, and talk for patients receiving high-dose chemotherapy and total body irradiation (TBI) as part of a bone marrow transplant procedure (Peterson and Cariello 2004).

XEROSTOMIA

ETIOLOGY.   Dry mouth is a very common complaint of patients with far-advanced cancer. Some have received radiation that has diminished their saliva production, and others are taking medication that is causing xerostomia as a side effect. Therapy is often effective in these patients and in those without a clear underlying cause.

PRACTICE POINTS: THERAPY FOR XEROSTOMIA

- Minimize the number of medications that produce xerostomia.
- Try sugar-free sour lemon drops or other sugar-free hard candy.
- Continue good routine oral hygiene, adding a fluoride-containing toothpaste for selected patients.
- Try pilocarpine (Salagen) or cevimeline (Evoxac) to ameliorate radiation-induced xerostomia.

I find it useful to review the patient's medications to see which could be contributing, and then discontinue these and if necessary substitute other agents that are less likely to induce this side effect. In addition to the antihistamines and anticholinergics, certain anticonvulsants, antipsychotics, hypnotics, beta-blockers, morphine, and diuretics can contribute to xerostomia. The more of these agents the patient is receiving, the more likely he is to develop xerostomia.

THERAPY.   Sugar-free sour lemon drops or other sugar-free hard candies are useful for patients with mild xerostomia. To prevent mouth pain and protect the teeth, I ask patients to avoid foods that contain sugar and encourage them to continue routine oral hygiene, supplemented, in some patients, with fluoride rinses. For those without cardiac contraindications, pilocarpine (Salagen) (5 to 10 mg t.i.d.) or cevimeline (Evoxac) (30 mg p.o. t.i.d.) an hour before meals is often very effective in inducing saliva production, especially for patients who have undergone radiation to the oral cavity or neck.

GASTROINTESTINAL PROBLEMS

ASCITES

Ascites is most common in patients with ovarian or breast cancer but also occurs in those with other genitourinary and gastrointestinal cancers and even in some with cancer of the lung. Ascites that is refractory to the usual diuretic measures (Aldactone [spironolactone] ± oral furosemide) can be difficult to manage. Adding oral hydrochlorothiazide or discontinuing oral furosemide and substituting intravenous furosemide infusions (100 mg over 24 hours) or Bumex (bumetanide) (0.5 to 2 mg/day p.o. or 0.5 to 1 mg IV—do not exceed 10 mg/day) may be effective. For other patients, not until their disease advances and their oral fluid intake diminishes does the ascites stabilize or decrease.

PERITONEOVENOUS SHUNTS.   If patients have only a few months to live, repeated paracentesis may be the most appropriate therapy. But for those patients with a reasonable life expectancy for whom ascites is a major problem, consider a surgical referral for percutaneous insertion of a peritoneovenous shunt (i.e., a Denver shunt or a LeVeen shunt) under local anesthesia in the operating room. These shunts were originally designed for patients with cirrhosis but have been useful in some patients with malignant ascites, particularly those with metastatic breast or ovarian cancer, who live a relatively long time.

The Denver shunt combines a venous catheter, a compressible pump with one-way valve(s), and a catheter that is placed into the ascites (Figure 7.1a). The portions of the catheters not in a vein or the ascitic fluid are tunneled subcutaneously, and the pump is also placed subcutaneously over ribs, to make it easier to compress (Figure 7.1b).

In response to the negative intrathoracic pressure induced by inspiration, ascitic fluid drains into the central venous circulation either through the one-way valve (the LeVeen shunt) or through a compressible valve system containing either a single- or double-valved shunt, depending on the viscosity of the ascites (the Denver shunt). Even more ascitic fluid can be moved into the central venous system if the patient uses an incentive spirometer.

For about 70 percent of patients with a Denver shunt, their ascites is resolved until death. The major complication, found to occur in about 25 to 30 percent of patients several months after shunt insertion, is reaccumulation of ascitic fluid due to obstruction of the one-way valve by the high protein content of malignant ascitic fluid. Other complications,

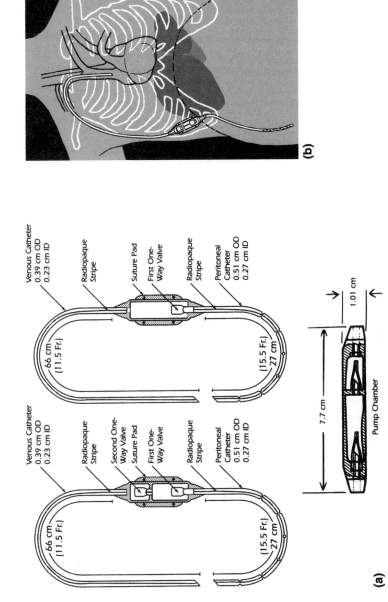

7.1 (a) Peritoneovenous Shunts and (b) Shunt Placement. From Denver Biomaterials, Inc.; with permission.

found in fewer than 10 percent of patients, included pulmonary edema responsive to diuretics and ascitic leaks, which stopped spontaneously. Fewer than 5 percent developed clinically significant disseminated intra-vascular coagulation, shunt infection (which required shunt removal), or superior vena cava occlusion (Faught et al. 1995). Cancer cell implants may occur at the venous anastomotic site, but they will not cause the shunt to fail or hasten the patient's death.

A surgical option for relief of ascites due to portal or hepatic vein ob-struction (not peritoneal carcinomatosis) is a transjugular intrahepatic portosystemic shunt (TIPS). These shunts are used mainly for patients with ascites from hepatic failure due to cirrhosis, but they have been ef-fective for patients with malignant ascites.

DIARRHEA

ETIOLOGY.   Diarrhea is less common than constipation or nausea and vomiting, but is found in 4 to 10 percent of terminally ill cancer patients. Common cancer-related etiologies include newly acquired lactose in-tolerance (e.g., after chemotherapy), drug effects (metoclopramide or excessive laxatives) or side effects (caffeine, theophylline, antibiotics), intermittent bowel obstruction, fecal impaction, sphincter incompe-tence (e.g., due to rectal cancer or spinal cord lesions), chronic radiation enteritis, infection, or products of neuroendocrine tumors. Small-cell lung cancers, for example, can produce vasoactive intestinal peptide (VIP), calcitonin, or gastrin. These and other substances from rarer tu-mors, such as gastrinomas, pheochromocytomas, medullary carcinoma of the thyroid, and especially malignant carcinoid, can cause volumi-nous diarrhea.

THERAPY.   Specific treatment for the conditions noted above is often effective. Even the diarrhea caused by the serotonin and substance P se-creted by carcinoids is often controllable with octreotide (150 to 300 μg SQ b.i.d. or over 24 hours by continuous infusion). Octreotide (500 μg IV or SQ every 8 hours) is also effective if used early in the treatment of diarrhea caused by acute graft-versus-host disease (Ippoliti et al. 1997). The use of simple subcutaneous pumps, or instruction of family mem-bers in the technique of subcutaneous injections, enables patients to be successfully treated at home.

When specific treatment is unavailable or is ineffective, patients can still be treated symptomatically. Rehydrate them orally using a solution of salted, sugared water such as Gatorade, and instruct the patient to avoid fats and milk products until the diarrhea resolves. For the diarrhea itself, use loperamide (Imodium), 4 mg initially then 2 mg after each loose stool, to a maximum of 16 mg / 24 hr. If this is ineffective, try tincture of opium, 15 to 20 drops orally every 4 hours.

NAUSEA AND VOMITING

ETIOLOGY. Nausea and vomiting are often amenable to therapy in cancer patients even when the cause is irreversible. In addition to chemotherapy and radiotherapy, causes of nausea and vomiting include disorders of the eighth nerve or vestibular apparatus, constipation, opioids, disease of the CNS, hepatic or renal failure, gastritis or gastric ulcer disease, gastric outlet or bowel obstruction, hyponatremia, or hypercalcemia.

PRACTICE POINTS: NONPHARMACOLOGIC THERAPY FOR PATIENTS WITH NAUSEA

- Provide frequent, small feedings of cold foods.
- Remove foods with unpleasant smell or visual appearance, even if they were prepared for other family members.
- Serve meals in pleasant, comfortable surroundings.
- Refer the patient for hypnosis or acupuncture.

THERAPY. Reversal of the underlying causes, whenever possible, is recommended. Constipation is a particularly common cause of nausea that can be overlooked, because patients assume they should not have many bowel movements if they are not eating as much. Management of constipation, including that induced by opioids, is reviewed in Chapter 5. For patients with other underlying causes, both nonpharmacologic and pharmacologic methods can be employed.

Families can provide frequent, small feedings of cold foods (which have less odor than warm foods) and remove foods whose sight or smell is unpleasant for the patient. Acupuncture, hypnosis, and progressive relaxation techniques have all shown some effectiveness.

Therapy can often be customized to treat the cause of the nausea (Table 7.3). Prochlorperazine (Compazine) prevents nausea that commonly occurs during the first few days of opioid therapy. Hyoscyamine (Levsin), scopolamine (Transderm Scōp), or meclizine (Bonine, Antivert)

Table 7.3   Pharmacologic Treatment of Nausea and Vomiting

Etiology of Nausea	Drug	Dose
KNOWN ETIOLOGY		
Initiation of opioid therapy	Prochlorperazine (Compazine®)	10 mg p.o. t.i.d. to q.i.d. or 25 mg b.i.d. p.r.
Vertigo	Hyoscyamine (Levsin®)	1–2 tsp. (elixir) or 1–2 tablets p.o./ sublingual/chewed q4h
	Scopolamine (Transderm Scōp)	1 patch q72h
	Meclizine (Bonine®, Antivert®)	25–50 mg t.i.d. p.o.
Delayed gastric emptying	Metoclopramide (Reglan®)	10–20 mg b.i.d. to q.i.d. p.o. or 1–5 mg/hr IV or SQ
Uremia, liver metastases	Haloperidol (Haldol®)	0.5–1 mg t.i.d. p.o., p.r., or SQ
	Prochlorperazine (Compazine®)	5–10 mg p.o. q4–6h or 25 mg p.r. b.i.d. or t.i.d.
Brain metastases	Dexamethasone	10 mg q.i.d. or 40 mg every morning p.o., p.r., or SQ
Anxiety	Lorazepam (Ativan®)	0.5 to 2 mg q4–6h p.o. or sublingual
	Hydroxyzine	25 to 100 mg t.i.d. or q.i.d. p.o.
Bowel obstruction	Octreotide (Sandostatin®)	150–300 µg SQ b.i.d. or 300–600 µg/24 hr continuous SQ infusion
UNKNOWN ETIOLOGY		
	Metoclopramide (Reglan®) +	10–20 mg p.o./SQ/IV q4h or 1 hr before meals +
	dexamethasone	10 mg p.o., p.r., or SQ b.i.d.
Refractory nausea	Dexamethasone +	10 mg p.o., p.r., SQ, or IV b.i.d. +
	metoclopramide (Reglan®) +	60–120 mg SQ or IV in 24 hr +
	Hydroxyzine	50–100 mg t.i.d. p.o., SQ, IV
	or	
	Diphenhydramine	25 mg t.i.d. to q.i.d. p.o., SQ, or IV
	Olanzapine (Zyprexa®, Zydis®)	2.5–5 mg p.o./sublingual q.h.s. to q.i.d.
Nausea still refractory	Ondansetron (Zofran®)	4–8 mg b.i.d. or t.i.d. p.o. or IV
	Granisetron (Kytril®)	1 mg b.i.d. p.o. or IV
	Haloperidol (Haldol®)	1–2 mg p.o. t.i.d. to q.i.d., 2–10 mg IV b.i.d. to t.i.d.
Other	Tetrahydrocannabinol (Marinol®)	2.5–10 mg p.o. b.i.d. to t.i.d.

are very helpful for patients with persistent nausea due to opioids or noninfectious inner ear problems; patients with these problems describe symptoms of motion sickness or may complain that the room is spinning. For gastroparesis not due to opioids, metoclopramide is effective orally (10 to 20 mg b.i.d. to q.i.d.) or by continuous subcutaneous or intravenous infusion (1 to 5 mg/hr). For patients with uremia or liver metastases, try haloperidol (Haldol) (0.5 to 1 mg t.i.d.), prochlorperazine (Compazine) (5 to 10 mg every 6 to 8 hours p.o. or 25 mg every 12 hours p.r.), or olanzapine (2.5 to 5 mg p.o. or sublingual b.i.d. to q.i.d.). For those with brain metastases, try dexamethasone (10 mg q.i.d. or 40 mg every morning if tolerated); and for those with anxiety, lorazepam (Ativan) (0.5 to 2 mg every 4 to 6 hours p.o. or sublingual) or hydroxyzine (Vistaril) (25 to 100 mg t.i.d. or q.i.d.).

TREATMENT-INDUCED NAUSEA AND VOMITING

Chemotherapy-induced nausea and vomiting plagues patients with cancer. Without adequate antiemetic therapy, 60 to 80 percent of patients receiving chemotherapy experience nausea and vomiting. Fortunately, over the past fifteen years advances in the understanding of treatment-related nausea and vomiting have changed the lives of cancer patients, their families, and the nurses and doctors who care for them. When I began my clinical practice, we were sometimes unable to give even curative chemotherapy, such as treatment for testicular cancer, because the available antiemetics were totally ineffective against the side effects induced by such drugs as cisplatin. Many of the cancer cures we now see are attributable to the revolution in the treatment of nausea and vomiting.

While nausea and vomiting continue to plague a minority of patients, we can now prevent both the immediate and the delayed nausea and vomiting in 75 percent of patients receiving the drugs that cause the worst symptoms, and we do much better with drugs that are less toxic (Berger and Clark-Snow 2001). Our patients and their families are suffering less, and our burden, as clinicians, is much lighter.

Certain patients are at significantly higher risk of developing nausea and vomiting when they receive chemotherapy. Patients at highest risk are those who are younger than 60 years of age, or have a history of motion sickness, or are women, particularly women who have had hyperemesis gravidarum (Gralla et al. 1999). Interestingly, alcohol seems to be protective, especially against the emesis induced by cisplatin therapy. Patients who have a history of alcohol intake of more than five alcoholic drinks per day (>100 g of alcohol) tend to have less nausea and vomiting than other patients receiving the same dose of drug and the same antiemetic protection (Berger and Clark-Snow 2001; Sullivan et al. 1983).

PATHOPHYSIOLOGY.   We still do not completely understand how chemotherapeutic agents induce nausea or vomiting. The most likely mechanism for acute and delayed chemotherapy-induced nausea and vomiting is stimulation of a neural network in the medulla oblongata called the central pattern generator. A number of neurotransmitters are thought to be involved, including serotonin, dopamine, and substance P. Drugs that block type 3 serotonin receptors (5-HT_3 receptors), dopamine (D_2) receptors, and neurokinin (NK_1) receptors are able to prevent most chemotherapy-induced nausea and vomiting (Gralla 2002). Vomiting that occurs within a day of receiving the chemotherapy is considered "acute," while that occurring from the second to fifth day after treatment is considered "delayed."

Patients can also develop "anticipatory" nausea and vomiting, as a classic conditioned response. Patients who develop nausea from chemotherapy learn to pair the clinic sights, smells, and sounds with the nausea and vomiting they experience there or shortly thereafter. Having motion sickness (Leventhal et al. 1988; Morrow 1984), being aware of tastes or odors during infusions, being generally anxious, and having acute or delayed chemotherapy-induced nausea or vomiting—all increase the odds of developing anticipatory nausea and vomiting (Andrykowski and Jacobsen 1993; Berger and Clark-Snow 2001).

RISK FACTORS FOR CHEMOTHERAPY-INDUCED NAUSEA AND VOMITING

- History of acute chemotherapy-related nausea or vomiting
- Emetogenicity of drug
- Age <50
- Female sex
- Hyperemesis gravidarum
- Low alcohol intake
- Motion sickness
- Generalized anxiety
- Lengthy infusions
- Awareness of tastes or odors during infusions

Unfortunately, patients with anticipatory nausea and vomiting do not need to be getting chemotherapy to become ill. Simply being in the clinic or even seeing people whom they associate with the clinic can cause them to vomit, even when they're nowhere near the oncology offices. Imagine the scene as I greeted a former patient I encountered unexpectedly at an airport. I watched her smile turn to distress as the conditioned reflex took over! I felt nearly as bad as she did.

THERAPY.   The best way to prevent both anticipatory and delayed nausea and vomiting is to eliminate the acute symptoms by giving aggressive preventive antiemetic therapy before and after the chemotherapy infusion. Fewer than 15 percent of patients who have no acute nausea and vomiting will develop delayed nausea or vomiting; 50 percent of those who do have acute problems will develop delayed vomiting, and 75 percent will have delayed nausea (Roila et al. 2002).

For patients who develop anticipatory nausea and vomiting, I use both nonpharmacologic and pharmacologic approaches. Nonpharmacologic therapies include hypnosis (Redd et al. 1982), progressive muscle relaxation with guided imagery (Buish and Tope 1992), systemic desensitization (Morrow and Morrell 1982), and distraction techniques (Redd et al. 1987). Lorazepam is a particularly useful agent for these patients. It causes amnesia for the events surrounding the chemotherapy and decreases anxiety (Laszlo et al. 1985).

I use the consensus guidelines to choose agents that will prevent

COMPARATIVE COSTS OF ANTIEMETIC DRUGS (FOR ONE CHEMOTHERAPY TREATMENT), 2003

Drug	Days Needed/Chemocycle	No. of Pills	Cost
Reglan (metoclopramide)	2.5	10	+
Compazine	2.5	10	+
Dexamethasone	2.5	10	+
Marinol (dronabinol)	2.5	10	++
Zofran (ondansetron)	3.3	10	++
Kytril (granisetron)	2.5	5	+++
Emend (aprepitant)	3	3	+++

Note: + = ~$10; ++ = ~$150; +++ = ~$250 to $350

or treat patients with acute or delayed nausea and vomiting caused by emetogenic chemotherapy (Koeller et al. 2002). The guidelines recommend basing the choice of antiemetic agent(s) on the emetogenic potential of the chemotherapy or radiotherapy regimen (Table 7.4), the side-effect profile of the antiemetic agent(s), and patient preferences and characteristics. For patients without prescription programs, the cost differences may dictate the outpatient regimen for the days following chemotherapy.

The side effects of the drugs often vary by age. Younger patients have a higher incidence of chemotherapy-induced nausea and vomiting. Therefore, even when they are receiving only moderately emetogenic therapy, we give younger patients a multidrug regimen normally used to prevent symptoms in patients receiving drugs of high emetogenicity (Johnson et al. 1997). Younger patients can tolerate cannabinoids (such as Marinol) better than can older patients and therefore find them more effective (Chang et al. 1979). But patients under 30 years of age receiving metoclopramide have a much higher risk of trismus or torticollis than patients over 30 (27 percent vs 2 percent) (Kris et al. 1983). Elderly patients, on the other hand, have a high risk of extrapyramidal side effects from metoclopramide, and they are more susceptible to the anticholinergic and sedating side effects of the diphenhydramine used to treat them (Johnson 1997). Metoclopramide at high doses, therefore, is too toxic for many patients and has been replaced by the 5-HT$_3$ receptor antagonists.

5-HT$_3$ Receptor Antagonists (Ondansetron, Granisetron, Palonosetron). The 5-HT$_3$ receptor antagonists are extremely effective for patients with acute nausea and vomiting. The most effective of these agents appear to be ondansetron, granisetron, and palonosetron. They are given orally or intravenously, usually along with dexamethasone, to patients receiving moderate or highly emetogenic chemotherapy (Koeller et al. 2002). When these agents are given along with dexamethasone, 75 percent of patients have no vomiting. The newest agent, palonosetron, blocks the 5-HT$_3$ receptor for as long as 40 hours, and may prevent delayed nausea and vomiting. Ondansetron also prevents emesis induced by single- or multiple-fraction radiation therapy (Roberts and Priestman 1993; Scarantino et al. 1992).

Ondansetron and the other 5-HT$_3$ receptor antagonists have far fewer side effects than metoclopramide. Reports of extrapyramidal reactions are very rare (Halperin and Murphy 1992). The side effects often seen

Table 7.4 Emetogenic Potential of Chemotherapeutic Agents

High

Carmustine ($>$250 mg/m^2)	Lomustine ($>$60 mg/m^2)
Cisplatin	Mechlorethamine
Cyclophosphamide ($>$1500 mg/m^2)	Pentostatin
Dacarbazine ($>$500 mg/m^2)	Streptozocin
Dactinomycin	

Moderate

Carboplatin	Hexamethylmelamine (p.o.)
Carmustine	Idarubicin
Cisplatin	Ifosfamide
Cyclophosphamide ($<$1500 mg/m^2)	Irinotecan
Cyclophosphamide (p.o.)	Melphalan
Cytarabine ($>$1 g/m^2)	Mitoxantrone ($>$12 mg/m^2)
Doxorubicin	Procarbazine (p.o.)
Epirubicin	

Low

Aldesleukin (IL-2)	Methotrexate (100 mg/m^2)
Asparaginase	Mitomycin
Cytarabine ($<$1 g/m^2)	Mitoxantrone ($<$12 mg/m^2)
Docetaxel	Paclitaxel
Doxorubicin ($<$20 mg/m^2)	Temozolomide
Etoposide (p.o.)	Thiotepa
Fluorouracil ($<$1000 mg/m^2)	Topotecan
Gemcitabine	

Minimal

Bleomycin	Trastuzumab
Capecitabine	Vincristine
Etoposide	Vinblastine
Methotrexate ($<$100 mg/m^2)	Vinorelbine
Rituximab	

Source: J. M. Koeller, M. S. Aapro, R. J. Gralla, S. M. Grunberg, P. J. Hesketh, M. G. Kris, and R. A. Clark-Snow, Antiemetic guidelines: creating a more practical treatment approach, *Supp Care Cancer* 10:519–522, 2002.

with metoclopramide (i.e., dystonic reactions, akathisia [severe restlessness, "ants-in-the-pants" feeling], sedation, and tardive dyskinesias) do not occur. Patients often develop constipation, and may develop mild headache and elevations in transaminases (Berger and Clark-Snow 2001).

Corticosteroids. We still do not understand how corticosteroids prevent nausea and vomiting. Some have suggested that corticosteroids relieve the cerebral edema induced by chemotherapeutic agents, such as cisplatin (Roila et al. 2002). Corticosteroids can be used either alone, when the chemotherapy has only low or moderate potential to cause vomiting, or as part of the regimen with metoclopramide or a 5-HT$_3$ antagonist (Berger and Clark-Snow 2001) or an NK-1 inhibitor. Dexamethasone and methylprednisolone are the best-studied agents, but no trials have demonstrated the superiority of one corticosteroid over another.

NK-1 Inhibitors. Substance P, a neurotransmitter that plays a key role in the transmission of the pain signal, can also cause vomiting, and it appears to play a role in chemotherapy-related nausea and vomiting. Its effects are mediated through NK-1 receptors. Agents that cross the blood-brain barrier and act as NK-1 inhibitors (e.g., aprepitant) are particularly effective in decreasing the delayed nausea and vomiting occurring after cisplatin chemotherapy (Campos et al. 2001). Aprepitant has few side effects itself. But it is an inhibitor of CYP3A4, and therefore may cause elevations of levels of dexamethasone and chemotherapeutic agents primarily metabolized by this route. Aprepitant can cause significant decreases in the prolongation of INR induced by warfarin. Aprepitant is added both on the day of chemotherapy and for two days after chemotherapy, as part of the regimen to prevent delayed nausea or vomiting (de Wit et al. 2003; Hesketh et al. 2003; Kris 2003).

Other Agents. For patients who are not responding to these drugs alone, adding haloperidol, droperidol, prochlorperazine, scopolamine, or the atypical antipsychotic olanzapine may be helpful (Berger and Clark-Snow 2001; Passik et al. 2002), as discussed earlier in this chapter. Many of these agents, however, have significant side effects. Haldol and droperidol produce dystonic reactions, akathisia, and occasionally hypotension. Transdermal scopolamine causes dry eyes and a xerostomia that can be intolerable. Olanzapine usually has very few side effects, but it does lower the seizure threshold and has been reported (rarely) to cause the neuroleptic malignant syndrome or insulin-resistant diabetes.

Combination Antiemetic Therapy.   For chemotherapeutic drugs with low or moderately low emetogenic potential, you may not need to give anything to prevent nausea, or you might give dexamethasone alone. For drugs of higher emetogenic potential, however, the guidelines recommend combinations of several antiemetic agents along with the agents mentioned above that are designed to treat anxiety, provide amnesia, or prevent known side effects.

The recommended combinations for acute nausea and vomiting include a 5-HT$_3$ receptor antagonist such as ondansetron, a corticosteroid such as dexamethasone, and an optional anxiolytic, such as lorazepam. If a patient has a number of risk factors that put her at high risk for developing delayed nausea and vomiting, or if a patient is receiving highly emetogenic combination chemotherapy that carries with it a significant incidence of delayed nausea and vomiting, aprepitant (an NK-1 inhibitor) might be included in the antiemetic combination to further lower the incidence of acute nausea or vomiting.

For patients at high risk for nausea and vomiting, it is very important to give antiemetic therapy for an adequate period before administering chemotherapeutic agents and to prescribe a regimen such as metoclopramide and dexamethasone for four to five days after chemotherapy to prevent delayed nausea and vomiting, as summarized below. Patients are at high risk if they are receiving one drug that is highly emetogenic

---

PREVENTION OF ACUTE AND DELAYED NAUSEA AND VOMITING

Emetogenic Risk	Day 1 Therapy	Day 2 to Day 4 or 5
High	Dex + 5-HT$_3$RA	Dex + metoclopramide
		or
		Dex + 5-HT$_3$ RA
	(+ aprepitant)	(+ aprepitant day 2, 3)
Moderate	Dex + 5-HT$_3$ RA	Dex

(From Koeller et al. 2002)

Note: Level of risk is based on emetogenicity of the drug and the presence of other risk factors discussed in the text. Aprepitant was not included in the guidelines, but they were written before aprepitant became available. Dex = dexamethasone; 5-HT$_3$ RA = 5-HT$_3$ receptor antagonist.

or two drugs that are moderately emetogenic. Patients who have several of the risk factors listed above can be treated as high risk even if they are receiving only low or moderately emetogenic agents.

BOWEL OBSTRUCTION

A surgical consultation is often indicated for patients with bowel obstruction because palliative surgery can be helpful for selected patients, often those who are not elderly and do not have ascites, previous radiation to the pelvis, or evidence of multiple sites of obstruction. Nasogastric intubation is sometimes required as a temporary measure before surgery, venting gastrostomy, or octreotide provide more definitive relief.

For many patients who are not candidates for surgery, symptoms caused by gastric outlet obstruction can be relieved by using a percutaneous endoscopic gastrostomy (PEG) tube for the venting gastrostomy. To control the associated cramping abdominal pain of patients whose intestinal obstruction is lower, an infusion of opioids, scopolamine (60 mg / 24 hr), and haloperidol (5 mg / 24 hr) has been recommended (Baines 1997). If this regimen does not control the nausea and vomiting

---

PRACTICE POINTS: TREATING BOWEL OBSTRUCTION IN PATIENTS WHO ARE NOT CANDIDATES FOR SURGERY

- Gastric outlet obstruction:
  —Venting gastrostomy (PEG); octreotide.
- Lower intestinal obstruction:
  —Initial: infusion of opioids, scopolamine (60 mg/24 hr) or scopolamine patch, and haloperidol (5 mg/24 hr) for nausea, vomiting, and cramping abdominal pain.
  —Refractory nausea/vomiting: if only a partial bowel obstruction or an ileus, add metoclopramide (1 to 2 mg/hr) and consider discontinuing haloperidol.
  —High-volume vomitus or refractory nausea/vomiting: (1) Discontinue scopolamine and haloperidol and add octreotide 300 to 600 µg/24 hr SQ or (2) discontinue haloperidol and increase rate of metoclopramide; add diphenhydramine (25 mg every 12 hours) and lorazepam (1 to 2 mg t.i.d.) p.r.n. to counter side effects.

and the patient has only a partial bowel obstruction or an ileus, the motility agent metoclopramide (1 to 2 mg/hr) can be added.

For patients with refractory nausea and vomiting or those with large volumes of vomitus, octreotide is a very effective agent. It inhibits secretion of growth hormone, gastrin, secretin, vasoactive intestinal peptide, pancreatic polypeptide, insulin, and glucagon, and blocks the secretion of gastric acid, pepsin, pancreatic enzymes, bicarbonate, and, probably most importantly for these patients, intestinal epithelial water and electrolytes.

A typical patient who would benefit from octreotide is someone with advanced ovarian cancer whose symptoms are due to recurrent bowel obstruction by tumor implants or adhesions. At doses of 150 to 300 μg subcutaneously, twice daily (or 300 to 600 μg / 24 hr continuous SQ infusion), octreotide has produced major improvements in these patients' lives. In about 3 days (range, 1 to 6 days), it eliminated the nausea and vomiting in all patients for whom it was tried and decreased the volume of nasogastric drainage dramatically. In one patient, the volume decreased from 2 liters to 100 ml. Over half of the treated patients improved enough that they could spend their last days at home (Mercadante 1994).

Nausea and Vomiting of Unclear Etiology

Symptomatic therapy is used to treat nausea of unclear etiology. Metoclopramide (Reglan) (10 to 20 mg p.o./SQ/IV every 6 hours or 1 hour before meals) is recommended as a first-line empirical nausea treatment. At this dose, it is associated with few side effects. If nausea persists, add dexamethasone (10 mg p.o. or SQ b.i.d.). Olanzapine is an atypical antipsychotic agent often used to treat delirium. This agent blocks the receptors of a number of neurotransmitters, including dopamine and serotonin. A series of case reports indicate that it is effective against nausea of unclear etiologies and does not cause extrapyramidal side effects. Doses start at 2.5 mg at bedtime and can be increased to 5 mg four times as needed.

If the patient remains nauseated 48 hours after the dexamethasone is added, continue the oral or subcutaneous dexamethasone and increase the metoclopramide dose, administering it as a continuous IV or SQ infusion of 60 to 120 mg over 24 hours. For patients who still do not have a satisfactory response, add a third drug: hydroxyzine (Vistaril) (50 to 100 mg t.i.d.), ondansetron (Zofran) (4 to 8 mg p.o. b.i.d. to t.i.d.), granisetron (Kytril) (1 mg p.o. b.i.d.), haloperidol (Haldol) (1 to 2 mg p.o. b.i.d. to q.i.d.), or diphenhydramine (Benadryl) (25 mg t.i.d. to q.i.d.). The latter is also useful for patients who develop extrapyramidal reactions from the infusion of metoclopramide. Ondansetron and granisetron have no associated extrapyramidal reactions but can induce constipation and a dose-related headache.

To give a combination of antiemetics subcutaneously, metoclopramide (30 mg) + haloperidol (Haldol) (1.5 mg) + promethazine (Phenergan) (6.25 mg) can be safely infused over 24 hours. Rectal combination preparations of these agents are also used.

For patients who do not mind the associated alterations in mental status, dronabinol (tetrahydrocannabinol) (Marinol) (2.5 to 10 mg p.o. b.i.d. to t.i.d.) can be a very effective oral antiemetic. Unfortunately, its absorption is somewhat variable.

RESPIRATORY PROBLEMS

Dyspnea

Dyspnea is frightening to patients with advanced cancer and to their families, who fear they will die a death of suffocation. It creates significant problems in about 40 percent of these patients. In the National Hospice Study (Reuben and Mor 1986), dyspnea was found to occur in as many as 70 percent of cancer patients at some time during their last six weeks of life. You may miss the dyspnea if you rely solely on observing tachypnea. In one study of hospice patients, 77 percent of patients reported dyspnea, but only 39 percent had their dyspnea charted (Thomas and von Gunten 2003).

PATHOPHYSIOLOGY.   Dyspnea is mediated by (1) J-receptors at the junction of capillaries and alveoli, which respond to alveolar fluid or to microemboli; (2) mechanoreceptors in the lungs, airways, and chest wall that respond to stretch; (3) peripheral chemoreceptors in the aorta and carotid bodies that respond to hypoxemia; and (4) central chemoreceptors that respond to increases in carbon dioxide. When the CO_2 rises to 75 mm Hg, endorphins are released centrally, causing the dyspnea to abate and the patient to become somnolent.

Patients experience dyspnea in one of three situations: when breathing requires more work (e.g., with interstitial lung disease or pleural effusions); when the patient is hypercapnic; and when the brain perceives less ventilation than it "expects" from the amount of work being done to provide the ventilation. The brain receives input on the work the muscles are doing, and "expects" a certain amount of return on the investment in terms of flow rate of air. When there is less air flow than expected, the patient experiences dyspnea.

ETIOLOGY.   In 25 percent of patients with dyspnea, no specific cause will be identified, but muscle weakness or anxiety may contribute. In the other 75 percent, a thorough physical exam and a few simple tests (e.g., chest x-ray, electrolytes, complete blood count, and pulse oximetry) are likely to reveal the cause of the dyspnea. The most common etiologies are pulmonary or cardiac pathology, ascites, anemia, and superior vena cava syndrome.

Pericardial effusions and tamponade are particularly subtle causes of dyspnea in cancer patients. Tumor infiltrating the pericardium causes it to become thick and rigid, and even a small amount of fluid can significantly impair cardiac filling. Because of the rigidity of the invaded pericardium, chest films may show a normal heart size even when tamponade is present. Thus I have a very high index of suspicion when a patient with known mediastinal disease—or, more commonly, with a left-side pleural effusion even after the fluid is drained—remains anxious and dyspneic.

Superior vena cava syndrome is most often seen in patients with lung cancer, though lymphoma and other cancers each cause about 10 percent of cases, with a smaller contribution from clotted indwelling central venous catheters. In addition to dyspnea, patients may have headache or blurred vision and appear plethoric, with facial, neck, and upper extremity edema in advanced cases. Chest films reveal disease in the right upper mediastinum, and radionuclide or MRI studies show compression of the superior vena cava with decreased flow.

THERAPY.   Anxious patients are likely to benefit from both pharmacologic and nonpharmacologic therapies. Lorazepam (0.5 to 2 mg every 4 to 6 hours p.o. or sublingual), clonazepam (0.5 to 1 mg p.o. at bedtime), or the other agents listed in Table 7.1 are helpful to decrease anxiety in the average patient. For very anxious patients or patients in an uncontrolled panic due to a perceived inability to breathe, give midazolam (0.2 to 0.5 mg IV very slowly), or morphine (5 to 10 mg IV or by nebulizer), or another opioid at an equivalent dose, or chlorpromazine (25 mg p.o. or IV). Relaxation techniques or formal hypnotic imagery may be very effective adjuncts. They can be taught to the patient by skilled practitioners, including members of the hospice team. Medical practitioners of hypnosis are listed in the directory of members of the American Society for Clinical Hypnosis (140 North Bloomingdale Road, Bloomingdale, IL 60108-1017; telephone: 630-980-4740; fax: 630-351-8490; e-mail: info@asch.net).

When possible, and as appropriate, reverse the specific medical cause of the dyspnea. Because dyspnea can be so distressing, I have recommended somewhat aggressive attempts to reverse the underlying process, even for patients with only months to live. About 70 percent of patients with superior vena cava syndrome, for example, will respond to radiation therapy for a median of about 3 months. High-dose corticosteroids are also usually included; they are tapered after a week if no benefit is observed or are tapered after the end of the radiation treatments. Blood transfusion may be tried for hypoxia due to anemia, and pericardiocentesis or pericardial window for pericardial effusion. Oxygen is indicated even for patients who retain CO_2 to maintain an oxygen saturation of 88 to 90 percent (pO_2 of 55 to 60 mm Hg).

Reversing obstruction of bronchi, blood vessels, or lymphatics also decreases dyspnea. External beam or endobronchial radiation therapy, laser treatments, cryotherapy, and stents all can reopen blocked bronchi. For some patients whose bronchial obstruction is not relieved in this way, radiation therapy still relieves the dyspnea, possibly by decreasing compression of the surrounding blood vessels and lymphatics. High-dose corticosteroids (e.g., Solu-Medral 80 mg IV three times daily) can help some patients with lymphangitic tumor spread.

Pleural effusions are a frequent cause of dyspnea in patients with lung or breast cancer, but can occur in patients with various kinds of cancer. For patients who are not physically active, symptoms can often be controlled with supplemental oxygen and/or opioids.

Others, however, will achieve relief only when the effusions are drained. Because the effusion reaccumulates within one month in 97 percent of treated patients, most patients with malignant effusions will need more than a simple thoracentesis. Sclerotherapy has been done with bleomycin (Moffett and Ruckdeschel 1992) and doxycycline, but talc slurries have been shown to be most effective (Shaw and Agrawal 2004). The chemotherapeutic drug mitoxantrone (40 mg) is another effective sclerosing agent. Infused after chest tube drainage, mitoxantrone induced a complete remission in all 20 patients in which it was used, and none experienced fluid reaccumulation in the ensuing two months (Morales et al. 1995).

Some patients have such extensive effusions or such a high rate of fluid production that the pleural space cannot be drained dry enough for a sclerosing agent to be effective; in others, despite adequate drainage, the lung will not reexpand. The quality of life of such patients may be severely impaired by the effusions or the collapsed lung. For those with a reasonable life expectancy (e.g., patients with breast cancer or lymphoma), a surgical procedure may be helpful.

Some surgeons believe that for patients who can tolerate general anesthesia, an open procedure is indicated; they can decide at surgery whether to use talc pleurodesis or to insert a pleural catheter. If, after the fluid is drained, the lung reexpands fully, the surgeon uses talc as an irritant. This has been successful in preventing recurrent effusions in over 90 percent of those undergoing such a procedure. If, however, the lung does not reexpand, the surgeon inserts a pleural catheter (Pleurx).

In one randomized trial, the Denver Pleurx Pleural catheter was as effective as a chest tube and sclerosis in improving dyspnea and quality of life in patients with malignant effusions (Putnam et al. 1999). The Pleurx catheter is a 15.5 French silicone catheter with a fenestrated length of 24 cm and a polyester cuff to reduce infection risk. The catheter's fenestrated end is situated in the pleural space, and several inches of its midportion, including the cuff, are tunneled subcutaneously, leaving the end of the catheter and valve exposed so that the patient can drain the fluid. Patients use a special drainage kit as often as their effusion requires.

In the trial, patients with these catheters went home much earlier (median length of hospitalization, 1 day vs 6.5 days; $p < .0001$). The patient drained the pleural fluid at home; spontaneous pleurodesis occurred in 46 percent (median time, 29 days). Complications of insertion occurred in 10 percent (10 of 96 patients). Three patients each had fever or pneumothorax, two had misplacement of the catheter, one had reexpansion pulmonary edema, and one had hypercapnic respiratory failure from oversedation. Late recurrences (21 percent), pain severity, and early inpatient complications (10 to 14 percent) were similar in both groups. Several subsequent reports have also confirmed the safety and utility of these catheters (Pollak 2002).

For the 25 percent of patients for whom no specific cause of dyspnea can be identified, symptomatic treatment is still possible. For these patients and for those in whom we cannot reverse the underlying cause, a variety of therapies will significantly relieve their distress (Table 7.5).

Something as simple as sitting in front of an open window or having a fan blowing air softly onto the face provides significant relief for some. For opioid-naive patients, low doses of hydrocodone or other opioid can be tried. The most useful treatment, even for patients taking high doses of systemic opioids, is oral or nebulized opioid. The opioid is often combined with dexamethasone. Typical starting doses are 2.5 to 5 mg of morphine given orally; or for nebulized therapy, 2.5 to 5 mg of preservative-free morphine or 1 mg of hydromorphone (Dilaudid) and 2 mg of dexamethasone in 2.5 ml of 0.9 percent saline every 4 hours as needed. If wheezing is present, albuterol (0.5 ml) can be added as well. The mixture is given by a nebulizer using room air or oxygen at 5 to 6 liters/min through an open face mask.

The opioid dose should be increased as needed until the dyspnea is relieved. Reports from the Leicestershire Hospice indicate that doses of up to 50 mg have been used. In some individuals, inhaled morphine causes bronchospasm (Ahmedzai 1997). Administration of the first dose should therefore be observed by a nurse or other clinician who can provide antiasthma treatment if needed.

For patients who develop these side effects, fentanyl, which does not induce bronchial histamine release, can be substituted for morphine. Nebulized fentanyl (25 µg in 2 ml of saline) was shown to improve oxygenation and decrease respiratory rate in a convenience sample of 35 cancer patients (i.e., all patients who agreed to participate in the trial) (Coyne et al. 2002). Ninety-one percent reported improvement in breathing within five minutes of the treatment, and that improvement lasted at least an hour. Small doses of nebulized opioids are thought to be effective because the opioids act directly on opiate receptors in the large airways. However, the Cochrane review found no benefit for nebulized opioids over other routes of delivery (Jennings et al. 2001).

COUGH

ETIOLOGY.   Cough, present in about 40 percent of patients with advanced cancer, is caused by many of the same disorders that cause dyspnea. It is mediated by stimulation of the vagus nerve by receptors in the pharynx, larynx, and upper airways and by airway opiate receptors.

Cough can occur in patients with postnasal drip, infection, heart failure, asthma / chronic obstructive lung disease, or esophageal reflux, or in those who are taking ACE inhibitors. Specific cancer-related causes include both obstruction of the airway and disorders of swallowing. Swallowing disorders can be due either to injuries of the ninth and tenth cranial nerves from tumor invasion or to carcinomatous meningitis. Because the normal pharyngeal muscle relaxation does not occur, such patients can aspirate their routine secretions, and cough can be their most troubling symptom.

THERAPY.   Specific therapies for the non-cancer-related causes listed above are usually very effective. Laser or radiation therapy may resolve a distressing cough due to an airway obstruction. For those without an obstruction whose cough is productive, chest physical therapy, humidity, and suctioning can help.

Various pharmacologic agents for symptomatic treatment of cough are listed in Table 7.5. Hyoscyamine (Levsin) or scopolamine (Transderm Scōp) can decrease excessive secretions. For patients who cough because of tenacious mucus, nebulized saline, albuterol (0.5 mg in 2.5 mg of normal saline), or terbutaline have been helpful, while expectorants and mucolytics have not. Since ipratropium worsens this problem, discontinue it when possible.

When specific therapy is unavailable or ineffective, oral opioids are the most effective nonspecific therapies for cough. Sweet elixirs containing dextromethorphan or one of the opioids used for mild pain are recommended as initial therapy, but methadone syrup, if available, can be very useful.

For more resistant coughs, higher doses of oral or nebulized opioids (see Dyspnea, above) may be needed. In addition, nebulized anesthetics (e.g., 2 ml of 2 percent lidocaine in 1 ml of normal saline for 10 minutes) can be given up to three times a day. Unfortunately, the anesthetics cause patients to lose their gag reflex temporarily. To avoid aspiration, ask patients to fast for about one hour after a nebulized anesthetic treatment. Since some patients develop bronchospasm after nebulized anesthetics, the first dose should be taken under close observation.

Hemoptysis

While 50 to 70 percent of patients with lung cancer complain of hemoptysis, it is a problem for only about 25 percent of those admitted to hospice. But despite its relative rarity, hemoptysis is one of the most frightening symptoms that patients experience. Letting the family know what to do should the hemoptysis worsen and advising them to use red

Table 7.5 Symptomatic Treatment of Dyspnea, Cough, and Hiccups

Cause	Drug	Dose
Dyspnea from anxiety/panic	Lorazepam (Ativan®)	0.5–2 mg p.o. or sublingual q4–6h
	Clonazepam (Klonopin®)	0.5–1 mg p.o. h.s. or b.i.d.
	Midazolam (Versed®)	0.2–0.5 mg IV slowly or 0.1–3 mg/hr SQ
	Morphine[1]	5–10 mg IV, p.o., or by nebulizer
	Chlorpromazine (Thorazine®)	25 mg p.o., p.r., or IV
Dyspnea— other etiology	Hydrocodone	5 mg q4h p.o. or SQ; titrate upward as needed
	Morphine[1]	15 mg q4h p.o. or SQ; titrate upward as needed
	Morphine[1] + dexamethasone (nebulized)	2.5–5 mg morphine + 2 mg dexamethasone in 2.5 ml normal saline q4h
		Can add albuterol (0.5 ml) if wheezing is present
Cough	Dextromethorphan elixir	15–30 ml q6h p.o. p.r.n.
	Hyoscyamine (Levsin®)	1–2 ml (drops) or 1–2 tablets p.o./ sublingual/chewed q4h
	Glycopyrrolate (Robinul®)	0.1–0.2 mg IV t.i.d. to q.i.d.
	Scopolamine (Transderm Scōp®)	1–3 patches q72h
	Codeine	30–60 mg q4h p.o.
	Morphine[1]	5–20 mg q4h p.o.
	Albuterol	0.5 mg in 2.5 mg normal saline
	Nebulized lidocaine	2 ml of 2% lidocaine in 1 ml of normal saline, for 10 min
	Nebulized morphine[1] + dexamethasone	2.5–5 mg morphine + 2 mg dexamethasone
Hiccups	Metoclopramide (Reglan®)	10–20 mg t.i.d. or q.i.d. p.o., p.r., or 10 mg q4h IV
	Proton pump inhibitor	Dosing variable
	Chlorpromazine (Thorazine®)	25–50 mg IV once; then 25–50 mg t.i.d. p.o. or p.r.
	Haloperidol (Haldol®)	2–10 mg/day p.o. p.r., or 0.5–2 mg IV q4h
	Sertraline	50–100 mg/day p.o.
	Baclofen (Lioresal®)	5–10 mg p.o. b.i.d. to 20 mg t.i.d.
	Nifedipine	10–20 mg p.o. t.i.d.

[1]Other opioids may be substituted for morphine. Begin with equipotent dose of the other opioid and titrate to effect.

or dark-colored bedding and towels, on which the blood is less apparent, may lessen their anxiety. (For a discussion of the management of patients with massive hemoptysis, see Chapter 8.)

As in patients without cancer, hemoptysis in cancer patients may be due to bronchitis, pneumonia, or a pulmonary embolism. In patients with cancer of the head and neck or lung, however, it is often due to cancer recurrence. Even for patients who have previously received radiation treatment, small amounts of additional radiation can control the bleeding in almost 90 percent. Bronchial lavage with iced saline, topical epinephrine, topical fibrinogen-thrombin solutions, balloon tamponade, and laser therapy may also be helpful. Embolization of the portions of the bronchial artery involved has been found to be particularly effective for patients with bronchiectasis and inflammation, but over half of the cancer patients embolized also stopped bleeding (Hayakawa et al. 1992). The optimal therapy for a given patient, therefore, may depend both on the site of bleeding and on the radiation, pulmonary, and angiographic expertise that is available.

HICCUPS

Hiccups are embarrassing and exhausting and interfere with a patient's ability to eat, drink, and sleep.

ETIOLOGY.   Patients with gastroesophageal reflux disease (GERD) or gastric compression are at the greatest risk of developing intractable hiccups. Hiccups also may occur in patients whose vagus or phrenic nerves are injured (anywhere in their course) or who have certain metabolic derangements (especially uremia, but also hyponatremia or hypocalcemia). Patients can develop hiccups as a side effect of benzodiazepines, barbiturates, progesterone, anabolic steroids, intravenous corticosteroids, or, more rarely, chemotherapy (e.g., cisplatin) or hydrocodone. Occasionally, you will find a previously unidentified ear infection, pharyngitis, or esophagitis, which, if treated effectively, may end the hiccups, as may treating ascites, pneumonia, pleuritis, or pericarditis.

THERAPY.   The nonpharmacologic treatments are those we've all used: granulated sugar, drinking from the far side of a glass, rubbing the back of the neck with a cool cloth, holding one's breath, or doing a Valsalva maneuver while breath-holding. For selected patients with intractable hiccups, phrenic nerve block (e.g., with bupivacaine) or lysis may be required, but these treatments are rarely needed. Some pharmacologic treatments are listed in Table 7.5. Metoclopramide is usually very effective. Hiccups due to GERD respond to proton pump inhibitors. For patients who cannot take oral medications, give up to 10 mg intravenously every 4 hours; for those who can, start with 10 to 20 mg three to four times a day. Chlorpromazine (Thorazine) (25 to 50 mg IV, then p.o. or p.r. t.i.d.) is very effective (80 percent "cure"), but it causes significant postural hypotension. Haloperidol (Haldol) (2 to 5 mg p.o. or p.r. or 0.5 to 2 mg IV) is probably equally effective but safer in older patients. Nifedipine (10 to 20 mg p.o. t.i.d.), sertraline (50 to 100 mg/day p.o.), and baclofen (5 to 10 mg p.o. t.i.d.—may be increased as needed) are also effective.

SKIN PROBLEMS

Fungating Lesions

Fungating lesions from cancers growing out through the skin can cause embarrassment, shame, and profound loss of self-esteem, especially for patients who previously were proud of their appearance. Not only are they painful, but the associated discharge and odor can be so offensive that even family members find it hard to remain near the patient.

Primary skin cancers and cancers of the head and neck that become refractory to chemotherapy and radiation can cause fungating skin lesions, as can metastases. Patients with breast cancer are particularly prone to develop skin metastases on the chest wall or scalp, but they also occur in about 10 percent of those with renal cancer and 5 percent of those with other cancers. Chemotherapy and radiation should be considered when the metastases first appear, as these treatments can be very effective, especially in reducing bleeding. Surgery should also be considered as a palliative measure, especially in recurrent breast cancer and extensive melanoma metastases.

SYMPTOMATIC TREATMENT.   While these wounds rarely heal completely, symptomatic treatment is often effective for tumors that are refractory to specific modalities. Pain from ulcerating lesions has been successfully relieved using a morphine-infused IntraSite gel (0.1 percent w/w solution) placed on the ulcerated surface and covered with sterile gauze (Twillman et al. 1999). Skin care protocols and tables of wound care products are included in the *Oxford Textbook of Palliative Medicine, Principles and Practice of Supportive Care in Oncology* and *Handbook of Palliative Care in Cancer* (see General References in this chapter's bibliography). Hospitals and visiting nurse associations have policies and guidelines, as well. Specially trained advanced-practice nurses are also valuable resources in caring for patients with decubitus ulcers, tumor metastases, skin infections, and other chronic skin wounds. Sarah Kagan, M.S.N., C.R.N.P., a colleague of mine who is a geriatric nurse practitioner and wound care expert, and Ilene Fleisher and Diane Bryant, certified enterostomal therapy nurses, have generously contributed material for the recommendations that follow. For additional questions, use your visiting nurse association as a resource.

PRACTICE POINTS: CARE OF FUNGATING SKIN LESIONS

- Keep the wound clean.
- Gently debride it.
- Use antibiotics.
- Control bleeding.
- Control odor.
- Relieve pain.
- Apply the correct, layered dressing.

Wound Cleaning.   Keep the wound clean by irrigating it with sterile saline, lactated Ringer's, or homemade saline solution (1 tsp. of salt dissolved in 1 pint of boiled water), or by showering. For wounds that are colonized with anaerobic organisms, consider applying metronidazole intravenous solution by gentle irrigation (e.g., pouring or through an irrigation syringe) or by applying gauze sponges soaked in metronidazole gel.

Debridement.   Debride the wound gently, using continuous moist saline dressings. For dry but purulent tissue, use an enzymatic debriding ointment (e.g., collagenase, Accuzyme) or a gel such as Debrisan. Debrisan is composed of polysaccharide dextranomer granules, which can be poured in a clean, moist wound and covered with a semiocclusive dressing. The granules will draw the bacteria and dead cells up out of the wound.

For wet, heavily exudative wounds, with or without colonization or obvious infectious findings, use absorptive dressings, which include hydrofibers, collagen, and calcium alginates, hydrophilic foams, and cadexomers/polymers. These are widely available under many trade names, including Aquacel, Hydrofiber wound dressing, Kaltostat, Sorbsan, Iodosorb, and Allevyn. Avoid hypertonic saline dressings, which would, literally, put salt in the wound. To prevent the exudate from macerating the tissue, providing a medium for infection and embarrassing the patient, use absorbent foam topped by a thick gauze pad and an alginate dressing. The alginate dressings do not have to be removed; they wash off during bathing (von Gunten 2002).

Antibiotics.   Consider adding topical or systemic antibiotics. Aerobic bacteria can easily superinfect fungating tumors. *Staphylococcus aureus* and other common pathogens often respond to topical antibiotics such as triple antibiotic ointment or mupirocin. Gram-negative organisms may be more prominent in anogenital areas, and you may need to recommend silver sulphadiazine cream and potassium permanganate sitz baths to prevent recurrent infection. Anaerobes respond to topical metronidazole; fungus to Nizoral or other ketoconazole creams; and painful viral lesions to acyclovir ointment.

Control of Bleeding.   Widespread oozing can be controlled with a sucralfate paste, made by mashing a 1-g tablet in a small amount of water-soluble gel. Gauze soaked in 1:1000 epinephrine solution, Gelfoam soaked in thrombin, Avitene, topical thromboplastin (100 µg/ml), or Surgicell can also be used. Silver nitrate sticks should be reserved for isolated bleeding points. Nonadherent, moist dressings can often decrease oozing by diminishing the trauma associated with dressing changes.

Control of Odor.   Eliminate the bacteria that are causing the odor, which are mostly anaerobic. Despite its toxicity to the skin and newly budding capillaries, you may consider using a disinfectant solution such as quarter strength Dakin's or 1 percent chlorhexidine gluconate as a first measure. Unfortunately, while these solutions are not expensive, they can cause discomfort and are not always effective. Most cases also require more expensive therapies: metronidazole gel (0.75 percent) applied to the lesion, along with oral metronidazole (200 to 400 mg p.o. t.i.d.) if needed. Metronidazole has been shown to be totally effective in 50 percent and reasonably effective in an additional 45 percent of patients for whom it was used.

Topical aromatherapeutics can be mixed into a bland base (e.g., vitamin A and D ointment) to provide odor control and a sense of well-being. Essential oils for first-line, nontoxic use are lavender (soothing, deodorizing); tea tree oil (antimicrobial, cleansing); and peppermint (deodorizing, cleansing). These should be added to the base at 10 to 30 drops per ounce.

If cost is an issue or metronidazole gel is not available, try applying Maalox, which may also relieve burning. Natural remedies such as applying yogurt or buttermilk, which prevent growth of odor-forming bacteria, or powdered sugar or honey, which compete with the bacteria for water, have also been effective in controlling odor. The yogurt can also relieve burning. One-quarter percent menthol may also be added to a bland base for topical antipruritic use on intact skin.

Pain Relief.   A series of case reports suggests that topical opioids may relieve the pain of skin ulcers (Twillman et al. 1999). Morphine-infused IntraSite gel (0.1 w/w solution or 1 mg morphine / 1 ml IntraSite gel) is spread on a clean ulcer, then covered by a 4 × 4 inch gauze dressing; or the gel is placed on the dressing, which is then applied to the wound to cover the entire ulcerated wound surface. New gel is applied when dressings are changed (usually twice a day). In the study, the concentration of morphine was increased when needed to 0.15 percent. Eight of the nine patients with severe pain from these ulcers reported complete pain relief for the duration of the treatment. No side effects were noted. A double-blind placebo-controlled trial is planned.

Wound Dressing.   Wound dressings serve a number of purposes. They allow the removal of excess exudate, bacterial toxins, and dead skin cells; maintain a moist, clean environment; are relatively impermeable to bacteria; and provide comfort and protection from further injury. Unless the patient is neutropenic or there is a reason to use sterile technique, clean technique can be used, including clean gloves, for dressing changes at home.

For a dressing to accomplish all this, it must be made up of layers with different functions. The material closest to the skin should be sterile, should allow exudates to pass through it, and should not stick to the skin. Hydrocolloid dressings (Duoderm, Granuflex, hydrogel, Xeroform) are particularly useful if there is little exudate, because they are nonadherent and provide pain relief; alginate dressings (Kaltocarb, Kaltostat, Aquacel hydrofiber) are better for a large amount of exudate. The middle layer should be absorbent, and the outer layer should be a charcoal dressing (e.g., Carboflex) to absorb odor. To minimize trauma to the lesion, ask the family and the nurses to change the dressings only when they are no longer absorbent or are not controlling the odor. The best way to remove them is to soak them off.

Pressure Ulcers

Pressure ulcers in terminally ill cancer patients have the same causes as those in other bed-bound patients: pressure leads to ischemia of the skin due to injury to the vascular, lymphatic, and other interstitial transportation structures. Friction, maceration, and shear forces contribute to vulnerability to pressure injury. Pressure ulcers occur most often in areas of bony prominence, especially the ischium and sacrum.

PREVENTION.   Prevention of pressure ulcers is often possible, and we can educate the family in how it is done. Whenever possible, I try to arrange for a physical therapist to visit the patient's home to teach the health aides and family to provide the physical care the patient will need.

The goal is to minimize the time the patient lies or sits in one position, being particularly careful to relieve pressure over bony prominences. Multiple bed pillows can be used for the frequent repositioning. Bed cradles, elbow and heel pads, and wheelchair cushions are all useful in an individualized plan of care. Maintaining adequate nutrition and hydration are of course helpful, but not always possible in this population. Multivitamin and mineral tablets or supplemental vitamin C (1000 mg/day) and zinc (220 mg/day) can be added to the diet of those unlikely to obtain enough from food.

Of course, the chair or mattress on which the patient lies is of particular importance, especially if the patient is very old, thin, or immobile and therefore at high risk for developing pressure ulcers. It may be worthwhile to have a consultant evaluate the need for a pressure-relieving mattress. Some devices, for example, have air cells that alternately inflate and deflate. The choice of mattress will depend on the patient's needs and what the patient can afford. The AHCPR guidelines on prevention and treatment of pressure ulcers categorize the available options by efficacy. Medicare will pay for category I products for patients who have stage II to III ulcers and category II products for those with stage IV ulcers.

THERAPY.   As with fungating wound lesions, nursing protocols are available for the treatment of all stages of pressure ulcers; sources, including the 1994 AHCPR guideline on pressure ulcers, are given at the end of the chapter. Some general treatment principles are outlined below. Local care should be directed toward prevention and comfort. Topical care techniques described for fungating skin lesions can also be used for pressure ulcers in palliative care. New hope for resolution of pressure ulcers appeared in 2003 with the report of dramatic healing of grade 3 to grade 4 pressure ulcers of the foot by nerve growth factor applied directly to the ulcer (Landi et al. 2003). Terminally ill patients were excluded from this study, however.

Preventing Contamination; Minimizing Shear Forces. Polyurethane films or hydrocolloid dressings (e.g., Tegaderm, Duoderm) can be used as dressings for pressure ulcers that are neither necrotic nor infected and need only a moist environment to heal. As with dressings over fungating lesions, the caregiver or nurse should change these only when necessary.

PRACTICE POINTS: TREATING PRESSURE ULCERS

- Prevent contamination and minimize shear forces.
- Protect the wound and promote healing.
- Eliminate or control infection, and debride.

Protecting the Wound; Promoting Healing. If the pressure ulcers are infected or have necrotic tissue, sterile normal saline irrigation is needed, and enzymatic agents (Elase, Travase, Accuzyme, Santyl [collagenase], streptokinase) can remove the eschar. As with fungating lesions, hydrocolloid dressings (Duoderm, hydrogel xeroform, Granuflex) are used if there is little exudate; alginate dressings (Kaltocarb, Kaltostat, Aquacel hydrofibers) are used if there is a large amount.

Eliminating or Controlling Infection; Debridement. Polysaccharide dextranomer granules (Debrisan) can be poured in a clean, moist wound and covered with a semi-occlusive dressing. They will draw the bacteria and dead cells up out of the wound. Unlike the other dressings, this should be cleaned and reapplied daily until the wound is clean and appears to be healing. If odor is a problem, a charcoal dressing (Carboflex) will be needed.

PRURITUS

ETIOLOGY. It was formerly thought that itch and pain were mediated by the same receptors. This turns out not to be the case. Itch-specific nerves have been found in both the peripheral and central nervous systems (Oaklander et al. 2003). Injury to these nerves, such as occurs in herpes zoster infections—especially those of the face—can cause a pathologic itch rather than pain. Chemical mediators of pruritus include histamine (H_1, not H_2, receptors) and serotonin (5-HT_2 and 5-HT_3 receptors).

Why scratching relieves an itch is still not entirely understood, but inducing pain in the area of the itch eliminates the itching sensation. Scratching does activate myelinated A-delta sensory fibers, which temporarily stops the pruritus. Additionally, the common itching that accompanies epidural opioids arises from opioid-induced inhibition of only the pain pathways. And the pruritus that accompanies liver failure may be mediated by a similar selective blockade by endogenous opiates, because it responds to naloxone or naltrexone.

But the vast majority of pruritus in advanced-cancer patients is not due to injury of the "itch" nerves. Rather, it is caused by the same conditions and illnesses that occur in people without cancer: dry skin, allergic reactions to drugs, uremia, cholestasis, or psychological stress. In addition, the pruritus can be caused by opioids, skin involvement with cancer, or a paraneoplastic process, such as is seen in patients with Hodgkin's disease and cutaneous lymphomas. Patients with myeloproliferative disorders also itch. They have increased numbers of cutaneous mast cells that can be activated by heat or other stimuli to produce pruritus.

PRACTICE POINTS: RELIEVING PRURITUS
- Patients should bathe with lukewarm water and avoid bath products containing deodorants or perfumes.
- Skin should be kept moist and fingernails short.
- Cooling or anesthetic creams may be applied.
- Oral antihistamines or NSAIDs may be needed.

I generally advise any patient with pruritus to keep the skin moist by frequent lubrication, cut fingernails short, and avoid all bath products that contain perfumes or deodorants. The baths themselves should be lukewarm, or oatmeal baths can be tried. Cooling the skin with menthol-containing creams (one-quarter percent menthol), camphor, peppermint, colloidal oatmeal lotions, or ice packs can provide symptomatic relief, as can calamine lotion or Caladryl (a combination of calamine lotion and Benadryl) and topical anesthetics (benzocaine, ELA-Max, EMLA). TENS machines have also been used by some patients to good effect.

Antihistamines (e.g., diphenhydramine [Benadryl]) will help when the cause of the itching is histamine release. If the pruritus results from biliary obstruction, internal stenting or radiation to obstructing nodes in the porta hepatis often relieves the pruritus for as long as the patient lives. If the obstruction cannot be relieved, cholestyramine (Questran), the SSRI paroxetine (Paxil), the 5-HT$_3$ receptor antagonist ondansetron, or methyltestosterone may be effective. Paroxetine is also helpful for patients with paraneoplastic or opioid-induced pruritus. Ondansetron is also effective for opioid-induced pruritus, and is also used for patients with myeloproliferative diseases such as polycythemia vera, as well as for those with renal failure. Mirtazapine, which is an H$_1$, 5-HT$_2$, and 5-HT$_3$ receptor antagonist, has also been reported to relieve pruritus in patients with cholestasis, advanced Hodgkin's and non-Hodgkin's lymphomas, and renal failure.

PRACTICE POINTS: SYMPTOMATIC THERAPY OF PRURITUS

Etiology	Therapy
Histamine release	Diphenhydramine
Cholestasis	Cholestyramine; paroxetine; ondansetron; mirtazapine; methyltestosterone
Paraneoplastic process	Paroxetine; mirtazapine
Opioids	Paroxetine, ondansetron, naloxone, naltrexone
Myeloproliferative process	Ondansetron
Renal failure	Ondansetron; mirtazapine

Doses: Diphenhydramine 25 to 50 mg p.o. every 8 hours; paroxetine 10 to 20 mg/day p.o.; ondansetron 8 mg p.o. b.i.d. to t.i.d.; mirtazapine 15 mg p.o. h.s.; methyltestosterone 25 mg sublingual b.i.d. for 7 to 10 days.

Oral antihistamines are probably the best nonspecific relievers of pruritus, but they may cause excessive daytime sedation. If sedation occurs, try a combination of antihistamine and pseudoephedrine. NSAIDs are occasionally useful because prostaglandins at least partially mediate pruritus. Opioids, on the other hand, are not: as discussed above, they may induce pruritus. Naloxone infusions (0.2 μg/kg/min) can, in fact, alleviate the pruritus due to primary biliary cirrhosis, but controlled trials have not been performed in cancer patients. Paroxetine

(Paxil), an antidepressant that is an SSRI (like fluoxetine [Prozac]), was effective in five patients with pruritus arising from a variety of etiologies. Dosing ranged from 5 to 30 mg/day (Zylicz et al. 1998).

INSOMNIA

To meet the official criteria for insomnia, a patient must have either difficulty falling asleep (i.e., taking more than 30 minutes) or difficulty staying asleep (when in bed trying to sleep, actually asleep less than 85 percent of the time) (Savard and Marin 2001). This problem must occur at least three times a week and must affect the patient's function in the daytime. Patients may have transient insomnia (lasting a month or less), short-term insomnia (1 to 6 months), or chronic insomnia (longer than 6 months). Insomnia occurs in one-third to one-half of people with advanced cancer. These patients usually do not report difficulty falling asleep, but they have trouble staying asleep.

The sleeplessness can often be more troublesome to the patient's family than to the patient, but, whether patients recognize it or not, lack of sleep can be contributing to their distress in a number of ways. At a minimum, they will feel much as we did when, as residents, we were up all night on call. But in addition, sleep deprivation may exacerbate pain and increase a patient's chance of becoming depressed.

ETIOLOGY. Patients who are terminally ill have numerous reasons for sleepless nights. Among them are many of the problems I have already discussed—pain, depression, anxiety, delirium, dyspnea, nocturnal hypoxia, nausea and vomiting, or pruritus, or hot flashes from estrogen deficiency. Medications that can cause insomnia include corticosteroids and antiemetics (prochlorperazine, metoclopramide, 5-HT$_3$ receptor antagonists) (Savard and Marin 2001). Patients' sleep-wake cycle may be somewhat reversed, because they are inactive and napping much of the day and then not sleepy at night. If they are severely iron-deficient or uremic, are taking tricyclic antidepressants, or have a peripheral neuropathy, they may also be wakened by restless leg syndrome. For some people, very small doses of caffeine or alcohol may be enough to keep them awake at night.

THERAPY. Insomnia may be treated either nonpharmacologically or with medications.

**PRACTICE POINTS: NONPHARMACOLOGIC THERAPY
FOR INSOMNIA**

- Psychological, legal, or spiritual counseling for concerns contributing to insomnia
- Eliminating daytime naps
- Going to bed at a set time
- If awake 30 minutes later, doing some relaxing activity in or out of bed
- Instruction in biofeedback, relaxation therapy, or hypnosis

---

When appropriate, I ask patients to consider professional counseling. I find that sleepless patients are somewhat more willing to explore some of the psychological, financial, and spiritual implications of their illness and to accept help in resolving them. A visit from the lawyer to finalize a will, from the hospice team to reassure the patient that his family will be supported through his final days, or from the rabbi or parish priest can often solve the problem and end the sleepless nights.

If these efforts are not sufficient, I next recommend techniques developed by sleep experts for patients without cancer. I encourage patients not to nap during the day and to remain out of bed as long as possible. I suggest that they go to bed and get up at a set time, no matter how tired they are. And I recommend that, if they do not fall asleep within thirty minutes, they engage in some relaxing activity, either out of or in bed. Progressive muscle relaxation or other forms of relaxation therapy, biofeedback, and hypnosis using imagery have been shown to be helpful as a component of short-term management, particularly for patients who cannot get to sleep or cannot regain sleep after they've awakened in the night. If they are willing, I teach patients these techniques and give them a tape that they can play to help them relax and fall asleep.

Medications can alleviate insomnia when these other approaches are ineffective (Table 7.6). Data from controlled trials indicate that benzodiazepines, antidepressants, zolpidem (Ambien), and, in one trial, melatonin are effective agents. I try to choose an agent that specifically addresses the cause of the insomnia. I have already discussed the treatment of pain, anxiety, and depression. For patients who develop nighttime delirium that is keeping them and their families awake, oral queti-

Table 7.6   Pharmacologic Treatment of Insomnia

Cause	Drug	Dose
Anxiety	Lorazepam (Ativan®)	0.5–2 mg p.o. h.s.
	Clonazepam	0.5–1 mg p.o. h.s.
Delirium	Olanzapine (Zyprexa®)	2.5–5 mg p.o. h.s.
	Haloperidol (Haldol®)	0.5–2 mg p.o. up to 10 mg p.o. in p.m.
	Quetiapine (Seroquel®)	25–50 mg p.o. h.s.
Menopausal symptoms	Venlafaxine (Effexor®)	37.5–75 p.o. b.i.d.
Restless leg syndrome		
Idiopathic	Dopamine agonists	
	Pramipexole (Mirapex®)	0.125 mg/day p.o.; increase by 0.125 mg q. 2–3 days as needed
	Levodopa-carbidopa (Sinemet®)	25/100 mg; 1–2 tabs. qhs
Painful	Gabapentin (Neurontin®)	100–300 mg p.o. h.s.
Other	Clonazepam (Klonopin®)	0.5–1 mg p.o. h.s.
Unknown	Oxazepam (Serax®)	10–20 mg p.o. h.s.
	Temazepam (Restoril®)	15–30 mg p.o. h.s.
	Trazodone (Desyrel®)	50–100 mg p.o. h.s.
	Zolpidem (Ambien®)	5–10 mg p.o. h.s.

Source: C. J. Early, Restless leg syndrome, *New England Journal of Medicine,* 348: 2103–2109, 2003.

apine (Seroquel) is useful. For older patients, start with 25 mg at bedtime; younger patients can tolerate initial doses of 50 mg at bedtime. Olanzapine (Zyprexa) (2.5 to 5 mg p.o. at bedtime) or haloperidol (e.g., Haldol) (beginning at 0.5 to 2 mg p.o. and increasing as needed to 5 mg), given before the onset of the agitation and repeated if needed during the night, are usually very effective. For those with restless leg syndrome, I use clonazepam 0.5 to 1 mg orally, or gabapentin 100 to 300 mg orally.

When you cannot determine the cause of the insomnia, oxazepam (Serax), 10 to 20 mg, or temazepam (Restoril), 15 to 30 mg, are usually effective, because they help people stay asleep. Initial doses should be low for the older or the cachectic patient or for those taking the medication sublingually, as blood levels are higher when the drug is taken by this route. Some older patients develop paradoxical agitation from benzodiazepines. Trazodone may be useful for them.

WEAKNESS AND FATIGUE

Fatigue is even more prevalent than pain in patients with metastatic cancer, but much less research has been done to define its pathophysiology, etiology, or effective therapy. The NCCN cancer-related fatigue treatment guidelines (version 1.2003) define fatigue as a "persistent, subjective sense of tiredness related to cancer or cancer treatment that interferes with usual functioning. Compared with the fatigue experienced by healthy individuals, cancer-related fatigue is more severe, more distressing, and less likely to be relieved by rest." A number of fatigue assessment tools are used by those doing research on the epidemiology, etiology, and therapy of fatigue. These researchers have documented that half of the patients being treated for acute leukemia or non-Hodgkin's lymphoma have severe fatigue, and almost all patients receiving chemotherapy or radiotherapy (96 percent) or in the terminal phases of cancer suffer from fatigue.

The treatment guidelines include recommended screening and evaluation protocols, and separate intervention guidelines for patients under active treatment, undergoing long-term follow-up, or at the end of life. The screening guidelines are similar to those for patients with pain, which is also a subjective experience and can be validly quantified. The guidelines recommend, as for pain, assessment on a 0 to 10 scale ("No fatigue" to "Worst fatigue imaginable"), expert multidisciplinary evaluation, and education and training of professionals and family members. Patients who scored greater than 7 were found to have a "dramatic decrease in physical functioning." The NCCN guidelines recommend further evaluation for any patient with a fatigue level of >4.

Identifiable, and sometimes even reversible, causes of fatigue can be found for some patients (Table 7.7), though the mechanism(s) by which they produce fatigue is not known. Pain, anxiety, depression, and insomnia are important causes of generalized weakness and fatigue. Drug side effects; pulmonary, renal, hepatic, or cardiac failure; infection; under- or overactive adrenal or thyroid function; and certain neurologic problems—all can present as generalized weakness, and the weakness may resolve if the causes can be reversed.

If no specific cause of fatigue is identified, or the therapy is ineffective, I would try the psychostimulant methylphenidate. The NCCN guidelines support its use, and a preliminary report of patient-adjusted dosing in a nonrandomized trial suggested benefit for a majority of

Table 7.7   Treatment of Weakness and Fatigue

Cause	Drug/Procedure	Dose
Anemia	Transfuse	
Renal failure	Erythropoietin (Epogen®) + iron	50–150 U/kg SQ t.i.w.
Cancer/treatment related	Erythropoietin (Procrit®) + iron	40,000–60,000 U SQ q. week
	Darbepoetin-α (Aranesp®) + iron	200–300 µg q 2 weeks SQ
Hypercalcemia	Pamidronate (Aredia®)	60–90 mg IV over 2 hr
	Zoledronic acid (Zometa®)	4 mg IV over 15 min
	Calcitonin	4–8 IU/kg SQ or IM q6–12h
	Gallium nitrate	100–200 mg/m²/day IV over 5 days
Hyponatremia		
SIADH	Demeclocycline (Declomycin®)	300 mg p.o. b.i.d. to q.i.d. until Na⁺ normal; 600–900 mg/24 hr p.o. maintenance
Adrenal replacement with tumor	Hydrocortisone + fludrocortisone (Florinef®)	20 mg every morning, 10 mg every evening + 0.05–0.15 mg/day p.o.
Hypokalemia from ectopic ACTH	Octreotide (Sandostatin®)	100–500 µg b.i.d. SQ
	Aminoglutethimide (Cytadren®) Metyrapone Mitotane (Lysodren®)	Consult with oncologist/endocrinologist
Hypoglycemia		
Insulinoma	Glucagon	Consult with endocrinologist
Mesenchymal tumors	Debulking surgery	
Anorexia	Adjust diet/supplements	
	Megestrol acetate (Megace®)	400 mg b.i.d. p.o.
	Dexamethasone	0.75–1.5 mg q.i.d. p.o., IV
	Prednisone	5 mg t.i.d. p.o.
	Methylprednisolone	16 mg b.i.d. p.o.
	Dronabinol (Marinol®) (δ-9-tetrahydrocannabinol)	2.5–7.5 mg t.i.d. p.o.
Anorexia and depression	Mirtazapine (Remeron®)	15 mg qhs
	Methylphenidate	2.5–10 mg p.o. 8 a.m. and noon

patients within seven days, and no serious side effects. Patients used up to 20 mg/day in divided doses. Modafinil (Provigil), an agent approved for narcolepsy, has not yet been assessed for its effect on fatigue. It is recommended for opioid-induced sedation (American Pain Society 2004). (*APS Guideline: Principles of Analgesic Use in the Treatment of Acute Pain and Cancer Pain*, 5th edition.)

EATON-LAMBERT SYNDROME

The Eaton-Lambert syndrome is a very rare complication of lung cancer that can cause weakness. Patients with this syndrome experience a sort of "reverse myasthenia": they get stronger, instead of weaker, as the day progresses. It affects the proximal muscles most prominently and sometimes remits when the cancer remits. It can persist, however, or recur. Plasmapheresis and agents that promote neurotransmitter release such as guanidine hydrochloride (125 to 500 mg p.o. t.i.d.) have been helpful.

ANEMIA

Blood transfusion was shown to improve strength in a group of anemic patients studied in palliative care units in the United Kingdom, but the mechanism is unclear (Gleeson and Spencer 1995). The patients' hemoglobin levels ranged from 4.9 g/dl to 10.7 g/dl before transfusion, but the degree of anemia did not correlate with improvement after transfusion. Those with a pretreatment hemoglobin level of >7.9 g/dl showed as much overall benefit as those with hemoglobin of ≤7.9 g/dl.

Patients whose anemia is caused only by renal insufficiency respond to erythropoietin (50 to 150 U/kg t.i.w.) and oral iron supplementation. Some patients with cancer or a diseased marrow (e.g., myelodysplasia) will also respond. Even patients who are on chemotherapy, whose disease is stable or in complete or partial remission, experience an improved quality of life for each gram/deciliter, with maximum effect between 11 and 12 g/dl. Erythropoietin did not, however, improve the fatigue or weakness of patients with progressive disease. For cancer patients who do not have progressive disease, whose anemia is otherwise unexplained, and whose hemoglobin level is <12 g/dl, a two-month trial of erythropoietin therapy may be warranted. The regimen is expensive and requires subcutaneous injections weekly, or every three weeks, of erythropoietin dosed according to a fixed or weight-based dosing regimen, along with supplemental oral iron for optimal response, even if total body iron stores are increased.

METABOLIC ABNORMALITIES

Cancer-related metabolic abnormalities that can present as weakness include hypercalcemia, hypomagnesemia, hyponatremia, hypokalemia, hyperglycemia, and hypoglycemia (Table 7.7).

HYPERCALCEMIA.   Hypercalcemia is a common complication of cancer. Prior to the widespread use of bisphosphonates to slow the development of metastases, it reportedly occurred in 10 to 40 percent of cancer patients at some time in the course of their illness. Subtle personality changes, fatigue, anorexia, or increased constipation may be the only presenting features, but many patients or their families will, on close questioning, report polyuria, nausea, increased sedation, difficulty concentrating, or symptoms typical of delirium. The severity of symptoms correlates more closely with the speed with which the hypercalcemia developed than with the absolute level of serum calcium. Mental status changes may not resolve for several weeks following normalization of serum calcium.

PRACTICE POINTS: CANCER-RELATED HYPERCALCEMIA

- Patients should be monitored for subtle signs and symptoms, especially nausea, increased constipation, and mental status changes.
- Severity of symptoms correlates with speed of development of hypercalcemia, not absolute level of calcium.
- Mental status changes may not resolve for several weeks following normalization of serum calcium.
- Adequate hydration and weight-bearing activity should be encouraged.
- Initial therapy is hydration and intravenous bisphosphonate, with furosemide only after the patient is fully rehydrated.
- Patients with refractory tumors or those who do not wish to receive tumor-directed therapy should be referred to hospice. Median survival is 30 days.

Hypercalcemia in patients whose disease is refractory to chemotherapy, or for whom no chemotherapy is planned, is associated with a median survival of only about one month. This grim prognosis should be taken into consideration when planning therapy for these patients; hospice care should be offered, if this has not yet been done. Treatment for symptomatic hypercalcemia can be covered by the hospice benefit.

Bony metastases may cause mild hypercalcemia, which can sometimes be reversed by hydrating the patient well and making sure she takes in adequate amounts of salt. Thiazide diuretics, which contribute to the hypercalcemia, should be discontinued. Activity is also helpful, since bone resorption from the metastases is increased when the patient is immobile and hypercalcemia can result.

In 80 percent of cancer patients with hypercalcemia, however, parathyroid hormone–related peptide is the cause. Specific pharmacologic therapy is usually required in addition to rehydration and furosemide diuresis. Pamidronate (Aredia) (60 to 90 mg IV over 2 hours) or zoledronic acid (Zometa) (4 mg IV over 15 minutes) given in the outpatient setting will reverse hypercalcemia caused by tumor production of parathyroid hormone–related peptide or by bone metastases within 24 to 48 hours. Pamidronate is preferred for patients with renal insufficiency. A normal calcium level is often maintained for several weeks to a few months. For patients with severe hypercalcemia, adding calcitonin (4 to 8 IU/kg SQ or IV every 6 to 12 hours) speeds normalization of the calcium levels. When the calcium level is normal, additional doses of intravenous pamidronate or zoledronic acid can be given, but after several months they tend to lose their effect. The second-line agent, plicamycin (25 μg/kg), is no longer available. Plicamycin sclerosed veins and led to serious tissue damage if it infiltrated the skin. It was given by someone skilled in administering sclerosing agents.

After repeated dosing, the effectiveness of plicamycin also waned. For selected patients, therefore, consider giving gallium nitrate. It can be given only once and requires a five-day continuous intravenous infusion (100 to 200 mg/m^2/day) with intensive hydration. It is expensive and may cause renal damage, but it reverses the hypercalcemia in 80 percent of cases. Unfortunately, as with the other agents, the hypercalcemia will eventually recur.

Corticosteroids are effective in reversing hypercalcemia only for patients with steroid-responsive tumors, such as multiple myeloma or some lymphomas, or the very rare lymphoma that is producing 1,25-dihydroxy vitamin D.

HYPOMAGNESEMIA.   This may be caused by diuretics or may persist as a residual side effect of chemotherapy with platinum derivatives. If you cannot modify the diuretic therapy, oral replacement with magnesium oxide (400 mg daily or b.i.d.) usually is effective.

HYPONATREMIA.   In patients with lung cancer, hyponatremia is most likely due to ectopic production of antidiuretic hormone (ADH). This syndrome of inappropriate antidiuretic hormone secretion (SIADH) can be treated by fluid restriction, but for patients with advanced cancer I prefer to give demeclocycline, an agent that induces pharmacologic diabetes insipidus. Begin with 300 mg/day twice a day, increasing to four times daily until the sodium normalizes. Maintenance doses are 600 to 900 mg/day orally. Escalating the dose slowly minimizes the gastrointestinal toxicity, and it is otherwise well tolerated and very effective.

Rarely, hyponatremia is due to Addison's disease. Metastases from some tumors (especially lung cancers) replace the adrenal gland and cause adrenocorticoid insufficiency manifested by hyponatremia and hyperkalemia. Oral hormone replacement with hydrocortisone (20 mg p.o. every morning and 10 mg p.o. every evening) plus fludrocortisone (Florinef) (0.05 to 0.15 mg p.o.) is usually adequate.

HYPOKALEMIA.   Hypokalemia may result from diuretics used to treat edema or, very rarely, from ectopic production of adrenocorticotropic hormone (ACTH). If octreotide, which suppresses production of ectopic ACTH, is not effective, one of a variety of agents that ablate the adrenals (i.e., aminoglutethamide, metyrapone, mitotane) can reverse the hypokalemia. Patients who undergo attempted pharmacologic adrenal ablation need careful monitoring and, if the procedure is successful, hormone replacement.

HYPERGLYCEMIA AND HYPOGLYCEMIA.   A common complication of the high-dose corticosteroid therapy needed by patients with spinal cord or brain metastases is *hyperglycemia,* which responds to standard diabetic regimens. *Hypoglycemia* resulting from insulin-producing islet cell tumors is rare, but other, non-islet cell tumors can also impair hepatic gluconeogenesis and cause hypoglycemia. One-fifth of these tumors are hepatomas, and about two-thirds are of mesenchymal origin (i.e., mesotheliomas, fibrosarcomas, leiomyosarcomas, neurofibrosarcomas, and hemangiopericytomas).

Frequent oral feedings of simple carbohydrates often help patients with insulin-producing tumors, but intravenous infusions of glucagon and/or glucose through indwelling central catheters or PICC lines may be required. For patients with large tumors of mesenchymal origin who require high-dose intravenous dextrose infusions to control their hypoglycemia, palliative debulking surgery should be considered.

ANOREXIA AND MALNUTRITION

Anorexia is a common complication of cancer, occurring in as many as 85 percent of people with advanced disease. If it is part of a syndrome of depression, accompanies an infection or a gastrointestinal disturbance, is from a metabolic derangement (e.g., hypercalcemia), or is a side effect of a drug that alters the taste of food (e.g., metronidazole), the anorexia may be reversible. But in many patients with advanced cancer, anorexia occurs with no definable cause. Symptomatic treatments include frequent and appetizing meals; supplements; appetite enhancers; and parenteral/enteral feeding (Table 7.7).

MEALS AND SUPPLEMENTS.   Exploring with the patient ways to make meals more appealing, and supplying booklets containing recipes and relevant nutritional information for patients with advanced cancer, can increase caloric intake by about 500 calories a day. For example, substitutes can be offered for meat, which is often distasteful: nuts or nut butters, or protein powders added to drinks such as milkshakes or blended fruit combinations containing, for example, ice, bananas, and orange juice. Patients can be advised to avoid eating large amounts of low-calorie foods and to change to a "grazing" style, eating several small meals a day. I usually ask patients to take a multivitamin pill so that they can eat what they want and not worry about maintaining a "balanced diet." Some patients may like nutritional supplements (e.g., Ensure, Sustacal, Resource), but others may prefer the taste of some of the powdered breakfast drinks dissolved in extra-rich milk for additional calories or, for those with lactose intolerance, in lactose-reduced milk.

There is no demonstrated benefit, however, to forcing meals or intake of these high-calorie supplements. Within a month after dietary counseling, most patients have returned to their previous caloric intake.

Several medications can act as *appetite enhancers*. Megestrol acetate (Megace) (400 mg b.i.d.) can improve appetite and cause weight gain, which may be important to patients who are concerned about their appearance. It usually does not improve strength, however, as there is no increase in muscle tissue; and, if the weight gain is excessive, it may even impair the patient's activity. A two-week trial is adequate; if there is no change in appetite or weight in that time, the agent can be discontinued. Megace can cause subclinical and, rarely, clinically apparent adrenal suppression, which manifests as adrenal insufficiency if the drug is discontinued. Stress corticosteroid doses should thus be given to patients recently withdrawn from Megace who develop a severe medical illness or are to undergo surgery.

Oxandrolone is an oral testosterone derivative that has been shown in several nonrandomized studies to increase weight in patients with HIV/AIDS. A recent prospective descriptive study demonstrated that in addition to increasing body weight, patients taking oxandrolone increased their body cell mass and their lean soft tissue mass. Patients took 10 mg orally, twice daily. Average weight increases were small (e.g., weight increase of 2.6 kg ± 3 kg; lean soft tissue mass increase of 3 kg ± 2.9 kg) but statistically significant, and were associated with improved quality of life (Earthman et al. 2002). A similar improvement in patients taking oxandrolone (10 mg p.o. b.i.d) was noted in an open-label study of 131 cancer patients who were losing weight. Results of a randomized double-blind placebo-controlled trial are not yet available (Tchekmedyian et al. 2003). Nandrolone is an androgenic anabolic steroid that has proved effective in reversing the weight loss of patients on dialysis or patients with AIDS, but there are not enough data on patients with cancer to recommend its use.

In randomized double-blind crossover trials, corticosteroids (e.g., 0.75 to 1.5 mg of dexamethasone q.i.d., 5 mg of prednisone t.i.d., or 16 mg of methylprednisolone b.i.d.) improved patients' appetites and food intake for a month or even two, but at the cost of significant side effects and no increase in weight or change in nutritional status.

Dronabinol (δ-9-tetrahydrocannabinol) (2.5 to 7.5 mg t.i.d.—also available by suppository) has been particularly effective in improving the appetites of patients with AIDS, but its side-effect profile limits the population that finds it useful. A prospective uncontrolled study of patients with advanced cancer showed that appetite was improved, but almost one-quarter of the patients could not tolerate the side effects of even the lowest dose (i.e., 2.5 mg b.i.d.). Mirtazapine (Remeron) at low doses (15 mg p.o. at bedtime) improves appetite. Olanzapine (Zyprexa) (2.5 to 5 mg p.o. at bedtime) decreases nausea and can improve appetite. No data are available on whether either of these drugs produces a weight gain.

Adenosine triphosphate (75 μg/kg IV infusion for 30 hours every 2 to 4 weeks) helped patients with stage 3B or 4 non–small cell lung cancer maintain their body composition and minimally increase their weight. The study was randomized but not blind or placebo-controlled (Agteresch et al. 2002).

Cyproheptadine and hydrazine sulfate, though initially promising, are no longer recommended. No significant increases in appetite, food intake, or weight were noted in several randomized placebo-controlled trials.

ENTERAL/PARENTERAL FEEDING.   This is most useful early in the course of illness, when patients are undergoing surgery, chemotherapy, or radiation therapy. If a patient cannot eat or absorb food because of gastrointestinal disease resulting from cancer or its treatment, I often recommend invasive techniques to provide nutrition, especially if the process is expected to respond to therapy.

Some patients undergoing radiation treatment for lung cancer, for example, may be aspirating because of recurrent laryngeal nerve paralysis. Others may be receiving combination chemo-radiotherapy for cancer of the head and neck or to relieve an esophageal obstruction. Such patients are very likely to benefit from a nasogastric feeding tube or a feeding gastrostomy or jejunostomy for several months until the paralysis or obstruction resolves. Continuous feeding (e.g., over 12 hours in the evening and while the patient sleeps) is usually well tolerated and, unlike bolus feeding, does not induce diarrhea. If diarrhea does occur, it can usually be managed by diluting the hypertonic preparations or changing to a supplement with a different formulation.

The tubes are placed in the patient either in the hospital or in a short-procedure unit, and the family is taught how to use them. Often, patients can give themselves the feedings, usually by continuous drip while they sleep. I find it helpful to arrange for a home nursing visit to ensure that everyone is using the equipment correctly and knows when to call with problems.

Parenteral nutrition similarly benefits patients who cannot use the enteral route, but whose cancer is otherwise stable or slowly progressive. Parenteral nutrition, however, is not indicated in the vast majority of cancer patients. Though patients will often take in more calories and gain weight, routine use of parenteral nutrition does not decrease chemotherapy-induced complications, prolong life, or reduce perioperative morbidity or postoperative mortality. Selected populations (e.g., bone marrow transplant recipients, severely malnourished patients, and those undergoing hepatectomy for hepatocellular carcinoma) may benefit.

Patients with far-advanced cancer are unlikely to benefit either from a feeding tube or from parenteral nutrition. They rarely complain of hunger or thirst, and small amounts of water or food satisfy them. Nevertheless, they may ask for enteral or parenteral nutrition because they associate their lack of food or water intake with their weakness or lethargy. Unfortunately, while malnutrition can contribute to weakness, reversing malnutrition does not lead to marked increase in strength or energy in patients with extensive, refractory disease. The reasons for this are unclear.

Rarely, even after I explain this, some patients or their families are still interested in enteral or parenteral nutrition. For some families, this is because they harbor one of the hidden concerns I discussed earlier: feelings of personal rejection because the patient does not want to eat; a sense that the patient has given up and will be abandoning them when they are not ready to let her go; or a feeling that the patient does not love them enough to continue the fight.

Others may not fully understand the implications of receiving an enteral device and being fed with tube feedings. The complications that may ensue from enteral feeding via feeding tube, gastrostomy, or jejunostomy are listed below (adapted from Ahronheim 1996).

Problems Related to the Feeding Device or Its Placement
- Discomfort
- Dislodgment
- Nasal, esophageal, gastric, or intestinal erosions or perforations
- Bleeding
- Peritonitis
- Abdominal wall leakage or cellulitis
- Ileus or bowel obstruction
- Pneumothorax
- Complications of the anesthesia required for placement
- Initiation of restraints on patient mobility

Problems Related to the Solutions Infused
- Electrolyte disturbance
- Bloating
- Regurgitation
- Aspiration
- Diarrhea

When patients and their families understand both the limited benefits and the magnitude of the problems enteral feeding can cause, it becomes much less attractive.

Parenteral feeding is likewise fraught with complications both during catheter insertion (e.g., pneumothorax, hemorrhage) and later (e.g., bacterial and fungal infections, catheter occlusion and migration leading to superior vena cava syndrome). It has not been shown to prolong life for these patients, but studies are more than ten years old. Until more studies are done, I suggest helping patients carefully weigh the burdens and benefits of this therapy.

COPING STRATEGIES

When the weakness is not reversible, it is useful to give the patient and his family some strategies for dealing with it.

PRACTICE POINTS: HELPING PATIENTS COPE WITH WEAKNESS AND FATIGUE

- Encourage patients to spend time out of bed.
- Advise patients to obtain equipment that will help them maintain mobility.
- Encourage patients to continue the activities that are most important and to relinquish others.
- Encourage sensory, intellectual, and interpersonal stimulation.
- Provide emotional support to family members who are distressed by the patient's symptoms.

Patients may mistakenly think that going to bed for a time will help them regain their normal strength, as it did in the past when they had another illness. It is important to advise them to minimize the time they spend in bed so as to maximize their remaining strength. Exercise was effective in reducing fatigue in a series of breast cancer patients undergoing chemotherapy (Miaskowski and Portenoy 2002). Selected patients may benefit from physical therapy consultation.

Patients can maintain mobility by renting the portable equipment that is now available: walkers, wheelchairs, lift-chairs, electric hospital beds, tray-tables, and commodes or shower chairs. Many insurance companies cover these rentals, and eligible veterans can use them free of charge.

Commonsense advice like planning for short rest periods during the day, limiting trips, and delegating exhausting chores can be surprisingly helpful. It is often hard for people to relinquish these tasks, especially if the tasks helped define their role in the family. You or your staff can often assist patients in identifying which of these tasks are most important to them and which they wouldn't mind delegating: cooking, for example, may be more important than shopping; reading the bedtime story as satisfying as giving the nighttime bath.

For those who are bedridden, sensory, intellectual, or interpersonal stimulation is still important. Listening to music, reading, or drawing can be encouraged. Or you can urge the family to take out of the library, rent, or purchase books on tape or videos, or encourage other family members or friends or hospice volunteers to drop by to reminisce, play games, or read to the patient.

A friend of mine was even more imaginative. One Saturday, she turned her mother's hospital room into a picnic site complete with a hamper and Italian delicacies. On another occasion, for a holiday meal, she brought formal linens and tableware and arranged a conference call so her mother could join the rest of the family in the festivities.

It helps me to remember that, in most cases, the weakness is not troublesome to the patient, who often is living a very satisfying life despite what others may see as disabling limitations. Families are much more likely to be suffering because of the changes in the patient than is the patient himself. The family members are often the most in need of our help.

ROLE OF HOSPICE PROGRAMS

Patients in hospitals, nursing homes, or inpatient hospice facilities have 24-hour nursing and physician coverage to help alleviate their symptoms. But about 20 percent of patients prefer and are able to be cared for, and to die, at home. Their families, who provide much of their care, often find this a particularly difficult time. Families of patients dying of cancer share a number of needs (Cherny et al. 1996). They include:

- Comfort for the patient
- Information and communication
- Evaluation of the family's needs and resources

- Education about care
- Emergency provisions
- Review of how the family is coping
- Care of the family when the patient is unconscious
- Preparation of the family for the dying process
- Conflict resolution

The members of a hospice team can help physicians to meet all these needs. Hospice nurses and social workers are superb problem-solvers who have developed detailed treatment strategies that are usually very effective in managing the complex symptoms of patients with advanced cancer. As I discussed in Chapter 3, hospice teams anticipate family concerns, and analyze and develop solutions for patients' and families' psychological, social, financial, and spiritual needs. Medical and nursing care are also expertly delivered. Nurses from the team make the needed assessments, and they educate the family in techniques of care and ensure that the appropriate medications, supplies, and services are obtained to provide optimal patient comfort.

Hospice nurses make routine home visits as often as needed and are a source of information and of communication from the family to the physician or other caregivers. Some patients require only weekly visits; others may need a nurse daily; and a few will need 24-hour nursing. Nurses bring medications and supplies, including emergency provisions, prepare the family for the dying process, and help support the family if the patient becomes unconscious.

Hospice programs have nurses available 24 hours a day, and a nurse will make a home visit at any time for emergencies. Hospice nurses serve the very important role of being with the family at the bedside as the patient dies, adjusting the patient's medications, and reassuring the family that everything possible is being done; they will also talk with the family immediately after the death to offer comfort and to assess and attempt to alleviate any persistent concerns.

The Medicare hospice benefit pays for all these services: personnel, medications, durable medical equipment, supplies, and any other authorized services needed to provide patient comfort (e.g., a surgical consultation to debride a wound). Some people are reluctant to elect this benefit because they misunderstand several of its provisions. For example, patients may think they have to give up their private physician. That is not true: patients can continue to see their own physician, who is allowed to bill for professional services separately under Medicare Part B, as before. And patients can be hospitalized if they develop a problem requiring an inpatient stay for management of a symptom, such as rapidly escalating pain or severe delirium. Hospice programs are required to offer four levels of care: routine home care, continuous home care (24-hour nursing), respite care, and inpatient care. And hospice programs have contracts with local hospitals so that they can continue to provide continuous care at whatever site the patient requires it.

Portions of the hospice services are available to patients without the Medicare hospice benefit. Private insurance, managed care plans, and Medicaid programs offer a variety of hospice benefits, and the indigent will be cared for as well. Your local hospice agencies, some of which are nonprofit, others for-profit, will be happy to inform you of the range of services they can provide. If you have other questions, contact the Hospice Association of America (228 7th Street SE, Washington, DC 20003; telephone: 202-546-4759).

ROLE OF THE PALLIATIVE CARE TEAM

But some patients may not feel "ready" for a hospice program. Others may have become accustomed to an intensity of supportive care (e.g., total parenteral nutrition, or transfusions) that they or their family feel contributes significantly to their quality of life. These services may not be available from the local hospice programs. In such circumstances, palliative care teams can work with the primary oncology team and the home nursing agency that offers a "bridge" to hospice, to meet the needs of patients and their families.

Like hospice teams, palliative care teams address all the domains of distress of patients with cancer and their families. While some palliative care teams are involved only with patients near the end of life, others work with patients at any point along their disease trajectory (diagnosis, relapse, or terminal care). They can provide both consultation and primary clinical care. Most teams are hospital based, but a few provide care to outpatients in physicians' offices, in home consultations, or in concert with a hospice run by the same organization (Billings and Pantilat 2001; Gazelle et al. 2001; Nelson and Walsh 2003).

Unfortunately, the majority of hospitals and academic centers do not have palliative care services. As shown by data from a 1998 American

Hospital Association (AHA) survey, only 36 percent of AHA members had a palliative medicine service and only 15 percent an end-of-life service (Pan et al. 2001). In 2000, a survey U.S. teaching hospitals (26 percent were part of or associated with a medical school; 53 percent had only residency training programs) revealed that only 18 percent had a palliative care consultation service, 19 percent had an inpatient unit, and 22 percent had a hospice affiliation. While 49 percent had a pain service, only 23 percent of these had either a palliative care consultation service or an inpatient unit. An additional 20 percent were planning palliative care programs (Billings and Pantilat 2001).

The paucity of palliative care teams likely relates more to the economics of supporting them than to questions about their efficacy, given that most such teams are hospital supported (Billings and Pantilat 2001). Recent descriptions of the work done by palliative care teams in the United States and elsewhere indicate that they are seeing significant numbers of patients in acute care facilities, some of which have separate inpatient palliative care units (Gazelle et al. 2001; Jenkins et al. 2000; Ng and von Gunten 1998; Pierucci et al. 2001; Santa-Emma et al. 2002; Smith et al. 2003; Virik 2002).

Palliative care teams almost always include nurses (usually nurse practitioners) and physicians (Billings and Pantilat 2001), and some also include social workers, chaplains, pharmacists, bereavement counselors, and volunteers (Billings and Pantilat 2001; Ng and von Gunten 1998). These multidisciplinary or interdisciplinary teams offer assessment and management of physical and psychological causes of distress, patient and family education, and counseling, problem solving, and support for the family. If the patient and family do not have access to an oncology social worker as part of their primary team, the palliative care team's social worker can be of particular help for patients in the last months.

Reports on the efficacy of these teams are mostly from uncontrolled studies, but they do indicate positive effects on patients' physical symptoms, improved satisfaction, and, with a palliative care unit, decreased hospital costs and resource utilization (Gazelle et al. 2001; Manfredi et al. 2000; Smith et al. 2003). A systematic quantitative review of the impact of palliative care teams on the end-of-life experiences of patients and their families found evidence for a small benefit; the benefit of team care was strongest when the team was working with patients in their homes (Higginson et al. 2003).

The palliative care team is a useful partner to the primary oncology team in both the inpatient and the outpatient setting. The palliative care team often gets to know the patient and family early in the course of the disease, when asked to help manage a difficult symptom. With the benefit of having worked with the patient and family over weeks to months, the palliative care team can more easily assist the primary oncology team during difficult family meetings, and remain to answer questions that the patient or family may have forgotten to raise with the primary oncologist. Palliative care team members can be there, as well, if you have to break "really bad" news, recommend stopping chemotherapy, discuss hospice care, or explore goals and values so as to help your patients and their families determine their wishes regarding resuscitation. Also important is the support the palliative care team can offer you and your staff in dealing with the emotional toll these situations exact. The team can even arrange services of remembrance to help acknowledge and work through the grief associated with this work.

Finally, palliative care teams benefit the institutions within which they work, helping to increase staff morale, decrease staff turnover, and enhance staff expertise in palliative and end-of-life care. Palliative care teams based in academic medical centers and in teaching hospitals affiliated with these centers also provide training and perform research in palliative medicine (von Gunten 2002). Both through consultations and through formal and informal didactic sessions, palliative care teams offer education about the palliative care needs of patients undergoing active therapies, as well as offering insight into the stresses of patients and families as they make the transition to care without chemotherapy (Abrahm 2000; Oneshuck et al. 1997; Sheldon and Smith 1996; von Gunten et al. 1995). The teams collaborate in joint problem-solving to arrive at integrated solutions, a practice not often observed in standard medical training (Beninghof and Singer 1992; Billings and Block 1997; Boaden and Leaviss 2000; Browne et al. 1995; James and MacLeod 1993; Nash and Hoy 1993).

In palliative care teaching rounds and seminars, medical students, residents, and fellows learn how to work within an interdisciplinary group and how to provide comprehensive care across care sites (inpatient, outpatient, home). This instruction can remedy the deficits of a medical education and training that leave clinicians ill-prepared to alleviate the suffering of patients with advanced disease, or of their families (Billings and Block 1997; Ferrell et al. 1999).

SUMMARY

Patients with far-advanced cancer can experience a number of distressing symptoms, which may or may not include pain. The causes of these problems often can be reversed, even in very frail patients. And even when we cannot reverse the cause of the problem, there is usually a very effective symptomatic treatment available.

In this chapter I have reviewed the major problem areas affecting patients with far-advanced cancer: anxiety and depression, infections and other lesions of the oral cavity; ascites, diarrhea, nausea, and vomiting; dyspnea, cough, hemoptysis, hiccups; fungating skin lesions, pressure sores, and pruritus; sleeplessness; and weakness and fatigue. I also reviewed the role of hospice programs and of palliative care teams.

Bibliography

GENERAL REFERENCES

Berger AM, Portenoy RK, Weisman DE. 2002. *Principles and Practice of Supportive Care in Oncology,* 2nd ed, Philadelphia: Lippincott-Raven.

Doyle D, Hanks G, Cherny N, Calman K (eds). 2004. *Oxford Textbook of Palliative Medicine,* 3rd ed. Oxford: Oxford University Press.

Fallon M, O'Neill W (eds). 1998. *ABC of Palliative Care.* London: BMJ Publishing Group.

Holland JC. 1998. *Psycho-Oncology.* New York: Oxford University Press.

National Comprehensive Cancer Network (NCCN). 2003. The NCCN Clinical Practice Guideline: Distress Management (Version 1.2003). *JNCCN* 1:344–374; Version 1.2005; www.nccn.org.

Storey P, Knight CF, Schonwetter RS. 2003. *Pocket Guide to Hospice/Palliative Medicine.* Glenview, Ill.: American Academy of Hospice and Palliative Medicine.

Waller A, Caroline NL. 1996. *Handbook of Palliative Care in Cancer.* Boston: Butterworth-Heinemann.

ANXIETY AND DEPRESSION

Block SD. 2000. Assessing and managing depression in the terminally ill patient. *Ann Intern Med* 132:209–218.

Breitbart W, Bruera E, Chochinov H, Lynch M. 1995. Neuropsychiatric syndromes and psychological symptoms in patients with advanced cancer. *J Pain Symptom Manage* 10:131–141.

Breitbart W, Payne D, Passik SD. 2004. Psychological and psychiatric interventions in pain control. In *Oxford Textbook of Palliative Medicine,* 3rd ed, Doyle D, Hanks G, Cherny N, and Calman K (eds). Oxford: Oxford University Press.

Chochinov HM, Wilson KG, Enns M, Lander S. 1997. Are you depressed? Screening for depression in the terminally ill. *Am J Psychiatry* 154:674–676.

Derogatis LR, Morrow GR, Fetting J. 1983. The prevalence of psychiatric disorders among cancer patients. *JAMA* 249:751–757.

Endicott J. 1984. Measurement of depression in patients with cancer. *Cancer* 53:2243–2249.

Massie MJ, Popkin MK. 1998. Depressive disorders. In *Psycho-Oncology,* Holland JC (ed). New York: Oxford University Press.

Musselman DL, Lawson DH, Gumnick JF, et al. 2001. Paroxetine for the prevention of depression induced by high dose interferon alfa. *N Engl J Med* 344:961–966.

Noyes R, Holt CS, Massie MJ. 1998. Anxiety disorders. In *Psycho-Oncology,* Holland JC (ed). New York: Oxford University Press.

Rozans M, Dreisbach A, Lertora JJL, Kahn MJ. 2002. Palliative uses of methylphenidate in patients with cancer: a review. *J Clin Oncol* 20:335–339.

Stark D, Kiely M, Smith A, et al. 2002. Anxiety disorders in cancer patients: their nature, associations, and relation to quality of life. *J Clin Oncol* 20:3137–3148.

ORAL CARE

De Conno F, Sbanotto A, Ripamonti C, Ventafridda V. 2004. Mouth care. In *Oxford Textbook of Palliative Medicine.* 3rd ed, Doyle D, Hanks G, Cherny N, Calman K (eds). Oxford: Oxford University Press.

Regnard C, Fitton S. 1989. Mouth care: a flow diagram. *Palliat Med* 3:67–69.

Sonis ST. 2004. A biological approach to mucositis. *J Support Oncol* 2:21–32.

Toth BB, Chambers MS, Fleming TJ, et al. 1995. Minimizing oral complications of cancer treatment. *Oncology* 9:851–858.

Waller A, Caroline NL. 1996. Oral complications and mouth care. In *Handbook of Palliative Care in Cancer.* Boston: Butterworth-Heinemann.

CANDIDA

Greenspan D. 1994. Therapy of oral candidiasis. *Oral Surg Oral Med Oral Pathol* 78:211–215.

TREATMENT-INDUCED MUCOSITIS

Peterson DE, Cariello A. 2004. Mucosal damage: a major risk factor for severe complications after cytotoxic therapy. *Semin Oncol* 31:35–44.

XEROSTOMIA

Chambers M, Toth B, Martin C, et al. 1997. Assessment of salivary flow improvement in cancer patients with oral pilocarpine as treatment for analgesia-induced xerostomia. *Proc Am Soc Clin Oncol* 6:50a.

Ellershaw JE, Sutcliffe JM, Saunders CM. 1995. Dehydration and the dying patient. *J Pain Symptom Manage* 10:192–197.

Jacobs CD (ed). 1996. Medical advances in the treatment of xerostomia. *Oncology* 10(suppl):3–20.

Johnson JT, Ferretti GA, Nethery WJ, et al. 1993. Oral pilocarpine for post-irradiation xerostomia in patients with head and neck cancer. *N Engl J Med* 329:390–395.

GASTROINTESTINAL PROBLEMS

Ascites

Burger JA, Ochs A, Wirth K, et al. 1997. The transjugular stent implantation for the treatment of malignant portal and hepatic vein obstruction in cancer patients. *Ann Oncol* 8:200–202.

Faught W, Kirkpatrick JR, Kreport GV, et al. 1995. Peritoneovenous shunt for gynecologic malignant ascites. *J Am Coll Surg* 180:472–474.

Kichian K, Bain VG. 2004. Jaundice, ascites, and hepatic encephalopathy. In *Oxford Textbook of Palliative Medicine*, 3rd ed, Doyle D, Hanks G, Cherny N, Calman K (eds). Oxford: Oxford University Press.

Rossle M, Ochs A, Gulberg V, et al. 2000. A comparison of paracentesis and transjugular intrahepatic portosystemic shunting in patients with ascites. *N Engl J Med* 342:1701–1707.

Wickremesekera SK, Stubbs RS. 1997. Peritoneovenous shunting for malignant ascites. *N Z Med J* 110:33–35.

Constipation/Diarrhea

Billings JA. 1985. Constipation, diarrhea, and other GI problems. In *Outpatient Management of Advanced Cancer: Symptom Control, Support, and Hospice-in-the-Home.* Philadelphia: JB Lippincott.

Ippoliti C, Champlin R, Bugozia N, et al. 1997. Use of octreotide in the symptomatic management of diarrhea induced by graft-versus-host disease in patients with hematologic malignancies. *J Clin Oncol* 15:3330–3354.

Mercadante S. 1995. Diarrhea in terminally ill patients: pathophysiology and treatment. *J Pain Symptom Manage* 10:298–309.

Mercadante S. 2002. Diarrhea, malabsorption, and constipation. In *Principles and Practice of Supportive Oncology*, 2nd ed, Berger AM, Portenoy RK, Weissman DE (eds). Philadelphia: Lippincott-Raven.

Waller A, Caroline NL. 1996. Diarrhea and rectal discharge. In *Handbook of Palliative Care in Cancer.* Boston: Butterworth-Heinemann.

Nausea and Vomiting/Bowel Obstruction

Baines M. 1997. Nausea and vomiting, and intestinal obstruction. *BMJ* 315:1148–1150.

Baumrucker SJ. 1998. Management of intestinal obstruction in hospice care. *Am J Hosp Palliat Care* July/Aug:232–235.

Billings JA. 1986. Nausea and vomiting. In *Outpatient Management of Advanced Cancer: Symptom Control, Support, and Hospice-in-the-Home.* Philadelphia: JB Lippincott.

Bruera E, Seifert L, Watanabe S, et al. 1996. Chronic nausea in advanced cancer patients: a retrospective assessment of a metoclopramide-based antiemetic regimen. *J Pain Symptom Manage* 11:147–153.

Currow DC, Coughlan M, Fardell B, Cooney NJ. 1997. Use of ondansetron in palliative medicine. *J Pain Symptom Manage* 13:302–307.

Dundee JW, Yang J. 1983. Prolongation of the anti-emetic action of P6 acupuncture by acupressure in patients having cancer chemotherapy. *J R Soc Med* 83:360–362.

Fainsinger R, Spachynski K, Hanson J, Bruera E. 1994. Symptom control in terminally ill patients with malignant bowel obstruction. *J Pain Symptom Manage* 9:12–18.

Hammond DC (ed). 1990. *Handbook of Hypnotic Suggestion and Metaphors.* New York: WW Norton.

Lichter I. 1993. Results of antiemetic management in terminal illness. *J Palliat Care* 9:19–21.

Mercadante S. 1994. Assessment and management of mechanical bowel obstruction. In *Topics in Palliative Care*, vol 1, Portenoy RK, Bruera E (eds). Oxford: Oxford University Press.

Mercadante S. 1994. The role of octreotide in palliative care. *J Pain Symptom Manage* 9:406–411.

NCCN Antiemesis Practice Guidelines. Version 1. 2005. www.nccn.org.

Srivastava M, Brito-Dellan N, Davis MP, et al. 2003. Olanzapine as an antiemetic in refractory nausea and vomiting in advanced cancer. *J Pain Symptom Manage* 25:578–582.

TREATMENT-INDUCED NAUSEA AND VOMITING

Aapro MS, Thuerlimann B, Sessa C, et al., on behalf of the Swiss Group for Clinical Cancer Research (SAKK). 2003. Randomized double-blind trial to compare the clinical efficacy of ondansetron with metoclopramide, both combined with dexamethasone in the prophylaxis of chemotherapy-induced delayed emesis. *Ann Oncol* 14:291–297.

Andrykowski MA, Jacobsen PB. 1993. Anticipatory nausea and vomiting with cancer chemotherapy. In *Psychiatric Aspects of Symptom Management in Cancer Patients*, Breitbart W, Holland JC (eds). Washington, D.C.: American Psychiatric Press.

Berger AM, Clark-Snow RA. 2005. Nausea and vomiting. In *Cancer: Principles and Practice of Oncology*, 7th ed, DeVita VT, Hellman S, Rosenberg SA (eds). Philadelphia: JB Lippincott.

Buish TG, Tope DM. 1992. Psychological techniques for controlling the adverse side effects of cancer chemotherapy: findings from a decade of research. *J Pain Symptom Manage* 7:287.

Campos D, Pereira JR, Reinhardt RR, et al. 2001. Prevention of cisplatin-induced emesis by the oral neurokinin-1 antagonist, MK-869, in combination with granisetron and dexamethasone or with dexamethasone alone. *J Clin Oncol* 19:1759–1767.

Chang AE, Shiling DJ, Stillman RC, et al. 1979. Delta-9-tetrahydrocannabinol as an antiemetic in cancer patients receiving high-dose methotrexate: a prospective randomized evaluation. *Ann Intern Med* 91:819.

de Wit R, Herrstedt J, Rapoport B, et al. 2003. Addition of the oral NK-1 antagonist aprepitant to standard antiemetics provides protection against nausea and vomiting during multiple cycles of cisplatin-based chemotherapy. *J Clin Oncol* 21:4105–4111.

Gralla RJ. 2002. New agents, new treatment, and antiemetic therapy. *Semin Oncol* 29(suppl 4):119–124.

Gralla RJ, Osoba D, Kris MG, et al. 1999. Recommendations for the use of antiemetics: evidence-based clinical practice guidelines. *J Clin Oncol* 17:2971 2994.

Halperin JHR, Murphy R. 1992. Extrapyramidal reaction to ondansetron. *Cancer* 69:1275.

Hesketh PJ, Grunberg SM, Gralla RJ, et al., the Aprepitant Protocol 052 Study Group. 2003. The oral neurokinin-1 antagonist aprepitant for the prevention of chemotherapy-induced nausea and vomiting: a multinational, randomized, double-blind, placebo-controlled trial in patients receiving high-dose cisplatin. *J Clin Oncol* 21:4112–4119.

Hesketh PJ, Kris MG, Grunberg SM, et al. 1997. Proposal for classifying the acute emetogenicity of cancer chemotherapy. *J Clin Oncol* 15:103–109.

Italian Group for Antiemetic Research. 1997. Ondansetron versus metoclopramide, both combined with dexamethasone, in the prevention of cisplatin-induced delayed emesis. *J Clin Oncol* 15:124–130.

Johnson MH, Moroney CE, Gay CF. 1997. Relieving nausea and vomiting in patients with cancer: a treatment algorithm. *Oncol Nurs Forum* 24:51.

Koeller JM, Aapro MS, Gralla RJ, et al. 2002. Antiemetic guidelines: creating a more practical treatment approach. *Support Care Cancer* 10:519–522.

Kris MG, Tyson LB, Gralla RJ, et al. 1983. Extrapyramidal reactions with high-dose metoclopramide. *N Engl J Med* 309:433.

Kris MG. 2003. Why do we need another antiemetic? Just ask. *J Clin Oncol* 21:4077–4080.

Laszlo J, Clark RA, Hanson DC, et al. 1985. Lorazepam in cancer patients treated with cisplatin: a drug having antiemetic, amnesic, and anxiolytic effects. *J Clin Oncol* 3:864.

Leventhal H, Easterling DV, Nerenz DR, Love RR. 1988. The role of motion sickness in predicting anticipatory nausea. *J Behav Med* 11:117.

Morrow GR. 1984. Susceptibility to motion-sickness and the development of anticipatory nausea and vomiting in cancer patients undergoing chemotherapy. *Cancer Treat Rep* 68:1177.

Morrow GR, Morrell BS. 1982. Behavioral treatment for the anticipatory nausea and vomiting induced by cancer chemotherapy. *N Engl J Med* 307:1476.

Navar RM, Einhorn LH, Passik SD, et al. 2005. A phase II trial of olanzapine for the prevention of chemotherapy-induced nausea and vomiting: a Hoosier Oncology Group Study. *Support Care Cancer.*

Passik SD, Kirsh KL, Theobold DE, et al. 2003. A retrospective chart review of the use of olanzapine for the prevention of delayed emesis in cancer patients. *J Pain Symptom Manage* 25:485–488.

Redd WH, Andresen GV, Minagawa RY. 1982. Hypnotic control of anticipatory emesis in patients receiving cancer chemotherapy. *J Consult Clin Psychol* 50:14.

Redd WH, Jacobsen PB, Die-Trill M, et al. 1987. Cognitive/attentional distraction in the control of conditioned nausea in pediatric cancer patients receiving chemotherapy. *J Consult Clin Psychol* 55:391.

Roberts JT, Priestman TJ. 1993. A review of ondansetron in the management of radiotherapy-induced emesis. *Oncology* 50:173.

Roila F, Donati D, Tamberi S, Margutti G. 2002. Delayed emesis: incidence, pattern, prognostic factors and optimal treatment. *Support Care Cancer* 10:88–95.

Scarantino CW, Ornitz RD, Hoffman LG, Anderson RF Jr. 1992. Radiation-induced emesis: effects of ondansetron. *Semin Oncol* 6(suppl 15):19.

Sullivan JR, Leyden MJ, Bell R. 1983. Decreased cisplatin induced nausea and vomiting with alcohol ingestion. *N Engl J Med* 309:796.

RESPIRATORY PROBLEMS

DYSPNEA

Ahmedzai S. 1997. Nebulized drugs in palliative care. *Thorax* 52:575–577.

Bottomley DM, Hanks GW. 1990. Subcutaneous midazolam infusion in palliative care. *J Pain Symptom Manage* 5:259–261.

Chan KS, Sham MMK, Tse DMW, Thorsen AB. 2004. Palliative medicine in malignant respiratory diseases. In *Oxford Textbook of Palliative Medicine*, 3rd ed, Doyle D, Hanks G, Cherny N, Calman K (eds). Oxford: Oxford University Press.

Corner J, Plant H, Hern RA, Bailey C. 1996. Non-pharmacological intervention for breathlessness in lung cancer. *Palliat Med* 10:299–305.

Coyne PJ, Viswanathan R, Smith TJ. 2002. Nebulized fentanyl citrate improves patients' perception of breathing, respiratory rate, and oxygen saturation in dyspnea. *J Pain Symptom Manage* 23:157–160.

Dudgeon DJ, Rosenthal S. 1996. Management of dyspnea and cough in patients with cancer. *Hematol Oncol Clin North Am* 10:157–172.

Gleeson C, Spencer D. 1995. Blood transfusion and its benefits in palliative care. *Palliat Med* 9:307–313.

Hansen-Flaschen J. 1997. Advanced lung disease: palliation and terminal care. *Clin Chest Med* 18:645–655.

Jennings AL, Davies AN, Higgins JP, Broadley K. 2001. Opioids for the palliation of breathlessness in terminal illness. *Cochrane Database Syst Rev* 4:CD002066.

LeGrand SB, Khawam EA, Walsh D, Rivera NI. 2003. Opioids, respiratory function, and dyspnea. *Am J Hospice Palliat Care* 20:57–61.

Pollak JS. 2002. Malignant pleural effusions: treatment with tunneled long-term drainage catheters. *Curr Opin Pulm Med* 8:302–307.

Putnam JB, Light RW, Rodriguez RM, Ponn R, Olak J, Pollak JS, Lee RB, Payne DK, Graeber G, Kovitz KL. 1999. A randomized comparison of indwelling pleural catheter and doxycycline pleurodesis in the management of malignant pleural effusions. *Cancer* 86:1992–1999.

Reuben DB, Mor V. 1986. Dyspnea in terminally ill cancer patients. *Chest* 89:234.

Ripamonti C, Bruera E. 1997. Dyspnea: pathophysiology and assessment. *J Pain Symptom Manage* 13:220–232.

Simon PM, Schwartzstein RM, Weiss JW, et al. 1990. Distinguishable types of dyspnea in patients with shortness of breath. *Am Rev Respir Dis* 142:1009–1014.

Thomas JR, von Gunten CF. 2003. Management of dyspnea. *Support Oncol* 1:23–34.

Waller A, Caroline NL. 1996. Dyspnea. In *Handbook of Palliative Care in Cancer*. Boston: Butterworth-Heinemann.

Pleural Effusions

Moffett MJ, Ruckdeschel JC. 1992. Bleomycin and tetracycline in malignant pleural effusions: a review. *Semin Oncol* 19(2 suppl 5):59–63.

Morales M, del Carmen Exposito M. 1995. Control of malignant effusions with intrapleural mitoxantrone. *Support Cancer Care* 3:147–149.

Petrou M, Kaplan D, Goldstraw P. 1995. Management of recurrent malignant pleural effusions: the complementary role of talc pleurodesis and pleuroperitoneal shunting. *Cancer* 75:801–805.

Ponn RB, Blancaflor J, D'Agostino RS, et al. 1991. Pleuroperitoneal shunting for intractable pleural effusions. *Ann Thorac Surg* 51:605–609.

Shaw P, Agrawal R. 2004. Pleurodesis for malignant pleural effusions. *Cochrane Database Syst Rev* 1:CD002916.

Tsang V, Fernando HC, Goldstraw P. 1990. Pleuroperitoneal shunt for recurrent malignant pleural effusions. *Thorax* 45:369–372.

COUGH

Sutton P, et al. 1998. Use of nebulised saline and nebulised terbutaline as an adjunct to chest physiotherapy. *Thorax* 43:57–60.

Trochtenberg S. 1994. Nebulized lidocaine in the treatment of refractory cough. *Chest* 105:1592–1593.

HEMOPTYSIS

Hayakawa K, Tanaka F, Torizuka T, et al. 1992. Bronchial artery embolization for hemoptysis: immediate and long-term results. *Cardiovasc Intervent Radiol* 15:154.

Lipchik RJ. 2002. Hemoptysis. In *Principles and Practice of Supportive Oncology,* 2nd ed, Berger AM, Portenoy RK, Weissman DE (eds). Philadelphia: Lippincott-Raven.

HICCUPS

Regnard C. 2004. Dysphagia, dyspepsia and hiccup. In *Oxford Textbook of Palliative Medicine,* 3rd ed, Doyle D, Hanks G, Cherny N, Calman K (eds). Oxford: Oxford University Press.

Smith HS, Busracamwongs A. 2003. Management of hiccups in the palliative care population. *Am J Hospice Palliat Care* 20:149–154.

Walker P, Watanabe S, Bruera E. 1998. Baclofen, a treatment for chronic hiccup. *J Pain Symptom Manage* 16:125–132.

Waller A, Caroline NL. 1996. Hiccups. In *Handbook of Palliative Care in Cancer.* Boston: Butterworth-Heinemann.

Wilcock A, Twycross R. 1996. Midazolam for intractable hiccup. *J Pain Symptom Manage* 12:59–61.

SKIN PROBLEMS

PRESSURE ULCERS / ULCERATING LESIONS

Allman RM, Walker JM, Hart MK, et al. 1987. Air-fluidized beds or conventional therapy for pressure sores. *Ann Intern Med* 107:641–648.

Beckett R, Coombes TH, Frost MR, et al. 1980. Charcoal cloth and malodorous wounds. *Lancet* II:594.

Bergstrom M, Bennett MA, Carlson SE, et al. 1994. Treatment of pressure ulcers. *Clinical Practice Guideline, No. 15.* Rockville, Md.: U.S. Department of Health and Human Services, Public Health Service, Agency for Health Care Policy and Research. AHCPR publication 95-0652.

Brennan S, Leaper D. 1985. Antiseptics and wound healing. *Br J Surg* 72:780–782.

DeConno F, Ventafridda V, Saita L. 1991. Skin problems in advanced and terminal cancer patients. *J Pain Symptom Manage* 6:247–256.

Foltz AT. 1980. Nursing care of ulcerating metastatic lesions. *Oncol Nurs Forum* 7:8–13.

Grocott P, Dealey C. 2004. Skin problems in palliative care: nursing aspects. In *Oxford Textbook of Palliative Medicine,* 3rd ed, Doyle D, Hanks G, Cherny N, Calman K (eds). Oxford: Oxford University Press.

Landi F, Aloe L, Russo A, et al. 2003. Topical treatment of pressure ulcers with nerve growth factor: a randomized clinical trial. *Ann Intern Med* 139:635–641.

Seiler W, Stahelin H. 1985. Decubitus ulcers: treatment through five therapeutic principles. *Geriatrics* 9:30.

Twillman RK, Long TD, Cathers TA, Mueller DW. 1999. Treatment of painful skin ulcers with topical opioids. *J Pain Symptom Manage* 17:288–292.

von Gunten CF. 2002. Three common issues in the palliative care of advanced head and neck cancer: skin, nutrition, and pain. In *ASCO Educational Book,* 38th Annual Meeting. Alexandria, Va.: American Society of Clinical Oncology.

Waller A, Caroline NL. 1996. Pressure sores. In *Handbook of Palliative Care in Cancer.* Boston: Butterworth-Heinemann.

Waller A, Caroline NL. 1996. Smelly tumors. In *Handbook of Palliative Care in Cancer.* Boston: Butterworth-Heinemann.

Wood DK. 1980. The draining malignant ulceration: palliative management in advanced cancer. *JAMA* 224:820–822.

PRURITUS

Bergasa NV, Talbot TL, Alling DW, et al. 1992. A controlled trial of naloxone infusions for the pruritus of chronic cholestasis. *Gastroenterology* 102:544–549.

Davis MP, Frandsen JL, Walsh D, et al. 2003. Mirtazapine for pruritus. *J Pain Symptom Manage* 25:288–291.

Goldman BD, Koh HK. 1994. Pruritus and malignancy. In *Mechanisms and Management of Pruritus,* Bernard JD (ed). New York: McGraw-Hill.

Larijani GE, Goldberg ME, Rogers KH. 1996. Treatment of opioid-induced pruritus with ondansetron: report of four patients. *Pharmacotherapy* 16:958–960.

Muller C, Pongratz S, Pidlich J, et al. 1998. Treatment of pruritus in chronic liver disease with the 5-hydroxytryptamine receptor type 3 antagonist, ondansetron: a randomized placebo-controlled, double-blind crossover trial. *Eur J Gastroenterol Hepatol* 10:865–870.

Oaklander AL, Bowsher D, Galer B, et al. 2003. Herpes zoster itch: preliminary epidemiological data. *Pain* 4:338–343.

Raderer M, Muller C, Scheithauer W. 1994. Ondansetron for pruritus due to cholestasis (letter). *N Engl J Med* 330:1540.

Schworer H, Hartmann H, Ramadori G. 1995. Relief of cholestatic pruritus by a novel class of drugs: 5-hydroxytryptamine type 3 (5HT-3) receptor antagonist: effectiveness of ondansetron. *Pain* 61:33–37.

Waller A, Caroline NL. 1996. Pruritus. In *Handbook of Palliative Care in Cancer.* Boston: Butterworth-Heinemann.

Zylicz Z, Smits C, Krajnik M. 1998. Paroxetine for pruritus in advanced cancer. *J Pain Symptom Manage* 16:121–124.

INSOMNIA

Earley CJ. 2003. Restless legs syndrome. *N Engl J Med* 348:2103–2109.

Kupfer DJ, Reynolds CF. 1997. Management of insomnia. *N Engl J Med* 336:341–346.

NIH Technology Assessment Panel on Integration of Behavioral and Relaxation Approaches into the Treatment of Chronic Pain and Insomnia. 1996. Integration of behavioral and relaxation approaches into the treatment of chronic pain and insomnia. *JAMA* 276:313–318.

Savard J, Marin CM. 2001. Insomnia in the context of cancer: a review of a neglected problem. *J Clin Oncol* 19:895–908.

WEAKNESS AND FATIGUE

GENERAL REFERENCES

American Pain Society. 2004. *Principles of Analgesic Use in the Treatment of Acute Pain and Cancer Pain*. Glenview Ill.: American Pain Society.

Bruera E, Driver L, Barnes E, et al. 2003. Patient-controlled methylphenidate for cancer-related fatigue: a preliminary report. *Proc ASCO* 22:737.

Miaskowski C, Portenoy RK. 2002. Assessment and management of cancer-related fatigue. In *Principles and Practice of Supportive Oncology*, 2nd ed, Berger AM, Portenoy RK, Weissman DE (eds). Philadelphia: Lippincott-Raven.

National Comprehensive Cancer Network (NCCN). 2004. NCCN Clinical Practice Guidelines in Oncology: Cancer-Related Fatigue (version 1.2004). www.nccn.org.

Strasser F, Bruera ED. 2002. Update of anorexia and cachexia. *Hematol Oncol Clin N Am* 16:589–617.

Wang XS, Giralt SA, Mendoza TR, et al. 2002. Clinical factors associated with cancer-related fatigue in patients being treated for leukemia and non-Hodgkin's lymphoma. *J Clin Oncol* 20:1319–1328.

EXERCISE

Courneya KSS, Friedenreich CM. 1999. Physical exercise and quality of life following cancer diagnosis: a literature review. *Ann Behav Med* 21:171–179.

Pinto BM, Maruyam NC. 1999. Exercise in rehabilitation of breast cancer survivors. *Psychooncology* 8:191–206.

EATON-LAMBERT SYNDROME

Caracini A, Martini C, Simonetti F. 2004. Neurological problems in advanced cancer. In *Oxford Textbook of Palliative Medicine*, 3rd ed, Doyle D, Hanks G, Cherny N, Calman K (eds). Oxford: Oxford University Press.

ANEMIA

Danna RP, Rudnick SA, Abels RI. 1990. Erythropoietin therapy for the anemia associated with AIDS and AIDS therapy and cancer. In *Erythropoietin in Clinical Applications: An International Perspective*, Garnick MB (ed). New York: Marcel Dekker.

Eschbach JW, Egrie JC, Downing MR, et al. 1987. Correction of anemia of end-stage renal disease with recombinant human erythropoietin. *N Engl J Med* 316:73–78.

Gabrilove JL, Cleeland CS, Livington RB, et al. 2001. Clinical evaluation of once-weekly dosing of epoietin alfa in chemotherapy patients: improvements in hemoglobin and quality of life are similar to three times weekly dosing. *J Clin Oncol* 19:2875–2882.

Glaspy J, Bukowski R, Steinberg D, et al. 1997. Impact of therapy with epoietin alpha on clinical outcomes in patients with nonmyeloid malignancies during cancer chemotherapy in community oncology practice. *J Clin Oncol* 15:1218–1234.

Gleeson C, Spencer D. 1995. Blood transfusion and its benefits in palliative care. *Palliat Med* 9:307–313.

Hesketh PJ, Arena F, Patel D, et al., 2004. A randomized controlled trial of darbopoietin alfa administered as a fixed or weight-based dose using a front-loading schedule in patients with anemia who have nonmyeloid malignancies. *Cancer* 100: 859–868.

National Comprehensive Cancer Network. NCCN Clinical Practice Guidelines in Oncology: Anemia. Version 2.2004. www.nccn.org.

Ramakrishnan R, Cheung WC, Wacholtz MC, et al. 2004. Pharmakokinetics and pharmodynamics modeling of recombinant human erythropoietin after single and multiple doses in healthy volunteers. *J Clin Pharmacol* 9:991–1002.

METABOLIC ABNORMALITIES

General References

Bower M, Cox S, 2004. Endocrine and metabolic complications of advanced cancer. In *Oxford Textbook of Palliative Medicine*, 3rd ed, Doyle D, Hanks G, Cherny N, Calman K (eds). Oxford: Oxford University Press.

Hypercalcemia

Bower M, Stein RC, Hedley A, et al. 1991. The use of nasal calcitonin spray in the treatment of hypercalcemia of malignancy. *Cancer Chemother Pharmacol* 28:311–312.

Kovacs CS, MacDonald SM, Chik CL, Bruera E. 1995. Hypercalcemia of malignancy in the palliative care patient: a treatment strategy. *J Pain Symptom Manage* 10:224–232.

Morton AR, Ritch PS. 1998. Hypercalcemia. In *Principles and Practice of Supportive Oncology*, Berger AM, Portenoy RK, Weissman DE (eds). Philadelphia: Lippincott-Raven.

Thiébaud D, Jacquet AF, Burckhardt P. 1990. Fast and effective treatment of malignant hypercalcemia: combination of suppositories of calcitonin and single infusion of 3-amino 1-hydroxypropylidene-1-biphosphate. *Arch Intern Med* 150:2125–2128.

Warrell RP, Jr, Israel R, Frisone M, et al. 1988. Gallium nitrate for acute treatment of cancer-related hypercalcemia: a randomized double-blind comparison to calcitonin. *Ann Intern Med* 108:669–674.

Ectopic ACTH

Bertagna Z, et al. 1989. Suppression of ectopic ACTH secretion by the long-acting somatostatin analogue octreotide. *J Clin Endocrinol Metab* 68:988–991.

UNKNOWN OR IRREVERSIBLE CAUSES

Bruera E, Driver L, Barnes E, et al. 2003. Patient-controlled methylphenidate (PCM) for cancer-related fatigue: a preliminary report. *Proc ASCO* 22:2965.

Hanna AR, Sledge GW, Mayer ML, et al. 2003. Preliminary results of a phase II trial of methylphenidate in patients with breast carcinoma. *Proc ASCO* 22:727.

ANOREXIA AND MALNUTRITION

General References

Agteresch HJ, Rietveld T, Kerkhofs LGM, et al. 2002. Beneficial effects of adenosine triphosphate on nutritional status in advanced lung cancer patients: a randomized clinical trial. *J Clin Oncol* 20:371–378.

Billings JA. 1986. Anorexia and nutritional care. In *Outpatient Management of Advanced Cancer: Symptom Control, Support, and Hospice-in-the-Home*. Philadelphia: JB Lippincott.

Bruera E, Sweeney C. 2004. Pharmacologic interventions in cachexia and anorexia. In *Oxford Textbook of Palliative Medicine*, 3rd ed, Doyle D, Hanks G, Cherny N, Calman K (eds). Oxford: Oxford University Press.

Earthman CP, Reid PM, Harper IT, et al. 2002. Body cell mass repletion and improved quality of life in HIV-infected individuals receiving oxandrolone. *J Parenter Enteral Nutr* 26:357–365.

Tchekmedyian S, Fesen M, Price LM, Ottery FD. 2003. Ongoing placebo-controlled study of oxandrolone in cancer-related weight loss. *Proc ASTRO* 57:S283–284.

Watanabe S, Bruera E. 1996. Anorexia and cachexia, asthenia, and lethargy. *Hematol Oncol Clin North Am* 10:189–206.

Megace

Jatoi A, Loprinzi CL. 2002. Cancer anorexia/weight loss. In *Principles and Practice of Supportive Oncology*, Berger AM, Portenoy RK, Weissman DE (eds). Philadelphia: Lippincott-Raven.

Leinung MC, Liporace R, Miller CH. 1995. Induction of adrenal suppression by megestrol acetate in patients with AIDS. *Ann Intern Med* 122:843–845.

Loprinzi CL, Kugler JW, Sloan JA, et al. 1999. Randomized comparison of megesterol acetate versus dexamethasone versus fluoxymesterone for the treatment of cancer anorexia/cachexia. *J Clin Oncol* 17:3299–3306.

Loprinzi CL, Michalak JC, Schaiad DJ, et al. 1993. Phase III evaluation of four doses of megestrol acetate as therapy for patients with cancer anorexia and/or cachexia. *J Clin Oncol* 11:762–767.

Simons JP-FHA, Aaronson NK, Vansteenkiste JF, et al. 1996. Effects of medroxy-progesterone acetate on appetite, weight, and quality of life in advanced-stage non-hormone-sensitive cancer: a placebo-controlled multicenter study. *J Clin Oncol* 14:1077–1084.

Corticosteroids

Bruera E, Roca E, Cedaro L, et al. 1985. Action of oral methylprednisolone in terminal cancer patients: a prospective randomized double-blind study. *Cancer Treat Rep* 69:751–754.

Moertel C, Schutt AG, Reiteneier RJ, Hahn RG. 1974. Corticosteroid therapy of preterminal gastrointestinal cancer. *Cancer* 33:1607–1609.

Needham PR, Daley AG, Lennard RF. 1992. Steroids in advanced cancer: survey of current practice. *BMJ* 305:999.

Willox J, Corr J, Shaw J, et al. 1984. Prednisolone as an appetite stimulant in patients with cancer. *BMJ* 288:27.

Dronabinol (δ-9-Tetrahydrocannabinol)

Beal JE, Olson R, Laubenstein L, et al. 1995. Dronabinol as a treatment for anorexia associated with weight loss in patients with AIDS. *J Pain Symptom Manage* 10:89–97.

Voth EA, Schwartz RH. 1997. Medicinal applications of δ-9-Tetrahydrocannabinol and marijuana. *Ann Intern Med* 126:791–798.

Cyproheptadine

Kardinal C, Loprinzi CL, Schaid DJ, et al. 1990. A controlled trial of cyproheptadine in cancer patients with anorexia and/or cachexia. *Cancer* 65:2657–2662.

Hydrazine Sulfate

Kosty MP, Fleishman SB, Herndon JE, et al. 1994. Cisplatin, vinblastine, and hydrazine sulfate in advanced non-small-cell lung cancer: a randomized placebo-controlled, double-blind phase III study of the Cancer and Leukemia Group B. *J Clin Oncol* 12:1113–1120.

Loprinzi CL, Goldberg RM, Su JQ. 1994. Placebo-controlled trial of hydrazine sulfate in patients with newly diagnosed non-small-cell lung cancer. *J Clin Oncol* 12:1126–1129.

Loprinzi CL, Kuross SA, O'Fallon JR, et al. 1994. Randomized placebo-controlled evaluation of hydrazine sulfate in patients with advanced colorectal cancer. *J Clin Oncol* 12:1121–1125.

ENTERAL/PARENTERAL FEEDING AND HYDRATION

Ahronheim JC. 1996. Nutrition and hydration in the terminal patient. *Clin Geriatr Med* 12:379–391.

Ellershaw JE, Sutcliffe JM, Saunders CM. 1995. Dehydration and the dying patient. *J Pain Symptom Manage* 10:192–197.

McCann RM, Hall WJ, Groth-Junker A. 1994. Comfort care for terminally ill patients: the appropriate use of nutrition and hydration. *JAMA* 272:1263–1266.

Shike M. 1996. Nutrition therapy for the cancer patient. *Hematol Oncol Clin North Am* 10:221–234.

COPING STRATEGIES

Miaskowski C, Portenoy RK. 2002. Assessment and management of cancer-related fatigue. In *Principles and Practice of Supportive Oncology*, 2nd ed, Berger AM, Portenoy RK, Weissman DE (eds). Philadelphia: Lippincott-Raven.

HOSPICE

Billings JA. 1986. *Outpatient Management of Advanced Cancer: Symptom Control, Support, and Hospice-in-the-Home*. Philadelphia: JB Lippincott.

Cherny NI, Coyle N, Foley KM. 1996. Guidelines in the care of the dying cancer patient. *Hematol Oncol Clin North Am* 10:261–286.

Harris NJ, Dunmore R, Tsheu MJ. 1996. The Medicare hospice benefit: fiscal implications for hospice program management. *Cancer Manage* 3:6–11.

ROLE OF THE PALLIATIVE CARE TEAM

Abrahm JL. 2000. The palliative care consultation team as a model for palliative care education. In *Topics in Palliative Care*, vol 4, Portenoy RK, Bruera E (eds). Oxford: Oxford University Press.

Beninghof A, Singer A. 1992. Transdisciplinary teaming: an inservice training activity. *Teaching Exceptional Children* winter:58–61.

Billings JA, Block S. 1997. Palliative care in undergraduate medical education. *JAMA* 278:733–743.

Billings JA, Pantilat S. 2001. Survey of palliative care programs in the United States. *J Palliat Med* 4:309–314.

Boaden N, Leaviss J. 2000. Putting teamwork in context. *Med Educ* 34:921–927.

Browne A, Carpenter C, Cooledge C, et al. 1995. Bridging the professions: an integrated and interdisciplinary approach to teaching health care ethics. *Acad Med* 70:1002–1005.

Elsayem A, Swint K, Fisch MJ, et al. 2004. Palliative care inpatient service in a comprehensive cancer center: clinical and financial outcomes. *J Clin Oncol* 22:2008–2014.

Ferrell BR, Carron AT, Lynn J, Keaney P. 1999. End of life care in medical textbooks. *Ann Intern Med* 130:82–86.

Gazelle G, Buxbaum R, Daniels E. 2001. The development of a palliative care program for managed care patients: a case example. *J Am Geriatr Soc* 49:1241–1248.

Higginson IJ, Finlay IG, Goodwin DM, et al. 2003. Is there evidence that palliative care teams alter end-of-life experiences of patients and their caregivers? *J Pain Symptom Manage* 25:150–168.

Homsi J, Walsh D, Nelson KA, et al. 2002. The impact of a palliative medicine consult service in medical oncology. *Support Care Cancer* 10:337–342.

James CR, MacLeod RD. 1993. The problematic nature of education in palliative care. *J Palliat Care* 9:5–10.

Jenkins CA, Shulz M, Hanson J, Bruera E. 2000. Demographic, symptom and medication profiles of cancer patients seen by a palliative care consult team in a tertiary referral hospital. *J Pain Symptom Manage* 19:174–184.

Manfredi PL, Morrison RS, Morris J, et al. 2000. Palliative care consultations: how do they impact hospitalized patients? *J Pain Symptom Manage* 20:166–173.

Nash A, Hoy A. 1993. Terminal care in the community—an evaluation of residential workshops for general practitioner / district nurse teams. *Palliat Med* 7:5–17.

Nelson KA, Walsh D. 2003. The business of palliative medicine—part 3: the development of a palliative medicine program in an academic medical center. *Am J Hospice Palliat Care* 20:345–352.

Ng K, von Gunten CF. 1998. Symptoms and attitudes of 100 consecutive patients admitted to an acute hospice / palliative care unit. *J Pain Symptom Manage* 16:307–315.

Oneschuk D, Fainsinger R, Hanson J, Bruera E. 1997. Assessment and knowledge in palliative care in second year family medicine residents. *J Pain Symptom Manage* 14:265–273.

Pan CX, Morrison RS, Meier DE, et al. 2001. How prevalent are hospital-based palliative care programs? Status report and future directions. *J Palliat Med* 4:315–324.

Pierucci RL, Kirby RS, Leuthner SR. 2001. End-of-life care for neonates and infants: the experience and effects of a palliative care consultation service. *Pediatrics* 108:653–660.

Santa-Emma PH, Roach R, Gill MA, et al. 2002. Development and implementation of an inpatient acute palliative care service. *J Palliat Med* 5:93–100.

Sheldon F, Smith P. 1996. The life so short, the craft so hard to learn: a model for postbasic education in palliative care. *J Palliat Care* 10:99–104.

Smith TJ, Coyne P, Cassel B, et al. 2003. A high-volume specialist palliative care unit and team may reduce in-hospital end-of-life care costs. *J Palliat Med* 6:699–705.

Virik K, Glare P. 2002. Profile and evaluation of a palliative medicine consultation service within a tertiary teaching hospital in Sydney, Australia. *J Pain Symptom Manage* 23:17–25.

von Gunten CF. 2002. Secondary and tertiary palliative care in US hospitals. *JAMA* 287:875–881.

von Gunten CF, von Roenn JH, Gradishar W, Weitzman S. 1995. A hospice / palliative medicine rotation for fellows training in hematology-oncology. *J Cancer Educ* 10:200–202.

The Last Days . . . and the Bereaved

THE DYING PATIENT

The last few days of life pose special problems for cancer patients, their families, and even the physicians caring for them. General practitioners, for example, have been found to suffer from "the end of the doctor-patient relationship, feelings of uselessness and failure, increased awareness of their own mortality, and the presence of 'questions without answers'" (Schaerer 1993). And taking care of dying patients has been found to be a major contributor to burnout among medical oncologists (Whippen and Canellos 1991). As difficult as this is for us, we must find a way to deliver the care that these patients and their families require.

If you have never before cared for a dying patient, you may feel you have nothing to offer. But that is far from the truth. Both the patient, if he or she is awake, and the family will welcome your visits and ongoing care. Don't worry about being blamed for what is happening, and let your instincts guide you in offering the patient and the family the respect and comfort you owe them.

COMPONENTS OF CARE

What do patients feel they need for a "good death"? Many patients would say:

- Optimizing physical comfort
- Maintaining a sense of continuity with one's self
- Maintaining and enhancing relationships
- Making meaning of one's life and death
- Achieving a sense of control
- Confronting and preparing for death
  (From Block 2001, 2900)

How can we help patients achieve these goals? Dr. Ned Cassem, a talented psychiatrist and teacher who has worked extensively with dying patients, articulates nine components essential to care of the dying (Cassem 1991):

Components of Care of the Dying

- Clinical competence
- Comfort
- Compassion
- Consistency and perseverance
- Cheerfulness
- Equanimity
- Visits from children
- Family cohesion and integration
- Communication

Of these components, the key for me has been acquiring the *clinical competence* to relieve a patient's physical and psychological distress. When I know I have decreased a patient's distress to a tolerable level, the other pieces fall naturally into place. I find I can, with compassion, hold his hand, talk with him or call him regularly, be cheerful, and manifest an equanimity that I truly feel. Children's visits with the patient become enjoyable, and family cohesion is enhanced by the lowered levels of stress. It becomes much easier for the family to be near the dying patient and, if they wish, to be present at the time of death.

SUPPORTING THE FAMILY

Whenever possible, as the final days approach I try to have family meetings, with the patient present, to review the implications of allowing the patient to die at home. Along with the nurses and social workers who are on our teams, we need to help caregivers locate additional home care resources or, if the patient and caregiver prefer, locate an acceptable nursing facility. For family members planning to provide the care at home, hospital beds, commodes, and home health aides may be among the equipment and services required. Caregivers are particularly prone to becoming exhausted and frustrated if they are trying to provide this care alone, and we must validate their need for help.

Because time is now short, we need to talk clearly with caregivers about their changing roles. They have generally been acting as the eyes and ears of the oncology team, to monitor for early warning signs as the patient rode the roller coaster typical of chemotherapy treatments. Families may not even realize that this monitoring of blood counts and being hypervigilant for any signs of deterioration have become second nature to them. They need to know that they can now relinquish those tasks without exposing the patient to danger, and that they have equally important tasks to work on in the time that remains. Patients will have stories to tell, meaning to make, legacies to leave—and may need help with these and with maintaining a sense of purpose. We can encourage patients and their families to work with hospice programs that can aid in these tasks. Communication, in fact, is key to our support of the patient's family members throughout their ordeal.

PRACTICE POINTS: COMMUNICATION DURING THE LAST DAYS

- Have a family meeting to discuss what is likely to happen next.
- Call frequently to give support and adjust the medical regimen.
- Mention that patients often need family permission to "let go" and reassurance that the survivors will be "OK."
- Tell the family Dr. Byock's "Five Things" (Byock 1997): I forgive you; forgive me; I love you; thank you; and good-bye.
- Provide written reminders: "Don't call 911"; "Signs and symptoms of dying"; "Who to call for help"; "What to do when death occurs."
- Assuage ethical or religious concerns about symptom management.
- Revisit the benefits of hospice care.

When a patient who is not enrolled in a hospice program is dying at home, I make every effort to call the patient and the family two or three times a week, increasing the frequency for the last few weeks. I think that the calls are particularly helpful for the caregivers, who are under a tremendous burden. I can answer their questions, provide emotional support, praise their efforts, and demonstrate my continuing concern. I also have the opportunity to modify the patient's treatment regimen frequently to ensure the best possible control of symptoms during these last days.

PRACTICE POINTS: "THE TRANSITIONAL PHASE"
- Increased somnolence
- Loss of appetite
- Weakness
- Confusion
- Falls
- Incontinence

(From Doyle-Brown 2000)

Family members often want to know how they will recognize that the last days are approaching. Some want to know how to focus their care. Over the course of the patient's illness, after all, they have frequently needed to be enthusiastic coaches; without their urging, the patient would not have bounced back as readily from what proved to be temporary setbacks. But if the patient is dying this time, they say, their goals as caregivers would change. Other family members have only a few weeks to be with the patient full-time. Vacation, sick, and even family leave days are limited, as is the time for which another person can assume the caregiver's other obligations.

What are the signs of what Doyle-Brown (2000) has termed "the transitional phase," before the patient becomes bed-bound, and what effects do they have on the family? Characteristics that denote the beginning of this phase include: increased sleep, almost total loss of appetite, and then weakness. Some caregivers mistakenly believe that the patient has some control over this phase, and they may be angry at the patient, thinking, "He's giving up!" As I discussed in Chapter 3, repeated rejection of specially prepared food is particularly distressing. Caregivers may have great difficulty allowing confused patients to remain as independent as they think they can still be. Some patients are not fully convinced that they need help, until they have fallen or become incontinent.

When it seems appropriate, I remind the caregivers that it is important to give the patient "permission" to die. I learned this many years ago from one of my residents. One day on rounds, John gently told me that a patient of mine, Mr. Garabaldi, was "holding on" because he didn't want to let me down—that I was the only one Mr. Garabaldi hadn't told that he wanted to die. I immediately reassured Mr. Garabaldi that he would not be disappointing me, that I knew he had been fighting for a long time, and that I understood his need to rest. His relief was obvious, and he died within the week.

Up until that point, I had no idea how important it was for me to tell someone explicitly that he can "let go." It does not matter whether the patient can respond verbally or indicate in any way that he has heard me; it still needs to be said. I now share this insight with family members and urge them to give this kind of permission to their loved one. And I ask them to tell the dying person not to worry about them, that they will be "OK."

Dr. Ira Byock, in *Dying Well*, lists an additional "Five Things" that both the dying patient and the family members need to hear: I forgive you; forgive me; thank you, I love you; good-bye. Some families say these things more easily than others, but almost all eventually will be able to say one or more. This seems to promote a feeling of peace in both family members and patients.

WRITTEN REMINDERS.   In addition to calling families and patients, the hospice program gives the families written reminders to post by the phone. Hospice programs provide numerous stickers with their phone number. They can be reached 24 hours a day, 7 days a week. Some states have "out-of-hospital" DNR forms. For clinicians who practice in states where such forms are not available, I would include among the reminders, "When [the patient] dies, don't call 911." I explain that if they call 911, the paramedics who arrive will be obliged to try to resuscitate the patient. In addition, I encourage someone in the family to inform the local ambulance company that the patient has an advance directive and does not want to be resuscitated. We have even sent the ambulance company a copy of the directive to keep in its files. Then, if 911 is called by mistake when the patient dies, the paramedics will know not to institute cardiopulmonary resuscitation.

I also include in the reminders my office and home telephone numbers. If hospice is not being used, I ask the family members to call me when the patient dies and I ask them to write down the phone number of the funeral home they plan to use and to tell the funeral director that I will be responsible for completing the death certificate.

THE FAMILY'S ETHICAL CONCERNS ABOUT PAIN MANAGEMENT.   Despite my reassurances to the contrary, a major source of concern for family members is giving pain medicine to someone who is dying. They fear that in trying to relieve pain, they might inadvertently be hastening death. Even though they cannot relieve the person's suffering in any other way, they may have religious concerns—often because they are not aware of the writings of their religious leaders on this subject.

I discussed in Chapter 2, and it is worth reiterating here, that Catholicism, Orthodox Judaism, and Islam all encourage the relief of suffering, even if there is a chance that, as a secondary effect, the person may die sooner than if the pain medicine were withheld. This is the so-called doctrine of double effect. The Catechism is very clear on this point: intent is the key. Unlike Roman Catholicism, Islam and Orthodox Judaism do not have one spokesperson, but in recent writings, the majority of opinions from clerics of both faiths are identical to that of the Roman Catholic hierarchy: if the intent of the caregiver or the physician is to relieve the patient's pain, the caregiver should give whatever medication is required. These three religions are also in concert about the right of the patient to refuse artificial means of prolonging life (e.g., respirators) or other therapies that will be of no benefit.

REFERRAL TO A HOSPICE PROGRAM.   Even if the patient or the family has previously resisted accepting the referral, I make every effort to engage hospice services for dying patients, including those dying in hospitals or in long-term care facilities. Patient care plans can be modified and streamlined, and physical, psychological, and spiritual symptoms can be addressed. Hospice personnel begin to prepare the family for the loss, help with other social or spiritual concerns, and offer continued assistance through bereavement programs after the death.

In a period as short as the few days or week before death, hospice care can be an enormous source of comfort to families and professional caregivers, particularly when they have never witnessed a "natural" death. The team members have "been there," can explain what is likely to happen, and can provide expert symptom management during the last hours or days. For patients at home, hospice staff will provide practical instruction in how the family can help with toileting, feeding, massage, and giving medications. As dying approaches, hospice personnel provide suggestions for answering the patient's questions and written materials that explain how the family or the personnel in inpatient or long-term care facilities can determine that death is imminent.

SUPPORTING THE INPATIENT WARD TEAM

When one of our patients is dying in the hospital, we feel the additional obligation of helping the primary oncology team, the house staff, and the ward staff (nurses, clerks, social workers) cope not only with the patient's and family's needs but with their own feelings of distress. The dying process often brings ward personnel close to patients and their families, even if this is the first time they have met.

To allay feelings of guilt and anxiety, we review with all team members the history of the illness, the limits of the treatments that remain, the burdens of those treatments, and, when appropriate, the limits the patient has placed on further supportive measures. We also remind them that, despite our best efforts, patients still die and that it is no one's fault. This can be very comforting. Even more helpful is suggesting things they can do that will enhance the patient's last days and further the healing process of the survivors.

Not uncommonly, however, house staff are the undeserving target of a patient's or a family's anger, as in the case of Mr. Champion.

PRACTICE POINTS: SUPPORTING THE INPATIENT WARD TEAM

- Remind the team of medicine's limitations in the face of illness that is refractory to treatment.
- Relieve anxiety and unwarranted guilt; explain patient/family anger.
- Develop a plan of care through which they will minimize patient and family suffering.
- Dispel misconceptions and praise their efforts.
- Record/update advance directives regarding elective intubation and resuscitation.
- To enable a truly informed choice, give realistic prognoses and realistic descriptions of the burdens and benefits of remaining therapeutic options, including mechanical ventilation.

Mr. Champion

Mr. Champion underwent definitive therapy for lung cancer, but six months later he was admitted for bilateral malignant pleural effusions. He required bilateral chest tubes and sclerosis, was febrile from resistant pneumonia, and was significantly malnourished. Despite control of his pain, Mr. Champion was unable to clear his numerous secretions, was severely tachypneic, and became recurrently hypoxic. No pulmonary emboli or clots were present in his upper or lower extremities.

Although Mr. Champion had told his oncologist, Dr. Rydell, that he did not wish to be intubated electively or resuscitated if that meant he would have to be on a respirator, no advance directive was on his chart. Because of Mr. Champion's rapidly deteriorating pulmonary status, I asked Dr. Rydell to confirm and document that Mr. Champion did not wish to be electively intubated.

The next morning, nurses on the unit told me of the conversation they had overheard between a furious Mrs. Champion and the house staff. It went something like, "Why did you have to ask Dr. Rydell to talk about those things with my husband? Look what you've done to him. You took away all his hope! He was fine until you made us have that talk—now look at him!" She went on in this vein for some time, and the next day she would not speak with the physicians whom she blamed for her husband's ongoing deterioration.

After Dr. Rydell confirmed that Mr. Champion did not wish to be intubated, the team treated his progressive dyspnea symptomatically with pulmonary toilet, suctioning, oxygen, antibiotics, anxiolytics, and opioids. He died two days later, in no apparent distress. As we gathered around him, his wife asked the house staff's forgiveness "for what I said out there in the hall." She included the doctors in the prayers she led, and in the thank-you gift she sent to all the floor staff later in the week.

Not all house staff are so lucky. Mr. Champion's wife was able to understand that her anger had been misplaced and to apologize to the staff. Many families don't, and the interns, residents, students, and nurses caring for the patient add the family's unjust accusations to their own unwarranted feelings of guilt about the patient's death.

In other instances, a family member will insist that everything be done for the patient despite the imminence of death and the wishes of the rest of the family and the health care team. Dr. Cassem suggests that underlying such requests is a history of antagonism between the dying patient and the relative who wishes aggressive therapies—that the guilt from the lack of resolution of the estrangement leads to the request. A family meeting directed at clarifying "achievable" goals, with attention to the special needs of the distressed person, can be very helpful.

Be sure to support the house staff through these stressful situations. Explain that they are often the lightning rod for the family's or patient's helplessness, despair, and anger. Encourage them not to take family attacks personally, to continue their exertions on the patient's behalf, and to work to eliminate all sources of distress. During hospitalizations that lead to death, and after the death itself, dispel any misconceptions the staff may have about their "fault" for the death and praise the work they did to make the dying person as comfortable as possible. Praise coming from nurses who have shared in the care of the patient can be particularly healing. In turn, you can encourage the house staff to praise the nurses for the care they have delivered. This kind of support goes a long way toward enabling young physicians and ward staff to recover from the pain they experience when a patient dies and to allow themselves a feeling of satisfaction for a job well done.

RESUSCITATION STATUS. In Mr. Champion's case, as the crisis neared Dr. Rydell simply needed to confirm that Mr. Champion's wishes had not changed. Later, when intubation would have been needed to support him (his pH was 7.24, pCO_2 80 mm Hg, and pO_2 55 mm Hg on a 100 percent rebreathing mask), we all felt confident that in not intubating him, we were caring for Mr. Champion within the limits he had set.

Unfortunately, the 1995 SUPPORT study (of patients dying in teaching hospitals) indicates that physicians often do not know the wishes of their hospitalized patients suffering from life-threatening illnesses—only 47 percent were aware that their patients did not wish to be resuscitated. One-third of outpatients had not even told their physicians that they had an advance directive.

We should do all we can to inform ourselves of the wishes of patients with far-advanced disease while they are still well enough to make rational decisions, and we should communicate these directives to all members of their health care teams in or out of the hospital. If we are realistic when we inform our patients of the extent of their disease, the likelihood that the remaining treatments will add meaningfully to the time they have left, and the realities of mechanical ventilation and the odds of ever being weaned from it, we enable them to make informed decisions about resuscitation and preventive intubation. Difficult discussions will then not have to be initiated in crisis situations, and we will avoid resuscitating patients whose disease is essentially untreatable and who might have been able to die comfortably, saving both them and their families needless suffering.

SYMPTOM MANAGEMENT GUIDE

Symptom management in patients' last days can be challenging. The SUPPORT study also revealed that family members often felt the patient's symptoms were not adequately controlled. Family members thought that, among the conscious patients, 40 percent had unrelieved severe pain and, of those with lung cancer or an underlying malignant condition with superimposed multisystem organ failure, 70 percent had severe dyspnea and 25 percent had moderate anxiety or dysphoria (Lynn et al. 1997).

Pay particular attention to the patient's comfort during the last days. If possible, when the patient is dying in the hospital, be present for at least five to ten minutes three times a day. Even if the family is not there when you are, the nurses will report your visits and the visits in themselves are often a source of comfort for the family. Sit at the bedside and observe the patient for any signs of pain, delirium, excessive upper airway secretions ("death rattle"), or myoclonus. If you find them, correct them as suggested in the following pages. Ask family or friends who are there what they have observed, and answer their questions. Let them know they can touch and speak to the patient, as they may be afraid to do so if the patient is being supported by a number of machines or is attached to intravenous lines.

SYMPTOM COMPLEX OF DYING PATIENTS.   Data on the frequency of the various symptoms that occur in the last days to week before death are somewhat conflicting. Patients usually have multiple symptoms, with combinations of those listed below varying with the underlying disease process:

Symptom Complex of Dying Patients
- Pain
- Noisy or moist breathing
- Urinary incontinence or retention
- Restlessness, agitation
- Dyspnea, cough
- Nausea and vomiting, anorexia, dysphagia, xerostomia
- Delirium
- Fatigue
- Existential or spiritual distress
- Cooling of extremities
- Fecal incontinence

Up to 70 percent of patients with advanced cancer have pain, and this pain requires ongoing therapy until death. Noisy or moist breathing, urinary incontinence or retention, and restlessness and agitation are seen in almost half of patients who are actively dying.

MANIFESTATIONS OF "ACTIVE DYING": THE LAST 10 TO 14 DAYS
- Dehydration, tachycardia, followed by decrease in heart rate and blood pressure
- Perspiration, clammy skin, cool extremities; just before death, mottling
- Diminished breath sounds, irregular breathing pattern with periods of apnea or full Cheyne-Stokes respiration; grunt or moan with exhale
- Mouth droop; difficulty swallowing; loss of gag reflex with pooling of secretions, causing "death rattle"
- Incontinence of bladder or rectum
- Agitation ± hallucinations; stillness; patient is difficult to arouse

(From Pitorak 2003)

One in five patients will be short of breath, and about one in ten will have nausea and vomiting. The incidence of delirium in patients dying of advanced cancer is 88 percent (Lawlor et al. 2000). Manifestations of delirium include sweating, confusion, jerking, twitching, or plucking at bed sheets. Patients lose the ability to swallow and become much less interactive. It is as though they are living in a large mansion in which they gradually move to rooms that are farther and farther from the front door. Responding to voice or touch takes them much longer, and they may stop showing any response. Most families seem to understand that the patient is not personally rejecting them. I often say that it just takes too much energy for the patient to "come to the front door."

Some patients may experience existential or spiritual distress, but others articulate visions of spiritual peace. One night at midnight, an Indian patient I cared for asked her husband for "water from the Ganges." Until then, he had seemed not to understand how ill she was. But after the request, he realized she was dying. They were able to grieve together, talk, and say their last good-byes. She died the next morning. And an Irish patient spoke glowingly to me of "going to the Isle to meet my people." She could see them waving at her. Could I? Her eyes were closed as she added, "My job is to get there. They're waiting for me." She continued to speak, but in Gaelic. As I got ready to leave, I wished her a peaceful journey. To my surprise, without opening her eyes, she said, in English, "Thank you."

COMMONLY REQUIRED MEDICATIONS.   Most of the problems experienced by dying patients can be controlled by a limited number of medications given by the rectal, transdermal, or, if necessary, parenteral route (Table 8.1). Medications are usually needed for pain, for rattling secretions, and for terminal anxiety, agitation, or delirium. Some patients need treatment for dyspnea or a variety of other miscellaneous problems. For those few patients whose distress cannot be controlled any other way, it may be necessary to consider palliative sedation.

PAIN CONTROL.   If one uses the WHO guidelines for cancer pain relief (see Chapter 5), 50 percent of cancer patients near death will have no pain, 25 percent mild to moderate pain, and only 3 percent severe pain. Patients require close monitoring, and both opioids and nonopioid adjuvants are usually required.

If the patient is unable to take pills, buccal, sublingual, rectal, or transdermal opioids are usually effective. In some cases, however, subcutaneous or, when intravenous access is available, intravenous infusions will be needed. Concentrated morphine or oxycodone solutions (20 to 40 mg/ml) can be given hourly or every 2 hours and are often satisfactory. Rectal administration of sustained-release opioid preparations is not approved by the FDA, but studies indicate that morphine absorption from a sustained-release preparation placed in the rectal vault is equivalent to that from oral administration. If pain is a new problem and the patient is opioid-naive, institute therapy with 15 to 30 mg of sustained-release morphine rectally every 12 hours. Alternatively, place a fentanyl patch and administer a liquid or rectal opioid for the first 12 hours until the blood level of fentanyl is adequate for pain relief.

Adjuvants can also be given rectally or subcutaneously. Patients previously benefiting from oral NSAIDs can receive rectal indomethacin; patients taking a stable glucocorticoid dose for bone or nerve pain can receive subcutaneous dexamethasone. Rectal doxepin can replace oral tricyclic antidepressants.

Table 8.1   Treatment of Problems That Are Common in the Final Days

Problem	Agent	Dose
Baseline pain	Morphine/hydromorphone, oxycodone	Sublingual, SQ; individualized
	Fentanyl transdermal (Duragesic®)	Individualized
Breakthrough pain	Concentrated oxycodone or morphine solution	Individualized
Death rattle	Scopolamine	Transderm Scōp® 1–3 patches q3d; 0.1–2.4 mg / 24 hr SQ, IV
	Hyoscyamine (Levsin SL®)	0.125 mg sublingual t.i.d. to q.i.d.
	Glycopyrrolate (Robinul®)	0.1–0.2 mg IV t.i.d. to q.i.d.
	Atropine + morphine + dexamethasone	2 mg + 2.5 mg + 2 mg by nebulizer
	Atropine + furosemide	Atropine 1–2 mg IV + furosemide 20–40 mg IV
Anxiety	Lorazepam (Ativan®) or	1 mg p.o.or sublingual q2h
	Alprazolam (Xanax®)	0.25–2 mg p.o. t.i.d.
Delirium	Haloperidol (Haldol®)	2–4 mg p.o., SQ, IM, IV q. 30 min p.r.n. to total 20 mg / 24 hr
	Olanzapine (Zyprexa®, Zydis®)	2.5–5 mg p.o./sublingual qhs to b.i.d. plus p.r.n. q4h
	Chlorpromazine (Thorazine®)	25–50 mg p.o. q4–8h or 25 mg p.r. q4–12h; preferred for dyspnea
	Midazolam (Versed®)	2–3 mg load; 0.5–1 mg/hr SQ, IV; increase p.r.n. to 100 mg/24 hr
	Phenobarbital (Nembutal®)	120–200 mg p.r. q12–24h
Dyspnea due to anxiety/panic	Midazolam (Versed®)	0.5–1.0 mg IV slowly or 0.1–1.25 mg/hr SQ
	Morphine	5–10 mg sublingual, IV, or by nebulizer
	Chlorpromazine (Thorazine®)	25 mg p.o., p.r. q4–12h; or 12.5 mg IV q4–8h

As many as half of patients need an increase in opioid dose during their last days. If the calculated opioid dose is too large to be delivered by sublingual, transdermal, or rectal routes, if pain relief does not seem to be satisfactory using any of these routes, or if the routes are unac-

---

PRACTICE POINTS: MEDICATION FOR PAIN CONTROL WHEN PILLS CANNOT BE SWALLOWED

- Concentrated morphine/oxycodone (20 to 40 mg/ml), buccal or sublingual
- Sustained-release preparations, p.r.; Kadian pellets suspended in water, given through a feeding tube
- Adjuvants, p.r. (e.g., NSAIDs, acetaminophen, doxepin)
- Opioids and dexamethasone, subcutaneous injection or infusion

---

ceptable to the patient or the caregiver, give the opioid by subcutaneous infusion or, if intravenous access is available, by intravenous infusion. Both types of infusion can be delivered in the home with the aid of hospice or other home nurses. The starting opioid dose for a patient whose pain is well controlled should be the intravenous equivalent of the oral dose (see Table 5.5); if the pain is not under control, give a dose that is slightly higher than the equivalent dose.

DEATH RATTLE.   Patients are usually unaware of these loud respirations, but they can be very distressing for families. They occur in 60 to 90 percent of dying patients. Sometimes, simply repositioning the patient is helpful because he may breathe more easily in a lateral recumbent position than supine. Most patients benefit from one of the drying agents, such as hyoscyamine (Levsin SL); scopolamine in a gel, a transdermal patch, or by infusion; intravenous glycopyrrolate; nebulized atropine combined with morphine and dexamethasone, or intravenous atropine with furosemide.

Scopolamine has been reported to be efficacious in as many as 70 percent of patients. Patients whose death rattle is due to salivary secretions often respond to lower doses of scopolamine than those required for patients with excessive bronchial secretions. If you prescribe one of these agents, the patient will also need to have his mouth moistened periodically.

TERMINAL RESTLESSNESS.   Almost half of patients who are actively dying of cancer show signs of restlessness and agitation. They may toss and turn, moan, have muscle twitching or spasm, and only intermittently be awake. Even though patients may appear to be out of contact with the external world, they often seem to be reassured by familiar voices or by being touched.

The agitation is sometimes due to reversible physical problems, such as a full bladder, fecal impaction, pain, nausea, or trouble breathing due to hypoxia or poorly cleared secretions. Some patients may have developed delirium either as an opioid side effect or in response to increasing blood levels of opioid as renal or hepatic function deteriorates. These patients respond to a change in opioid or, if monitoring for pain can be done frequently, a decrease in opioid dose or a change to an immediate-release preparation given as needed. In other patients, unresolved spiritual, psychological, or social problems induce the distress. All members of the hospice team will reevaluate the patient with these issues in mind. They often can detect the cause of the problem and offer workable solutions.

PRACTICE POINTS: TREATMENT OF "DEATH RATTLE"
- Place the patient in the lateral recumbent position.
- Administer drying agents:
  —Hyoscyamine (Levsin SL), 0.125 mg sublingual t.i.d. to q.i.d.
  —Scopolamine
      Transderm Scōp, 1 to 3 patches every 3 days.
      Subcutaneous infusion, 0.1 to 2.4 mg / 24 hr.
  —Glycopyrrolate 0.1 to 0.2 mg IV t.i.d. to q.i.d.
  —Atropine
      By nebulizer, 2 mg atropine + 2.5 mg morphine + 2 mg dexamethasone.
      Atropine 1 to 2 mg IM + furosemide 20 to 40 mg IV.

Patients may need a mild sedative such as lorazepam (e.g., Ativan) or alprazolam (e.g., Xanax), spiritual reassurance, a visit from an estranged family member or friend, or just permission to "let go." When it is possible to arrange these, the anxiety often disappears entirely and the patient appears calm and peaceful.

Other patients, however, are agitated because they are delirious. Consider rehydration if you suspect severe dehydration. These patients usually respond to haloperidol (e.g., Haldol), olanzapine (Zyprexa, Zydis) or chlorpromazine. For patients with dyspnea, chlorpromazine, which is effective for both delirium and dyspnea, may be used as first-line therapy. Chlorpromazine is also more sedating than haloperidol,

---

PRACTICE POINTS: TREATMENT OF TERMINAL AGITATION

- Evaluate the patient for reversible physical problems: full bladder, fecal impaction, pain, nausea, hypoxia, secretions, opioid side effects (especially if there is decreased urine output), marked dehydration.
- Consider the need to change opioid, opioid dose, or opioid preparation (i.e., from sustained to immediate release given as needed).
- Consider rehydration (1 to 1.5 liters / 24 hr).
- Consider the need for psychological or spiritual counseling (e.g., for resolution of family estrangements or for permission to "let go").
- Medicate for anxiety
  —Lorazepam (e.g., Ativan), 1 mg p.o. or sublingual every 2 hours, or alprazolam (e.g., Xanax), 0.25–2 mg p.o. t.i.d.
- Medicate for mild delirium (see also Chapter 7).
  —Haloperidol (e.g., Haldol), 2 mg p.o., SQ, or IV, repeated at 30 minutes p.r.n. After an additional 30 minutes, double the dose, if needed, to a total of 20 mg / 24 hr.
  —Olanzapine (Zyprexa, Zydis), 2.5 to 5 mg p.o. b.i.d.; may give an additional 2.5 mg q4h p.r.n.
  —Chlorpromazine, 25 to 50 mg p.o. or p.r. every 4 to 8 hours; preferred for dyspneic patients or for those who would benefit from sedation.
  —Phenobarbital (Nembutal), 120 to 200 mg p.r. every 12 to 24 hours.
- Medicate for refractory delirium.
  —Midazolam 3-mg load followed by 0.5 to 1.0 mg/hr midazolam infusion; increase rate by 0.5 to 1 mg/hr until calm.
  —Pentobarbital 3 mg/kg IV load, followed by 1 to 2 mg/kg/hr IV. Not compatible with other drugs. Stable for only 12 hours.

---

and this extra sedation may be beneficial at this time. Phenobarbital suppositories (Nembutal) or pentobarbitol infusions are often helpful as well. Larger doses of midazolam (up to 100 mg / 24 hr) may be needed if there is a great deal of myoclonus.

DYSPNEA. Dying patients with dyspnea benefit from the same symptomatic therapies recommended for patients with less advanced disease (see Table 7.5). Aggressive treatment of panic due to perceived

---

**PRACTICE POINTS: TREATMENT OF DYSPNEA THAT IS
CAUSING PANIC**

- Morphine, 5 to 10 mg liquid sublingual or p.o., IV, or nebulized
- Chlorpromazine, 25 mg p.o. or p.r., or 12.5 mg IV
- Midazolam, 0.5 to 1.0 mg IV very slowly

---

breathlessness is particularly important for these patients, and hospice nurses often instruct families in how to administer the necessary morphine, chlorpromazine, or, for refractory panic, midazolam.

HYDRATION.   In a recent report from Oregon, most hospice patients who voluntarily refused food and fluids to hasten their death seemed to their hospice nurses to have had a "good death," and they did not complain of hunger or thirst (Ganzini et al. 2003). While patients are unlikely to be thirsty or hungry, they may have a dry mouth caused by opioids. A prospective study at St. Christopher's Hospice in London found no difference in the reports of thirst or dry mouth between dehydrated and normally hydrated dying patients (Ellershaw et al. 1995). Over 90 percent of all patients with these complaints, however, were receiving opioids. Thus it is not necessary to reverse the dehydration to relieve dry mouth; no controlled studies have shown that rehydration is effective. Moistening the mouth with gauze soaked in ice water or offering sips of water, ice chips, or fruit-flavored ice pops is usually all that is needed.

Parenteral hydration can actually cause increased distress by increasing urine output, inducing pulmonary or peripheral edema, or increasing ascites, pulmonary secretions, or nausea and vomiting from

---

PRACTICE POINTS: HYDRATION IN DYING PATIENTS

- Remember: thirst ≠ dehydration.
- Moisten lips with gauze soaked in ice water, or offer sips of water or plain or fruit-flavored ice chips.
- If parenteral hydration is chosen, do not exceed 1 to 1.5 liters/day to avoid increasing distress (e.g., increasing urine output, pulmonary secretions, nausea and vomiting, ascites, or pulmonary or peripheral edema).

---

increased gastric secretions. If you think parenteral hydration is indicated, try to limit replacement to a liter or a liter and a half a day, and use furosemide to manage overhydration.

MASSIVE HEMOPTYSIS (OR OTHER BLEEDING).   Massive hemoptysis is relatively rare, in one report occurring in 7 percent of about 500 patients hospitalized in a cancer hospital. In a dying patient, it will usually have been preceded by less extensive hemoptysis, giving you and the home care or hospice team the opportunity to prepare the patient and family. If you think the patient is likely to develop either a massive bleed (e.g., from a head and neck tumor near the carotids) or massive hemoptysis, suggest the family get dark-colored sheets, towels, and blankets to mask the blood. Because emergency intravenous access may be needed for patient sedation, consider insertion of a PICC line in patients without an indwelling venous access device.

The hospice nurse can leave a kit in the home that contains prefilled syringes of appropriate medication for a patient with massive hemopty-

---

PRACTICE POINTS: TREATMENT OF MASSIVE HEMOPTYSIS OR EXSANGUINATING BLEEDING

- Ask the family to purchase dark-colored towels, blankets, or sheets to mask the blood.
- When appropriate, insert a PICC line for emergency IV access.
- Ascertain whether the family feels comfortable giving medications IV, SQ, or p.r. and instruct them as appropriate in administering the following:
  —Rectal diazepam (10 mg), rectal lorazepam (2 mg), or IV midazolam (1 to 5 mg) from prefilled syringes.
  —Morphine IV or SQ from prefilled syringes.
   Dose for opioid-naive patient: 10 mg morphine.
   Dose for patient on opioids: the intravenous equivalent of the "rescue" opioid dose.
   Example. For a patient taking 600 mg SR morphine every 24 hours:
    Oral rescue: 60 mg; IV rescue: 20 mg (i.e., 60 mg / 3).
    Opioid dose for sedation: 20 mg IV morphine.
- Teach the family how to place the patient bleeding side down in the Trendelenburg position when bleeding occurs.

sis or an exsanguinating bleed. It includes morphine, to be given intravenously when possible, and a benzodiazepine. Midazolam (Versed) can be given intramuscularly or intravenously; diazepam or lorazepam (e.g., Ativan) can be given rectally. When the event occurs, the patient is placed bleeding side down, in the Trendelenburg position, and the medications noted above are given. If the nurses arrive in time, they can position the patient and administer these medications or start continuous infusions of morphine and/or midazolam, if necessary.

MISCELLANEOUS. For patients with catheters who are experiencing dysuria, lidocaine can be added to saline bladder irrigation. For patients with nausea or vomiting due to bowel obstruction, continue (or add) octreotide; for nausea or vomiting from other causes, metoclopramide plus haloperidol (e.g., Haldol) plus promethazine (Phenergan) can be safely infused subcutaneously or intravenously. Famotidine can be converted to a subcutaneous infusion if the patient had been getting relief from gastrointestinal symptoms when taking this. Myoclonus responds to midazolam. All these medications can be given in the home by the caregivers or by home care or hospice nurses.

PRACTICE POINTS: TREATMENT OF OTHER DISTRESSING PROBLEMS

- Catheter-induced dysuria: lidocaine bladder irrigation
- Nausea/vomiting
  —Due to bowel obstruction: octreotide, 150 to 300 µg SQ b.i.d. or 300 to 600 µg / 24 hr SQ infusion.
  —Due to other causes: metoclopramide 30 mg + haloperidol 1.5 mg + promethazine 6.25 mg, SQ or IV infusion over 24 hours.
- Myoclonus due to opioid toxicity: midazolam 5 mg loading dose (2 mg for patients over 60), then 10 to 100 mg / 24 hr IV infusion.

PALLIATIVE SEDATION. Palliative sedation is considered when, despite expert evaluation and management, a patient who is near death continues to experience intolerable physical, psychological, or spiritual/existential distress. Most often, the desire for palliative sedation arises when psychological or spiritual/existential concerns coexist with physical problems. Expert palliative care, pastoral consultation, and evaluation by a psychiatrist should be undertaken at this point. The consultants may identify previously inapparent problems that are amenable to therapy or may suggest ways to improve control of physical, psychological, spiritual, or existential symptoms. See Figure 8.1 for an algorithm that describes the assessment and management that should precede consideration of palliative sedation.

Unfortunately, the doses of opioid, neuroleptic, or benzodiazepine that will control pain, cough, dyspnea, seizures, or agitation may sedate the patient so profoundly that unconsciousness ensues. Some ethicists have invoked the doctrine of double effect, discussed above, to support such "palliative sedation." They argue that while harm is foreseen, no harm is intended by the sedation-induced unconsciousness; on the contrary, the physician has an obligation to help the patient and no alterna-

---

PRACTICE POINTS: PALLIATIVE SEDATION

- Indications: The patient is imminently dying and is experiencing suffering (physical, psychological, and/or spiritual/existential) that is refractory to expert attempts at management, including palliative care and psychiatric and spiritual consultation.
- Family counseling:
  —Obtain informed consent from the patient and family or, if necessary, from the health care proxy.
  —Ask, "Later, will you still feel that we did the right thing? Will you feel that anything should have been done differently?"
- Provide close monitoring by a nurse or physician.
- Initiate a medication regimen for reversible symptoms (e.g., pain); titrate to comfort: e.g., SQ or IV opioid infusions.
- For symptoms that are refractory to opioids or for patients with intolerable side effects, choose one of the following initial doses and titrate to comfort. (If the patient is thought to be experiencing ongoing pain, continue the opioid infusion while administering another agent.)

Midazolam	Bolus 0.5 mg; then 0.5–1.5 mg/hr
Lorazepam	0.5–1 mg/hr
Phenobarbital	130 mg q. 30 min to 1000 mg / 24 hr
Pentobarbital	3 mg/kg load, then 1–2 mg/kg/hr
Thiopental	3–5 mg/kg/hr

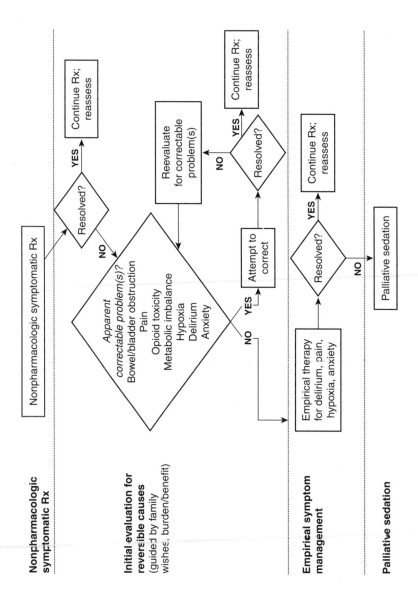

Nonpharmacologic symptomatic Rx

Initial evaluation for reversible causes
(guided by family wishes, burden/benefit)

Empirical symptom management

Palliative sedation

8.1   Agitation in the Last Days

tive ways remain to provide that help. Since the action meets both these conditions (i.e., no harm is foreseen and benefit will accrue), palliative sedation may be considered ethical. Others cite the Autonomy of the patient and Beneficence as the ethical underpinnings.

Some have gone as far as suggesting that "death-hastening or death-causing palliative analgesic administration" is obligatory in such settings (Cavanaugh 1996). Situations may occur, Cavanaugh suggests, when our obligation to relieve the patient's pain or suffering is greater than our obligation to avoid hastening or causing death. In such instances, he says, the use of opioids or other agents to induce sedation would become obligatory.

Discussions among the health care team, the patient, and family members usually achieve consensus on the need for and acceptability of sedation as a means of achieving symptom control. We should attempt to obtain formal informed consent either from the patient or from the health care proxy. In addition, Dr. Byock (1997) recommends that we try to ensure that families will not regret their decision after the patient dies. He asks them to imagine that, several months after the death, they are recalling the events immediately preceding it and asking themselves whether anything should have been done differently. If the answer is no, he proceeds with the agreed-upon plan. He finds that families who have had these conversations do not develop subsequent guilt or regrets.

If neither the specific therapies described above nor opioid infusions effectively relieve the distressing symptom, intravenous benzodiazepines or rectal, subcutaneous, or intravenous barbiturates can be used and will work. The benzodiazepine midazolam, while quite effective, is also quite costly. In exceptional circumstances, anesthesiologists can deliver propofol (Moyle 1995).

IMMEDIATELY AFTER THE DEATH

Studies indicate that many house officers are not trained in what to do after the patient dies (Ferris et al. 1998). If you are present at the death, or if you have been asked to "pronounce" the patient dead, offer your condolences to all others present before you leave the room. Such expressions can be very comforting. If you are invited to participate in a prayer, this is perfectly appropriate if you so wish. Encourage those present to spend as much time as they need to, to say or do whatever they need to say or do, including touching the body. Answer the family's questions, and if the family was not present at the death, review the dying process with them. Reassure them about pain control or other concerns they have about the patient's suffering.

If hugging comes naturally to you and seems to be called for now, this, and the tears that may accompany it, are also OK. Just be sure to mitigate the manifestations of your sorrow so that the family doesn't feel the need to take care of you. Also offer condolences to the nurses and other staff who have cared for the patient. If the family has shared with you praise for the care that the patient received, be sure to share this with the staff as well: "*Her family told me they were so appreciative of the wonderful care you gave her.*" Those of you who work with house staff can help them deal with their grief by allowing them to review the circumstances of the death, their feelings for the patient, and their contributions to the care of the patient. Studies indicate that interns, in particular, need this support (Redinbaugh 2003).

The nurses will be bathing and caring for the patient's body according to the patient's wishes. Some religions require special rituals after a person has died. These needs should be known prior to the death, and arrangement made to have the appropriate people informed. Some Jewish patients, for example, will direct that their body be bathed and prepared for burial by a specially trained group of men or women (the Chevra Kadosha). In the next part of this chapter I discuss more about what you and the team can do to help the bereaved family.

SUMMARY

The dying patient presents an increased burden for an already stressed family, especially when the patient is dying at home. But families who have been able to care for a dying loved one at home often express their profound satisfaction that they did everything they could. Even those who need to bring the patient to the hospital for the final few days or hours may feel an appropriate sense of pride and accomplishment.

Most family members have never seen anyone die and, while willing to do whatever is necessary to allow the patient to die at home, they are totally unprepared for the reality of that death. We and the home hospice teams can help them identity when the last days and weeks have come, and can often provide the expertise and support the family needs during the patient's final days.

THE BEREAVED

Our responsibilities to the patient and family continue after the patient's death as we try to help the bereaved survivors. To anticipate their needs and to develop a suitable support program for them, it is useful to understand the many dimensions and manifestations of grief and mourning. The writings of Dr. Colin Parkes, Dr. Therese A. Rando, and Dr. Holly Prigerson are superb resources for physicians or other clinicians wanting in-depth, scholarly, and clinically useful discussions of normal and complicated mourning. Their formulations are the foundation of the following discussion, and references to their works, as well as to those of others working in this area, are listed at the end of the chapter.

LOSS, GRIEF, AND MOURNING

Those who are bereaved are suffering from a number of losses. In addition to the loss of the loved one, secondary losses can occur, such as having to leave the family home or changing one's social standing from wife to widow. In addition, the death is likely to revive the pain of losses that occurred many years before. A father's death, for example, may evoke memories of a divorce or the death of a child. The bereaved also suffer from the loss of "what might have been"—a reconciliation that never happened, a father to walk with down the aisle, a twenty-first birthday party. At the time of the death, bereaved family members enter this maelstrom of loss and may need help sorting out the sources of their pain.

A survivor's grief is a "process of experiencing the psychological, behavioral, social, and physical reactions to the perception of loss" (Rando 1993). The intensity of a survivor's grief is predicated on a number of factors relating to the deceased and the survivor's relationship with the deceased, characteristics of the mourner, the nature of the death, and societal and cultural factors.

For example, being very attached to or very dependent on the deceased or having a great deal of ambivalence in one's feelings toward the deceased can exacerbate the grief, as can a personal history of clinical depression or difficulty in handling previous losses. A sudden or accidental death, suicide, or homicide also magnifies the grief experienced, while a good support system and religious rituals can lessen it.

DIFFERENTIATION BETWEEN GRIEF AND DEPRESSION. It can sometimes be challenging to distinguish between manifestations of grief and those of depression (Block 2001, Prigerson et al. 1996). Block explains that while survivors with grief have "somatic distress, sleep and appetite disturbances, decreased concentration, social withdrawal and sighing," they do not express "hopelessness, helplessness, feelings of worthlessness, guilt, or suicidal ideation." People with grief can still get pleasure at times, have only passive wishes "for death to come quickly," and look forward to the future. By contrast, for those with depression, "nothing is enjoyable" and the feelings are "constant, unremitting." Some may have "intense and persistent suicidal ideation and no sense of a positive future."

Depression responds better to pharmacologic therapy than does grief. Methylphenidate, SSRIs, and bupropion SR (sustained-release) all have been found to improve depression, and did not worsen grief intensity (Block 2001; Zisook et al. 2001). Prigerson has extensively studied patients with grief and depression, and she reports that in randomized trials of patients with complicated grief, these patients do not improve with tricyclic antidepressants or interpersonal psychotherapy (Prigerson and Jacobs 2001). They may respond, however, to crisis intervention, "guided mourning," or brief dynamic psychotherapy. Paroxetine (Paxil) was effective in reducing symptoms by ~50 percent in an open-label trial.

PHASES OF GRIEF AND MOURNING, AND PROCESSES OF MOURNING. Each bereaved person's loss is unique, as are the experience and manifestations of the grief and mourning. But many people pass through one or more identifiable stages of grief and the rebuilding of a life without the deceased. Dr. Rando describes three phases of grief and mourning and six processes of mourning experienced by most survivors who are able to reintegrate. The phases, which include periods of overlapping manifestations, are *avoidance, confrontation,* and *accommodation* (Rando 1993, p. 45):

Phases of Grief and Mourning, and the Six "R" Processes of Mourning

Avoidance Phase
1. *Recognize* the loss.
   Acknowledge the death.
   Understand the death.

Confrontation Phase

2. *React* to the separation.

   Experience the pain.

   Feel, identify, accept, and give some form of expression to all the psychological reactions to the loss.

   Identify and mourn secondary losses.

3. *Recollect* and *reexperience* the deceased and the relationship.

   Review and remember realistically.

   Revive and reexperience the feelings.

4. *Relinquish* the old attachments to the deceased and the old assumptive world.

Accommodation Phase

5. *Readjust* to move adaptively into the new world without forgetting the old.

   Revise the assumptive world.

   Develop a new relationship with the deceased.

   Adopt new ways of being in the world.

   Form a new identity.

6. *Reinvest*

During the *avoidance* phase, survivors may initially appear numb, confused, or dazed, but some form of denial usually follows as the reality of the death intensifies. A wide range of behaviors can be expected, from uncontrolled shrieking to an unnerving calm.

During the *confrontation* phase, the pain intensifies because the absence of the person who has died asserts itself repeatedly. The mourner begins to yearn for the one who is dead, and pangs of intense grief occur each time the deceased is sought and not found; denial dissolves and disorganization, depression, disinterest, and despair take its place (Parkes 1987). During this phase, the survivor commonly experiences a variety of feelings, behaviors, physical symptoms, spiritual concerns, and thoughts (listed in Figure 8.2; for a more complete list of psychological, behavioral, social, and physical responses, see Rando 1993).

The family must adjust to an environment without the person who has died. The role played by the deceased in the marriage, the family, and even the community may be increasingly revealed to the survivors as time goes on, and mourning may be needed for each loss. Ideally, the survivors will be able to cope with the increasing responsibilities, but

WHAT TO EXPECT

Recovery from the loss of someone you love is often a long and painful process. However, if you can make it through the pain, things will get better. Most people find that their grief lasts anywhere from six months to two years. Since each person is unique, you will progress at your own pace and in your own way.

Grief is often associated with certain feelings and physical symptoms. Some of these include:

Common Feelings/Behaviors
- Fear and anxiety
- Anger and guilt
- Depression and despair
- Separation and longing
- Sudden wave of psychic pain
- Confusion and inability to concentrate or make decisions
- Tearfulness and crying
- Sighing
- Restlessness
- Yearning
- Helplessness
- Relief
- Hope

Spiritual Responses
- Faith may be strengthened, altered, or abandoned

Common Physical Symptoms
- Decreased or increased appetite
- Decreased energy; weakness of muscles
- Nausea and diarrhea
- Decrease or increase in your sex drive
- Inability to sleep or sleeping too much
- Feeling something stuck in your throat
- Tightness in chest, breathlessness
- Oversensitivity to noise
- Vivid dreams
- Dry mouth

Common Thoughts
- Disbelief
- Preoccupation with "if only" and "what if" and with memories
- Sense of his/her presence
- "Who am I now?"

WHAT TO DO

1. Give yourself permission to feel loss and to grieve over the loss.
2. Recognize that your grief is unique.
3. Expect to have some negative feelings.
4. Accept the help of others; let people know how they can help you.
5. Give yourself time alone.
6. Engage in physical activity.
7. Read books about feelings of grief and the process of recovery.
8. Talk to others about your loss.
9. Attend community support groups.
10. Most important: Recognize that at some point your pain will lessen.

WHAT NOT TO DO

1. Avoid making major changes.
2. Try not to withdraw from social activities.
3. Avoid excessive smoking or drinking.

WHEN TO CALL

Please call:
- If you have any questions or would like further information.
- If you feel that you would like professional counseling.

8.2 What to Expect—for the Bereaved. From J. Abrahm, M. E. Cooley, and L. Ricacho, Efficacy of an educational bereavement program for families of veterans with cancer, *Journal of Cancer Education*, 10:207–212, 1995; with permission.

many may need assistance or training—for example, in household finance or managing children.

Accepting the reality of the loss and experiencing its pain are essential if the pain is to be overcome. It is very difficult for people to move beyond loss if they never allow themselves to feel it in some way that is appropriate for them. Family obligations and unspoken strictures against demonstrations of grief can further impair a survivor's ability to experience the pain of the loss adequately. Putting those feelings aside to deal with later or denying their existence altogether will only prolong or inhibit the process.

Eventually—and there is no useful timetable to determine when this will occur—most survivors reach the third phase, *accommodation*. Dr. Rando chose this word carefully. It does not imply closure or return to the premorbid state. Instead, it suggests passage to a state in which life will never be the same, but in which the survivor tacitly acknowledges that an accommodation must be made if he or she is ever to resume old relationships and responsibilities. And even more difficult is the decision to try to establish new ones and risk recurrent loss, to realize that loving someone new need not mean betraying the memory of the person who has died. The survivor must craft a new relationship with the deceased, a new identity, and a new role in society.

Throughout the confrontation phase, and even in the accommodation phase and for years after the death, survivors are likely to experience what Dr. Rando calls "subsequent temporary upsurges of grief" (Rando 1993). Precipitants for these recurrent pangs of grief include anniversaries, holidays, and seasonal changes; reaching the age at which the loved one died; having a child reach the age of the child who died; favorite shared activities and personal reminders (e.g., music, smells, favorite objects); and a new personal or public trauma that resurrects the pain of old losses, especially if the one who died was the person turned to in times of crisis. The severity of the grief can match that of the initial loss and can be frightening for survivors who had thought themselves beyond experiencing pain of that intensity.

INTERVENTIONS.   Given these roadmaps of what to expect, clinicians and researchers have devised interventions to ameliorate the suffering of survivors, and have demonstrated their value. Some take place in anticipation of the patient's death and were described in earlier chapters. These include skillfully communicating the diagnosis and terminal prognosis; providing emotional, psychological, and spiritual support as

well as physical comfort; and helping families to resolve outstanding issues. It is also important to provide support in the final days and make
the death as peaceful as possible.

A formal bereavement program usually takes place during the first
year after the patient's death; accommodation is usually well under way
by that time. After the formal program ends, the bereaved are welcome
to continue participation in any bereavement activities that have been
useful to them.

A SAMPLE BEREAVEMENT PROGRAM

Even families who are coping well benefit from support for this extended period after the patient's death. All home hospice teams provide
the year of bereavement care and welcome in their group programs
families who did not receive hospice services. In addition, you might
consider providing your own year-long bereavement program. Various
people in the office can participate, and it can be very rewarding for each
of them.

AT THE TIME OF DEATH: THE AVOIDANCE PHASE.   The program we use
begins immediately after the death. Family members are often in a state
of shock; their moods may swing wildly, changing from moment to mo-

---

PRACTICE POINTS: SUPPORTING THE SURVIVORS

- Reassure family members that their response to the patient's death is
  normal.
- Listen sympathetically if they wish to review the circumstances of
  the patient's death.
- Reassure the family that you will remain available to them to help
  them with the grieving process.
- During the first year following the patient's death, call and write to
  the family at regularly scheduled intervals; don't wait for them to get
  in touch with you.
- Offer to send educational materials on manifestations of grief, coping techniques, and professional resources, if the family wishes.
- Invite them to participate in a memorial service.
- Identify family members at high risk for prolonged, intense grief and
  arrange a referral for professional support even before the patient
  dies.

ment. This volatility may be frightening for them—to be detached and numb one minute and distraught the next—and we try to reassure them that this reaction is normal and that they should not worry about controlling themselves.

If I am sad, I let myself cry with them, or if they seem to need to talk things over, I ask leading questions to help them feel free to tell me their feelings. I find that they often want to review the circumstances of the death, to assure themselves that the person was not suffering and that everything that could have been done was done. I always try to find something for which I can praise them, such as their care of the patient or their advocacy role for him, and add how lucky he was to have had them there when he needed them. Even if I was not present at the death, I try to offer as much of this kind of reassurance and support as I can in the course of a telephone call.

INITIAL FOLLOW-UP CALL.   We next call the family within 24 to 48 hours of the death to offer our condolences and help. During this call, we can offer comfort and provide a listener for a retelling of the story of the death and the meaning of it for the bereaved. If necessary, we again reinforce the normality of the wide emotional swings or other symptoms of acute grief they may be experiencing. We listen empathetically and indicate our unconditional continued support. We end the conversation by asking whether we can keep in touch, and let them know we will be calling again in about a month. We also write them a letter about a week after the death (Figure 8.3). You and your house staff team can find a full discussion of the principles that underlie the writing of a good condolence letter in Fast Fact and Concept #22 on the End of Life / Palliative Education Resource Center website (www.eperc.mcw.edu).

If the family was involved with a hospice program, we remind them that all members of the hospice team are still available to them. Some survivors will have developed a close relationship with the hospice nurse, social worker, volunteer, or chaplain, and it may be easier for them to continue to work with someone familiar who knew the deceased.

FOUR TO SIX WEEKS AFTER THE DEATH: CONFRONTATION DISPLACES AVOIDANCE.   About a month after we send the letter, we call again and offer to send a variety of materials that might be helpful. We include a letter (Figure 8.3) and a list of readings, a description of grief, and a list of feelings and physical signs commonly experienced by those who are grieving, and what to do or not do about them (Figure 8.2).

Letter sent one week after death

Dear _____ :

We share your sadness about your loss of _____. We realize how hard it is when death occurs and want to let you know how important it is to be with family and friends at this time. If we can help you in any way, please call us at _____. Again, all of us in the Hematology/Oncology department send our deepest sympathy.

Sincerely,

Letter sent three to six weeks after death and repeated at six months

Dear _____ :

When we spoke on the phone, you said you would like more information to help you understand what you have been going through since _____ died. We have therefore enclosed information describing common feelings many people experience at the loss of a loved one as well as a list of books you could read that discuss these issues and a list of groups in your area that you could try for more support.

We realize that this is a hard time for you and we offer this information in the hope that it may be of some help. If you have any questions or want to talk with someone, please feel free to call us at _____ and ask for me.

Sincerely,

Holiday letter

Dear _____ :

We were thinking of you because we know that this time of year may be difficult, since this is the first time without _____ . Others around you may also be thinking of _____ at this time. We want you to know that it is OK to talk about your loved one, of your memories of those special times together.

Remember to take one day at a time. If you find yourself feeling anxious, depressed or lonely, please feel free to call. We all hope you find comfort and peace at this time. If there's anything we can do to help, please call.

Sincerely,

8.3 Letters to the Bereaved. From J. Abrahm, M. E. Cooley, and L. Ricacho, Efficacy of an educational bereavement program for families of veterans with cancer, *Journal of Cancer Education,* 10:207–212, 1995; with permission.

For example, at this point it is normal for bereaved family members or friends to experience sudden overwhelming grief, just as intense as it was initially, in response to familiar places or other reminders of the lost person ("subsequent temporary upsurge of grief"). Alternatively, they may be angry about having been left or may become depressed, and they commonly experience a period in which they just don't care about anything.

We also include a list of support groups in their area, including those hosted by the hospice, because talking about their loss with skilled bereavement counselors or others who have suffered similar losses can help in recovery. Groups such as Widow-to-Widow and, for parents who have lost a child, Compassionate Friends or Candlelighters (website: www.candle.org) can provide much-needed understanding and help with rebuilding a life. The circumstances of the death, or how the bereaved person was notified about it, may need to be repeated many times until the circumstances finally lose their ability to wound. The bereaved person may not feel comfortable "burdening" his or her friends or family with the story. But talking with a bereavement counselor or a therapist or with others in a similar situation may be acceptable and very helpful.

OTHER CONTACTS.   Because this has been shown to be a time of most need for bereaved families, we call again at six months and repeat our offer of various materials. Many families who have just begun the accommodation phase now find them very helpful. We also participate in and help plan memorial services. And in anticipation of a recurrence of grief, we send a letter at the first anniversary of the person's death, and we send the "holiday letter" (Figure 8.3) just before the winter holiday season, a few weeks before Thanksgiving. Survivors frequently respond to our offer to call, and they tell us how much they appreciate our continuing interest.

Initially we were somewhat concerned that these calls and letters might have an adverse effect, bringing up painful memories that had been successfully buried. But this was not the finding of a study we did to examine this question. A research nurse who had begun working with us after we started the program, and who did not know the patients or their families, conducted telephone interviews of the survivors, using a standardized questionnaire. She discovered that none of the survivors felt the interventions were harmful.

I think you and your staff will also find the process very rewarding. I have noticed that as I speak to survivors at longer and longer intervals, and begin to remember patients as they were before the terminal stages of their illness, it helps me achieve closure and makes it easier for me to move on.

COMPLICATED MOURNING

After the initial period of intense grieving, most families do very well. But others do not. For these families the bereavement process is very severe and prolonged. Many do not pass beyond the avoidance phase. Others are unable to reach any kind of accommodation with their loss. These survivors are experiencing what has been termed "complicated mourning."

WHO IS AT RISK?   A number of characteristics of the death itself and of the person who is bereaved and his or her relationship with the deceased can predict whether a survivor is likely to remain reasonably functional or is at high risk for severe psychological distress (Kissane 2004; Rando 1993; Raphael 1977):

Deaths That Prolong or Distort Normal Grief and Mourning
- Unexpected and sudden death, even in a patient with advanced disease
- Random, traumatic, violent, or mutilating death
- Death following a prolonged illness
- Death that seemed to be preventable

Many survivors of deaths with these characteristics exhibit what has been called the "unanticipated mourning" syndrome. Mourning is delayed or absent because denial is very strong, and survivors manifest symptoms typical of post-traumatic stress disorder. Such survivors have nightmares or hallucinations that replay the events preceding the death. They can experience anxiety or panic attacks in response to sights or sounds that remind them of the circumstances of the death.

Prigerson has reported that complicated grief symptoms can last for several years (Prigerson and Jacobs 2002). Survivors suffering from complicated grief are at increased risk for social dysfunction and for a number of adverse health consequences (such as cardiac events, cancer, and hypertension). She has refined a sensitive and specific diagnostic algorithm that identifies patients suffering from complicated grief.

FEATURES OF COMPLICATED GRIEF

Criterion 1: Extreme levels of three of the four "separation distress" symptoms: "(1) yearning or (2) searching for the deceased, (3) intrusive thoughts of the deceased, or (4) excessive loneliness since the death" *and*

Criterion 2: Extreme levels of four of the eight "traumatic distress" symptoms. "(1) purposelessness or feelings of futility about the future; (2) subjective sense of numbness, detachment, or absence of emotional responsiveness; (3) difficulty acknowledging the death; (4) feeling that life is empty or meaningless; (5) feeling that part of oneself has died; (6) shattered world view (e.g., lost sense of security, trust, control); (7) assumes symptoms or harmful behaviors of, or related to, the deceased person; and (8) excessive irritability, bitterness, or anger related to the death."

If both criteria 1 and 2 are met, if they last for six months or longer, and if they cause significant impairment of physical, social, or occupational function, the patient meets the algorithm's criteria for "complicated grief."

(From Prigerson and Jacobs 2001)

Persons who have been angry with or had an ambivalent relationship with the deceased suffer "conflicted grief." At the time of the death the survivor often feels nothing but relief, but months later, feelings of yearning, guilt, and loss become prominent. In contrast, persons with any of the other characteristics listed above suffer "chronic grief": the grieving is as intense at the end of a year as it was initially; no effort has been made toward accommodation to a life alone.

Characteristics of the Mourner or of the Relationship with the Deceased That Distort Normal Grief and Mourning

- An ambivalent relationship or one filled with anger
- Dependency, the survivor having played either the strong or the weak role
- Unresolved additional losses
- Additional stresses on the mourner
- A perceived lack of social support

BEREAVEMENT RISK ASSESSMENT TOOL.   In my practice, in addition to considering the factors reviewed above, I have used the Bereavement Risk Assessment Tool developed at St. Christopher's Hospice in London to determine who is at high risk (Figure 8.4). Families at high risk are those who score 15 or higher on this scale or those who, for whatever reason, the evaluator suspects are likely to cope either badly (requiring special help) or very badly (requiring urgent help). For example, people who have a number of young children at home, who are burdened by feelings of anger and self-reproach, who do not work outside the home, or who are clinging or pining could easily score above 15 on this assessment tool.

DETECTING COMPLICATED MOURNING.   Some survivors who did not appear to be at high risk before the patient died will nevertheless manifest signs of unresolved grief for months after the death. Some people, for example, may remain in denial, having failed even to begin grieving: they may never have seemed sad and may even have avoided the funeral. Others are unable to make decisions; they lose initiative; they are filled with guilt and self-reproach, exhibit self-destructive behaviors, and may ultimately develop a major depression beginning at the time of the death and recurring at important anniversaries (Block 1985).

Still others are unwilling to let go, refusing to allow any of the deceased's personal effects to be moved. They cannot discuss their lost relative without becoming very upset; but they repeatedly talk about their bereavement and feel it acutely, even if months have elapsed. Finally, some may be intensely angry—at the deceased, at the physicians, or at others who cared for the person who died.

TREATMENT.   Clinicians and researchers who have done extensive work in this area recommend that, to minimize psychological morbidity, we begin psychological support for family members who are at high risk even before the patient dies. For those at less risk, we should maintain close contact after the death and institute intensive support as soon as they manifest a need.

For some family members—for example those with unresolved anger, crises of faith, or guilt—ongoing spiritual counseling is very helpful. Others who have problems of self-reproach, dependency, or ambivalence toward the person who has died or will soon die may benefit from individual or group psychotherapy delivered by therapists experienced with the problems of the bereaved. With this treatment and appropriate medication, if needed, many troubled survivors are able to

PATIENT NAME _____ S/O NAME _____ DATE _____

A. Children <14 @ Home:	B. Occupation of Principal Wage Earner:	C. Anticipated Employment of Key Person:	D. Clinging or Pining:
0 None 1 One 2 Two 3 Three 4 Four 5 Five or more	1 Professional and executive 2 Semiprofessional 3 Office and clerical 4 Skilled manual 5 Semiskilled manual 6 Unskilled manual	0 Works full time 1 Works part time 3 Retired 4 Housewife 5 Unemployed	1 Never 2 Seldom 3 Moderate 4 Frequent 5 Constant 6 Constant, intense
E. Anger:	**F. Self-reproach:**	**G. Relationship Now:**	**H. How Person Will Cope:**
1 None (or normal) 2 Mild irritation 3 Moderate; occasional outburst 4 Severe; spoils relationships 5 Extreme; bitter	1 None 2 Mild, vague 3 Moderate 4 Severe 5 Extreme; major problem	1 Close, intimate 2 Warm supportive family 3 Family supportive, but live a distance 4 Doubtful 5 None of these	1 Well; normal grief and recovery without special help 2 Fair; may need no special help 3 Doubtful; may need special help 4 Badly; requires special help 5 Very badly; requires urgent help

8.4 Bereavement Risk Assessment Tool.   Total score >15 = high risk; score 4 or 5 on item H = urgent need. From C. Parkes and R. Weiss, *Recovery from Bereavement,* copyright © 1983 by Colin Murray Parkes and Robert S. Weiss; with permission of Basic Books, a member of Perseus Books, L.L.C.

maintain or regain their mental equilibrium. For an authoritative discussion of this topic, please see Dr. Rando's 1993 book *Treatment of Complicated Mourning.*

UNRESOLVED GRIEF. For the unfortunate remainder, however, the grief seems never to lessen. These men and women are inconsolable. We must remember that their feelings are not their "fault." It may well be that the very chemistry of their brains has changed and their world is now radically different. They are heart-broken, and, over time, some of them may find wisdom, if not ease, in their "heart-brokenness."

To these people, I offer my continuing support and sympathetic ear.

As well as I can, I bear witness. I listen to the stories they need to tell, try to understand their despair and the anger they need to express, and offer what small solace my attention can bring them. I understand that I am in a special position for them: I knew the person for whom they are grieving and I may be the only one to whom they feel free to talk about their feelings. I neither judge them nor presume to urge them to "get over it." But if at some point they feel trapped by their grief or overwhelmed by it, and if, on their own, they begin to look for ways to find some balance in their lives, they may feel less inhibition about turning to me for the help they will then need.

SUMMARY

The last service we can offer to patients and their families is to help the survivors recover from the loss. For a minority, our support will be needed for the rest of their lives. The majority, however, will heal, and though they will never be quite the same, they will be able to integrate the loss into their new identity and role in society.

The courage demanded of the bereaved is eloquently captured by the writer Fred Chappell in his novel *I Am One of You Forever,* in the chapter "The Telegram." It is a story full of magic and truth, in which the telegram that announces a tragic death cannot be discarded or destroyed. We hear from the son in the family:

Then one evening I pulled a chair to the table and sat down to stare at the telegram. *Let it do to me what it can,* I thought. It was just at dusk and the telegram was the brightest object in the room. I don't know how long I sat looking. The room darkened and stars appeared in the upper window panes. At last the telegram began to change shape. Slowly wrinkling and furling inward, it took the form of a yellow rose, hand-sized, with a layer of glowing yellow petals. It seemed to hover an inch or so above the tablecloth. It uttered a mournful little whimper then, a sound I had once heard a blind puppy make when it could not find its mother's warm flank. And with that sound it disappeared from my sight forever, tumbled spiraling down a hole in the darkness. I watched it go away and my heart lightened then and I was able to rise, shaken and confused, and walk from the room without shame, not looking back, finding my way confidently in the dark.

I think that my grandmother and mother and father each had to undergo this ritual, and I think that we each saw the telegram take a different transformation before it disappeared, but we never spoke of that either.

By supporting family members as they find the strength to face their grief, we fulfill our last obligation to the deceased and to the family.

Bibliography

THE DYING PATIENT

Block SD. 2001. Psychological considerations, growth, and transcendence at the end of life: the art of the possible. *JAMA* 285:2898–2905.

Breitbart W, Chochinov HM, Passick S. 2004. Psychiatric symptoms in palliative care. In *Oxford Textbook of Palliative Medicine*, 3rd ed, Doyle D, Hanks G, Cherny N, Calman K (eds). Oxford: Oxford University Press.

Bruera E. 1997. Research into symptoms other than pain. In *Oxford Textbook of Palliative Medicine*, 2nd ed, Doyle D, Hanks GWC, MacDonald N (eds). Oxford: Oxford University Press.

Byock I. 1997. *Dying Well: Peace and Possibilities at the End of Life*. New York: Riverhead Books.

Cassel CK, Omenn GS (eds). 1995. Caring for patients at the end of life. *West J Med* 163:223–305.

Cassem NH. 1991. The dying patient. In *Massachusetts General Hospital Handbook of General Hospital Psychiatry*, Cassem NH (ed). St Louis: Mosby–Year Book.

Cavanaugh TA. 1996. The ethics of death-hastening or death-causing palliative analgesic administration to the terminally ill. *J Pain Symptom Manage* 12:248–254.

Cherny NI, Coyle N, Foley KM. 1994. Suffering in the advanced cancer patient; a definition and taxonomy. *J Palliat Care* 10:57–70.

Cherny NI, Coyle N, Foley KM. 1996. Guidelines in the care of the dying cancer patient. *Hematol Oncol Clin North Am* 10:261–286.

Cherny NI, Portenoy RK. 1994. Sedation in the management of refractory symptoms: guidelines for evaluation and treatment. *J Palliat Care* 10:31–38.

Conill C, Verger E, Henriquez IL, et al. 1997. Symptom prevalence in the last week of life. *J Pain Symptom Manage* 14:328–331.

Cowan JD, Walsh D. 2001. Terminal sedation in palliative medicine—definition and review of the literature. *Support Care Cancer* 9:403–407.

Coyle N, Adelhardt J, Foley KM, Portenoy RK. 1990. Character of terminal illness in the advanced cancer patient: pain and other symptoms during the last four weeks of life. *J Pain Symptom Manage* 5:83–93.

Doyle-Brown M. 2000. The transitional phase: the closing journey for patients and family caregivers. *Am J Hospice Palliat Care* 17:354–357.

Ellershaw JE, Sutcliffe JM, Saunders CM. 1995. Dehydration and the dying patient. *J Pain Symptom Manage* 10:192–197.

Ferris TGG, Hallward JA, Ronan L, Billings JA. 1998. When a patient dies: a survey of medical housestaff about care after death. *J Palliat Med* 1:231–240.

Fine PG. 1999. Low-dose ketamine in the management of opioid nonresponsive terminal cancer pain. *J Pain Symptom Manage* 17:296–300.

Fish DN. 1991. Treatment of delirium in the critically ill patient. *Clin Pharmacol* 10:456–466.

Fürst CJ, Doyle D. 2004. The terminal phase. In *Oxford Textbook of Palliative Medicine*, 3rd ed, Doyle D, Hanks G, Cherny N, Calman K. (eds). Oxford: Oxford University Press.

Ganzini L, Goy ER, Miller LL, et al. 2003. Nurses' experiences with hospice patients who refuse food and fluids to hasten death. *N Engl J Med* 349:359–365.

Golf M, Paice JA, Feulner E, et al. 2004. Refractory status epilepticus. *J Palliat Med* 7:85–88.

Greene WR, Davis WH. 1991. Titrated intravenous barbiturates in the control of symptoms in patients with terminal cancer. *South Med J* 84:332–337.

Grond S, Zech D, Schug SA, et al. 1991. Validation of World Health Organization guidelines for cancer pain relief during the last days and hours of life. *J Pain Symptom Manage* 6:411–422.

Knight CF, Schonwetter RS. 2003. *Pocket Guide to Hospice/Palliative Medicine*. Glenview, Ill.: American Academy of Hospice and Palliative Medicine.

Lawlor PG, Gagnon B, Mancini IL, et al. 2000. Occurrence, causes and outcome of delirium in patients with advanced cancer: a prospective study. *Arch Intern Med* 160:786–794.

Lynch M. 2003. Palliative sedation. *Clin J Oncol Nurs* 7:653–665, 667.

Lynn J, Teno JM, Phillips RS, et al., for the SUPPORT Investigators. 1997. Perceptions by family members of the dying experience of older and seriously ill patients. *Ann Intern Med* 126:97–106.

McIver B, Walsh D, Nelson K. 1994. The use of chlorpromazine for symptom control in dying cancer patients. *J Pain Symptom Manage* 9:341–345.

Moyle J. 1995. The use of propofol in palliative medicine. *J Pain Symptom Manage* 10:643–646.

Pitorak EF. 2003. Care at the time of death: how nurses can make the last hours of life a richer, more comfortable experience. *Am J Nurs* 103:42–52.

Quill TE. 1996. *A Midwife through the Dying Process: Stories of Healing and Hard Choices at the End of Life*. Baltimore: Johns Hopkins University Press.

Quill TE, Lo B, Brock D. 1997. Palliative options of last resort: a comparison of voluntarily stopping eating and drinking, terminal sedation, physician-assisted suicide, and voluntary active euthanasia. *JAMA* 278:2099–2104.

Redinbaugh EM, Sullivan AM, Block SD, et al. 2003. Doctors' emotional reactions to recent death of a patient: cross sectional study of hospital doctors. *BMJ* 327:185.

Scavone JM, Greenblatt DJ, Goddard JE, et al. 1992. The pharmacokinetics and pharmacodynamics of sublingual and oral alprazolam in the post-prandial state. *Eur J Clin Pharm* 42:439–443.

Schaerer R. 1993. Suffering of the doctor linked with the death of the patients. *Palliat Med* 7(suppl 1):27–37.

Study to Understand Prognoses and Preferences for Outcomes and Risks of Treatment (SUPPORT). 1995. A controlled trial to improve care for seriously ill hospitalized patients. *JAMA* 274:1591–1598.

Truog RD, Berde CB, Mitchell C, Grier HE. 1992. Barbiturates in the care of the terminally ill. *N Engl J Med* 327:1678–1682.

Vachon MLS. 1987. Occupational stress in the care of the critically ill, the dying and the bereaved. Washington, D.C.: Hemisphere.

Vanio A, Auvinen A, with members of the Symptom Prevalence Group. 1996. Prevalence of symptoms among patients with advanced cancer: an international collaborative study. *J Pain Symptom Manage* 12:3–10.

Waller A, Caroline NL. 1996. Terminal care. In *Handbook of Palliative Care in Cancer.* Boston: Butterworth-Heinemann.

Wanzer SH, et al. 1989. The physician's responsibility toward hopelessly ill patients: a second look. *N Engl J Med* 320:844–849.

Whippen DA, Canellos GP. 1991. Burnout syndrome in the practice of oncology: result of a random survey of 1000 oncologists. *J Clin Oncol* 9:1916–1920.

Wilcock A, Twycross R. 1996. Midazolam for intractable hiccup. *J Pain Symptom Manage* 12:59–61.

THE BEREAVED

Abrahm JL, Cooley ME, Ricacho L. 1995. Efficacy of an educational bereavement program for families of veterans with cancer. *J Cancer Educ* 10:207–212.

Barry LC, Kasl SV, Prigerson HG. 2002. Psychiatric disorders among bereaved persons: the role of perceived circumstances of death and preparedness for death. *Am J Geriatr Psychiatry* 10:447–457.

Block SD. 1985. Coping with loss. In *Outpatient Management of Advanced Cancer: Symptom Control, Support, and Hospice-in-the-Home,* Billings JA. Philadelphia: JB Lippincott.

Chappell F. 1985. *I Am One of You Forever.* Baton Rouge: Louisiana State University Press.

Chappell F. 1996. *Farewell, I Am Bound to Leave You.* New York: Picador USA.

Chochinov H, Holland JC, Katz LY. 1998. Bereavement: a special issue in oncology. In *Psycho-Oncology,* Holland JC (ed). New York: Oxford University Press.

Kissane DW. 2004. Bereavement. In *Oxford Textbook of Palliative Medicine,* 3rd ed, Doyle D, Hanks G, Cherny N, Calman K (eds). Oxford: Oxford University Press.

Parkes CM. 1987. *Bereavement: Studies of Grief in Adult Life,* 2nd ed. Madison, Conn.: International Universities Press.

Parkes CM. 1998. Bereavement in adult life. *BMJ* 316:856–859.

Prigerson HG, Bierhals AJ, Kasl SV, et al. 1996. Complicated grief as a disorder distinct from bereavement-related depression and anxiety: a replication study. *Am J Psychiatry* 153:1484–1486.

Prigerson HG, Jacobs SC. 2001. Caring for bereaved patients: "All the doctors just suddenly go." *JAMA* 286:1369–1376.

Rando TA. 1984. *Grief, Dying, and Death: Clinical Interventions for Caregivers.* Champaign, Ill: Research Press.

Rando TA. 1993. *Treatment of Complicated Mourning.* Champaign, Ill: Research Press.

Raphael B. 1977. Preventive intervention with the recently bereaved. *Arch Gen Psychiatry* 34:1450–1454.

Worden JW. 1985. Bereavement. *Semin Oncol* 12:472–475.

Zisook S, Shuchter SR, Pedrelli P, Sable J, Deaciuc SC. 2001. Bupropion sustained release treatment for bereavement: results of an open trial. *J Clin Psychiatry* 62:227–230.

CLINICIAN BIBLIOGRAPHY

BOOKS

PALLIATIVE CARE

Berger, Ann M., Russell K. Portenoy, and David E. Weissman, eds. *Principles and Practice of Supportive Oncology*, 2nd ed. Philadelphia: Lippincott-Raven, 2002.

A superb text that includes useful reviews of all aspects of supportive oncology. It is particularly helpful for an American audience because the drugs recommended are available in the United States. It also offers very practical management suggestions and includes descriptions of the appropriate roles of invasive therapies for palliation. A must for every oncology fellowship program.

Billings, J. Andrew. *Outpatient Management of Advanced Cancer: Symptom Control, Support, and Hospice-in-the-Home*. Philadelphia: J. B. Lippincott, 1985.

An outstanding resource for clinicians. In addition to the Part One coverage of symptom control, Part Two, Psychosocial Support, and Part Three, Hospice-in-the-Home, present a unique, insightful approach to the concerns of dying patients and their families. Extensively referenced. (Out of print.)

Breitbart, William, and Jimmie C. Holland, eds. *Psychiatric Aspects of Symptom Management in Cancer Patients*. Washington, D.C.: American Psychiatric Press, 1993.

Much of the information is this volume is included in the newer Oxford Textbook of Palliative Medicine (listed below), but, as the title indicates, this 1993 book contains more information on specific psychiatric aspects. It is a clear, well-written volume. Of particular interest to those in primary care is the treatment of organic mental disorders and the chapter on the stress associated with caring for cancer patients.

Buckman, Robert. *How to Break Bad News: A Guide for Health Care Professionals*. Baltimore: Johns Hopkins University Press, 1992.

An insightful guide to the conversations of physicians with patients and their families: why patients thought physicians said what they did, and why patients responded in the ways they did. Valuable to clinicians and educators as well as students.

Christakis, Nicholas A. *Death Foretold: Prophecy and Prognosis in Medical Care.* Chicago: University of Chicago Press, 1999.

A brilliant discussion of the challenges of making and communicating prognoses; required reading for all who care for patients with advanced illness.

Doyle, Derek, Geoffrey W. C. Hanks, Nathan Cherny, and Kenneth Calman, eds. *Oxford Textbook of Palliative Medicine,* 3rd ed. Oxford: Oxford University Press, 2004.

A comprehensive, thoroughly referenced, useful textbook on all aspects of palliative care and care of dying patients. A standard in the field.

Fallon, M., and W. O'Neill, eds. *ABC of Palliative Care.* London: BMJ Publishing Group, 1998.

As the title suggests, a primer for those new to the field of palliative care.

Faulkner, Anne, and Peter Maguire. *Talking to Cancer Patients and Their Relatives.* Oxford: Oxford University Press, 1994.

This book contains a superb description of the components of the conversations that nurses and physicians must have with cancer patients. It is full of useful suggestions for how to deepen and improve these conversations so that we can discern what is troubling our patients and their families.

Gallagher-Allred, Charlotte R., and Madalon O'Rawe Amenta, eds. *Nutrition and Hydration in Hospice Care: Needs, Strategies, Ethics.* New York: Haworth Press, 1993 (paperback edition 1997).

A very clearly written, thorough discussion on the ethical, philosophical, and practical issues surrounding nutrition and hydration in patients who are near the end of life.

Holland, Jimmie C. *Psycho-Oncology.* New York: Oxford University Press, 1998.

This comprehensive text is an excellent resource for those interested in various aspects of psychological care not only of patients and their families, but of the medical personnel who care for them (nurses, house staff, etc.).

Houldin, Arlene D. *Patients with Cancer: Understanding the Psychological Pain.* Philadelphia: Lippincott, 2000.

Dr. Houldin is an insightful clinician who shares the lessons she has learned from years of counseling cancer patients.

Rolling Ferrell, Betty, and Nessa Coyle, eds. *Textbook of Palliative Nursing.* New York: Oxford University Press, 2001.

A state-of-the art discussion of the subject; required for all hospital libraries and those of palliative care programs.

Saunders, Cicely, Mary Baines, and Robert Dunlop. *Living with Dying: A Guide to Palliative Care*, 3rd ed. Oxford: Oxford University Press, 1995.

In just 56 pages, Dame Cicely, the founder of the modern hospice movement in England, provides a splendid overview of the essential elements of caring for dying cancer patients, their families, and the staff responsible for them.

Stone, Douglas, Bruce Patton, and Sheila Heen. *Difficult Conversations: How to Discuss What Matters Most*. New York: Penguin Books, 1999.

The lessons of this book, written for businesspeople by the group who wrote Getting to Yes, *are highly applicable to the conversations that must be undertaken in palliative care.*

PAIN AND SYMPTOM MANAGEMENT

Andrews, Tom. *The Hemophiliac's Motorcycle*. Iowa City: University of Iowa Press, 1994.

Eloquent evocations and narrative poems telling what it was like growing up with hemophilia in the pre–home care era, and then living in the peri-HIV era.

Barber, J., ed. *Hypnosis and Suggestion in the Treatment of Pain: A Clinical Guide*. New York: W. W. Norton, 1996.

This book includes an orientation to hypnotic evaluation and a discussion of the use of hypnosis in pain syndromes (including cancer pain) and in children and elders.

Irving, G. A., and M. S. Wallace, eds. *Pain Management for the Practicing Physician*. New York: Churchill Livingstone, 1997.

An excellent resource for physicians who want a general, practical text about pain—its anatomy, physiology, pharmacology, and treatment. This book provides descriptions and treatment algorithms for the most frequently encountered nonmalignant and malignant pain syndromes.

McGuire, Deborah B., Connie Henke Yarbro, and Betty Rolling Ferrell, eds. *Cancer Pain Management*, 2nd ed. Boston: Jones and Bartlett, 1995.

Edited by nurses who are leaders in this field, this book is an excellent source of information on all aspects of cancer pain assessment and management, including both pharmacologic and nonpharmacologic therapies for adults and children. Extensively referenced.

Parris, Winston C. V., ed. *Cancer Pain Management: Principles and Practice*. Boston: Butterworth-Heinemann, 1997.

This multi-author, comprehensive book is for those who want to know more about cancer pain management than is given in the Handbook of Palliative Care in Cancer *or the* AHCPR Management of Cancer Pain: Clinical Practice Guideline No. 9 *(both listed under Handbooks/Primers) but less than is given in the* Oxford Textbook of Palliative Medicine *(listed above). The authors include representatives of all the relevant disciplines who work with cancer patients in pain. The book includes more detail on neurolytic procedures than is found in many texts. Extensively referenced.*

Ripamonti, Carla, and Eduardo Bruera, eds. *Gastrointestinal Symptoms in Advanced Cancer Patients.* New York: Oxford University Press, 2002.

Twycross, Robert, ed. *Pain Relief in Advanced Cancer.* New York: Churchill-Livingstone, 1994.

A superlative, clinically relevant, comprehensive review of pain and suffering from one of the most experienced clinicians in the field of hospice and symptom management.

Wall, P. D., and R. Melzack, eds. *Textbook of Pain*, 3rd ed. New York: Churchill Livingstone, 1994.

An exhaustive textbook, authoritative and wide-ranging in scope, edited by two original thinkers who are among the modern founders of the field of pain research and management.

DEATH AND DYING

Blank, Linda L., ed. *Caring for the Dying: Identification and Promotion of Physician Competency.* Philadelphia: American Board of Internal Medicine, 1996. Available from Linda L. Blank, telephone: 215-446-3500, ext. 3567; American Board of Internal Medicine website: www.abim.org.

Two documents are available: (1) Educational Resource Document *(250 references and listings of other information resources) and (2)* Personal Narratives of Physicians Caring for Dying Patients.

Byock, Ira. *Dying Well: Peace and Possibilities at the End of Life.* New York: Riverhead Books, 1997.

Dr. Byock is a past president of the American Academy of Hospice and Palliative Medicine. In this book, he uses the narratives of the patients and families he has cared for to explore the possibilities for growth even at the end of life.

Byock, Ira. *The Four Things That Matter Most: A Book about Living.* New York: Free Press, 2004.

Expanding on themes raised in Dying Well, *Dr. Byock offers a continued meditation on how families and patients can communicate the important things to each other when the patient's time is short.*

Callahan, Daniel. *The Troubled Dream of Life.* New York: Simon & Schuster, 1993.

Dr. Callahan, of the Hastings Center, explores our "illusion," as he calls it, of control regarding our choices of how we die—our medical options, euthanasia, and "the pursuit of a peaceful death." He urges us to reframe how we perceive death—accepting it as a part of nature, rather than regarding it as a moral evil to be fought at any cost.

Corless, Inge B., Barbara B. Germino, and Mary A. Pittman. *A Challenge for Living: Dying, Death, and Bereavement.* Boston: Jones and Bartlett, 1995.

A compilation of essays by leaders in a variety of disciplines on the physical, psychosocial, and spiritual needs of the patient and the caregivers, as well as the needs of the bereaved. Each essay is referenced.

Curtis, J. Randall, and Gordon D. Rubenfeld, eds. *Managing Death in the Intensive Care Unit: The Transition from Cure to Comfort.* Oxford: Oxford University Press, 2001.

Dr. Curtis and colleagues have written a very useful series of essays that deal with the ethical and practical aspects of caring for dying patients in the ICU.

Diamant, Anita. *Saying Kaddish: How to Comfort the Dying, Bury the Dead, and Mourn as a Jew.* New York: Schocken Books, 1998.

Kuhl, David. *What Dying People Want: Practical Wisdom for the End of Life.* New York: Public Affairs, 2002.

Lief, Judith L. *Making Friends with Death: A Buddhist Guide to Encountering Mortality.* Boston: Shambhala, 2001.

Mojtabai, A. G. *Soon: Tales from Hospice.* Cambridge, Mass.: Zoland Books, 1998.

Parkes, C., and R. Weiss. *Recovery from Bereavement.* New York: Basic Books, 1983.

This book and that written by Therese Rando, listed below, provide clinicians with comprehensive discussions of bereavement and of the treatment of those who cannot seem to recover from the patient's death.

Quill, Timothy E. *Death and Dignity.* New York: W. W. Norton, 1993.

A thought-provoking book by the noted advocate of palliative care, patient dignity, and the patient's right to die. Chapters include Making Choices and Taking Charge, Reconsidering Medicine's Goals and Values, Medical Technology, Comfort Care and Its Limits, Physician Assisted Suicide, and Advance Directives. Includes a bibliography.

Rando, Therese A. *Treatment of Complicated Mourning.* Champaign, Ill.: Research Press, 1993.

This book and that written by C. Parkes and R. Weiss, listed above, provide clinicians with comprehensive discussions of bereavement and of the treatment of those who cannot seem to recover from the patient's death.

GENERAL INTEREST

American Cancer Society. *Guidelines on Support and Self Help Groups.* Atlanta: American Cancer Society, 1995.

A practical, working manual for those interested in developing various types of support or self-help groups sponsored by the American Cancer Society. Evaluation tools and references are included.

Atul, Gawande. *Complications: A Surgeon's Notes on an Imperfect Science*. New York: Picador, 2002.

A beautifully written book full of insight from a superb physician and teacher.

Aulisio Mark P., Robert M. Arnold, and Stuart J. Younger, eds. *Ethics Consultation: From Theory to Practice*. Baltimore: Johns Hopkins University Press, 2003.

A valuable resource for institutions that wish to train ethics consultants and start ethics committees. Of particular utility is the chapter on core competencies for health care ethics consultation.

Bandeira, Manuel. *Selected Poems* (bilingual ed., trans. David R. Slavitt). Riverdale-on-Hudson, N.Y.: Sheep Meadow Press, 2002.

Poems of love and death.

Bigby, Judyann, ed. *Cross-Cultural Medicine*. Philadelphia: American College of Physicians, 2003.

A very well-written and well-edited contemporary account of the issues that must be considered as clinicians care for patients from the variety of cultures within the United States. The book includes, but is by no means limited to, discussions on communicating about the illness and its prognosis and rituals surrounding dying patients.

Broyard, Anatole. *Intoxicated by My Illness*. New York: Fawcett Columbine, 1992.

Anatole Broyard, journalist and author, died of metastatic prostate cancer. This very moving, very lively collection of articles deals with a number of subjects of interest to physicians, including what he expected from his own physicians, as well as a discussion of other books about cancer. It also includes a short story that mirrors Broyard's experience as one of his parents died of cancer.

Cancer Care. *A Helping Hand: The Resource Guide for People with Cancer*, 2nd ed. Available from Cancer Care, Inc., 1180 Avenue of the Americas, New York, NY 10036-3602; telephone: 1-800-813-HOPE (4673) or 212-221-3300; e-mail: info@cancercare.org; website: www.cancercare.org.

A comprehensive and detailed listing of the growing number of services available across the country to people with cancer. In addition to the addresses, telephone and fax numbers, and e-mail addresses for hundreds of resources for people with cancer, each organizational listing contains a description of its mission and the services it provides.

Cassell, Eric. *The Nature of Suffering and the Goals of Medicine*. New York: Oxford University Press, 1991.

A seminal work from a physician and scholar who elucidates the unspoken assumptions that impede successful care of the dying in America today. He analyzes the structural, personal, and professional barriers that separate us from our patients and prevent us from un-

derstanding and appreciating their goals and values. He comprehensively yet concisely delineates the nature of suffering. All physicians caring for patients with acutely disabling or chronically advanced illness will benefit from the insights they can gain from this book.

Cassileth, Barrie R. *The Alternative Medicine Handbook: The Complete Reference Guide to Alternative and Complementary Therapies.* New York: W. W. Norton, 1998.

Dr. Cassileth is an internationally known expert on alternative medicine and unorthodox therapies. This book is an extremely valuable reference tool for those of us working with patients who seek these therapies in addition to those we offer—Dr. Cassileth suggests that this includes at least one-third to one-half of cancer patients.

Field, M. J., and C. K. Cassell, eds. *Approaching Death: Improving Care at the End of Life.* Washington, D.C.: Institute of Medicine, National Academy Press, 1997.

de Sponde, Jean. *Sonnets of Love and Death,* bilingual ed, trans David R. Slavitt. Evanston, Ill.: Northwestern University Press, 2001.

Hall, Donald. *Without.* New York: Houghton Mifflin, 1998.

Lynch, Thomas. *The Undertaking: Life Studies from the Dismal Trade.* New York: Penguin Books, 1997.

Pastan, Linda. *Carnival Evening: New and Selected Poems, 1968–1998.* New York: W. W. Norton, 1998.

The poem, "The Five Stages of Grief" is of special interest to those of us trying to understand how to help our bereaved patients.

Price, Reynolds. *A Whole New Life: An Illness and a Healing.* New York: Atheneum, 1994.

A cautionary tale for physicians by novelist and short story writer Reynolds Price, who had locally advanced cancer; he chastises us for what he terms our "clinical distance."

Remen, Rachel Naomi. *Kitchen Table Wisdom: Stories That Heal.* New York: Riverhead Books, 1996.

Remen, Rachel Naomi. *My Grandfather's Blessings: Stories of Strength, Refuge, and Belonging.* New York: Riverhead Books, 2000.

Rachel Remen is co-founder and medical director of the Commonweal Cancer Help Program. She has extensive experience in the clinical care of those who are suffering and facing life-threatening illnesses as well as in teaching undergraduate, graduate, and practicing physicians how to heal the pain of their own losses—and to become better physicians in the process. In both of these very readable, engaging books, she uses stories that teach by indirection and very powerfully convey her message.

Roth, Philip. *Patrimony.* New York: Simon & Schuster, 1991.

A wonderful revelation of Philip Roth's relationship with his father—their time together when Roth was a child and the years in which his father's life was profoundly altered by a rare brain tumor. Roth was the primary caregiver for his father during this time, and he writes about the experience as only he can.

Stone, John. *Where Water Begins: New Poems and Prose.* Baton Rouge: Louisiana State University Press, 1998.

Sulmasy, D. P. *The Healer's Calling: A Spirituality for Physicians and Other Health Care Professionals.* New York: Paulist Press, 1997.

Daniel Sulmasy is a philosopher, a health services researcher, a Franciscan Friar, and a medical oncologist. In this eloquent, thoughtful book he relates his "personal experience of being a man of faith engaged in the work of a health care professional" as a basis for our own self-explorations. Chapters include Spirituality and the Health Care Professional; Medicine, Love and the Art of Being Uncertain; The Wine of Fervent Zeal and the Oil of Compassion; God-Talk at the Bedside; Prayer and the Five Senses: A Physician's Meditation; Suffering, Spirituality, and Health Care; and Wounded Healers.

Webb, Marilyn. *The Good Death: The New American Search to Reshape the End of Life.* New York: Bantam, 1997.

Marilyn Webb is an investigative journalist who spent six years exploring this topic. In this almost 500-page volume, she shares the stories of patients and families for whom death provided either the opportunity for growth or unremitting pain, and explains the many factors that contributed to such different outcomes.

OTHER BOOKS OF INTEREST

Annas, G. J. *The Rights of Patients: The Basic ACLU Guide to Patient Rights,* 2nd ed. Carbondale: Southern Illinois University Press, 1989.

Benson, Herbert, with Marg Stark. *Timeless Healing: The Power and Biology of Belief.* New York: Scribner (Simon & Schuster), 1996.

Jonsen, A. R., M. Siegler, and W. J. Winslade. *Clinical Ethics,* 3rd ed. New York: McGraw-Hill, 1992.

Parris, Winston C. V. *Cancer Pain Management: Principles and Practice.* Boston: Butterworth-Heinemann, 1997.

Patt, Richard B. *Cancer Pain.* Philadelphia: Lippincott-Raven, 1996.

HANDBOOKS/PRIMERS/GUIDELINES

PALLIATIVE CARE

Hallenbeck JL. *Palliative Care Perspectives.* Oxford: Oxford University Press, 2003.

MacDonald, Neil, ed. *Palliative Medicine: A Case-Based Manual.* Oxford: Oxford University Press, 1997.

This book is designed for physicians who wish to teach principles of palliative medicine to medical students, residents, or fellows. Thirty symptom problems and psychosocial issues are addressed in carefully designed cases, along with relevant references.

National Consensus Project for Quality Palliative Care. *Clinical Practice Guidelines for Quality Palliative Care.* NHPCO Marketplace, Dept 929, Alexandria, VA 22334-0929; telephone: 800-646-6460; website: www.nhpco.org/marketplace

Storey, Porter. *Primer of Palliative Care,* 3rd ed. American Academy of Hospice and Palliative Medicine. Glenview, Ill.: AAHPM Press, 2004. Available from AAHPM, telephone: 703-787-7718; e-mail: aahpm@aahpm.org; website: www.aahpm.org.

A useful primer for managing the most distressing symptoms: pain, dyspnea, nausea and vomiting, anorexia, constipation, restlessness and delirium, and psychological, social, and spiritual distress. It contains a useful annotated bibliography of key references.

Storey, Porter, and Carol F. Knight. *Hospice/Palliative Care Training for Physicians: A Self Study Program.* American Academy of Hospice and Palliative Medicine. Dubuque, Iowa: Kendall/Hunt Publishing, 1996, 1997, 1998, 2003. Available from AAHPM, e-mail: aahpm@aahpm.org.

This eight-part UNIPAC series offers an excellent, modular, case-based study program for those interested in learning more about palliative care. Pre- and post-tests are included, and CME credit is available for each module. Volumes include: I. The Hospice/Palliative Medicine Approach to End-of-Life Care; II. Alleviating Psychological and Spiritual Pain in the Terminally Ill; III. Assessment and Treatment of Pain in the Terminally Ill; IV. Management of Selected Non-pain Symptoms in the Terminally Ill; V. Caring for the Terminally Ill: Communication and the Physician's Role on the Interdisciplinary Team; VI. Ethical and Legal Decision Making When Caring for the Terminally Ill; VII. The Hospice/ Palliative Medicine Approach to Caring for Patients with HIV/AIDS; VIII. The Hospice/ Palliative Medicine Approach to Caring for Pediatric Patients. Modules can be purchased individually or in sets (for a discount).

Storey, Porter, Carol F. Knight, and Ronald S. Schonwetter. *Pocket Guide to Hospice/Palliative Medicine.* Glenview, Ill.: American Academy of Hospice and Palliative Medicine, 2003.

Waller, Alexander, and Nancy L. Caroline. *Handbook of Palliative Care in Cancer.* Boston: Butterworth-Heinemann, 1996.

An extremely well-organized, useful, inexpensive handbook containing clear, succinct recommendations for evaluation and treatment of the multitude of physical and emotional symptoms experienced by patients with cancer. An excellent addition to the library of any clinician caring for cancer patients. Referenced.

PAIN

American Pain Society. *Principles of Analgesic Use in the Treatment of Acute Pain and Cancer Pain,* 5th ed. Glenview, Ill.: American Pain Society, 2003. Available from American Pain Society Publication Orders, 4700 W. Lake Avenue, Glenview, IL 60025-1485.

Gordon, Debra B., June L. Dahl, and Karen Kunz Stevenson, eds. *Building an In-stitutional Commitment to Pain Management: The Wisconsin Resource Manual for Improvement.* Madison: Wisconsin Cancer Pain Initiative, 1996.

Immunex Corporation. *A Guide to Pain Management in Advanced Prostate Cancer: Health Care Professional Edition.* Seattle: Immunex Corporation, 1997. Available from Immunex Corporation, telephone: 1-800-220-6302.

> *This free booklet, produced by the corporation that sells Novantrone, has a reasonable discussion of options for these patients; it contains a listing of pain management resources and copies of pain assessment tools. Included is a copy of the patient edition, which is also available separately.*

Miaskowski C, Cleary J, Burney R, et al. *Guideline for the Management of Cancer Pain in Adults and Children.* APS Clinical Practice Guidelines Series, No. 3. Glenview, Ill.: American Pain Society, 2005. www.ampainsoc.org.

> *This landmark publication is a consensus document prepared by the leading national pain experts from numerous clinical fields. It contains assessment and management guidelines, including pharmacologic and nonpharmacologic techniques, guidelines for treating the elderly, and assessment and management tools.*

DEATH AND DYING

Lynn J. and J. Harrold. *Handbook for Mortals: Guidance for People Facing Serious Illness.* New York: Oxford University Press, 1999.

> Handbook for Mortals *is a straightforward, clearly written manual that I give to patients and families who are facing a terminal prognosis. It includes practical suggestions and seeks to empower families to get the information they need from their health care providers. It is a valuable book also for nurses and physicians who are not familiar with the demands that caring for these patients place on them and on families as they try to navigate the health care system and care for the patients at home.*

Parkes, Colin Murray, Pittu Laungani, and Bill Young, eds. *Death and Bereavement across Cultures.* New York: Brunner-Routledge, 1997.

> *In the editors' words, this handbook "describes the rituals and beliefs of the major world religions; explains their psychological and historical context; shows how customs are changed by contact with the West, and considers the implications for the future." It also includes an exploration of mourning traditions throughout the world.*

SERIES

Bruera, Eduardo, and Russell K. Portenoy, eds. *Topics in Palliative Care.* Oxford: Oxford University Press, 1997, 1998 (2 vols), 2000.

UNIPAC Series. *Hospice/Palliative Care Training for Physicians: A Self-study Program.* Larchmont, N.Y.: Mary Ann Liebert, 2003.

JOURNALS

Issues Devoted to Palliative Care or Care of the Terminally Ill

Cherny, N. I., and K. M. Foley, eds. Pain and palliative care. *Hematology/Oncology Clinics of North America,* February 1996. Philadelphia: W. B. Saunders.

This issue gives a concise, comprehensive, up-to-date discussion of the important topics in palliative care and pain, edited by noted experts in this field. Extensively referenced.

Ferrell, Bruce A., ed. Pain management in the elderly. *Clinics in Geriatric Medicine,* August 2001. Philadelphia: W. B. Saunders.

Matzo, Marianne L., and Joanne Lynn, eds. Death and dying. *Clinics in Geriatric Medicine,* May 2000. Philadelphia: W. B. Saunders.

Excellent review of issues arising in the care of the terminally ill geriatric patient; not limited to cancer patients.

Rousseau, Paul C. Palliative care. *Primary Care: Clinics in Office Practice,* June 2001. Philadelphia: W. B. Saunders.

Relevant Medical Journals

These journals are for physicians interested in practical, useful articles discussing improvements in symptom management or hospice-related subjects. Authors include clinicians from a variety of medical and other clinical disciplines.

Alternative Medicine Alert. American Health Consultants, P.O. Box 71266, Chicago, IL 60691-9986; telephone: 1-800-688-2421; fax: 1-800-850-1232.

The American Journal of Hospice and Palliative Care. 470 Boston Post Road, Weston, MA 02193; telephone: 617-899-2702.

Innovations in End-of-Life Care. An on-line journal from Last Acts; highlights promising practices in end-of-life care; website: www2.edc.org.

The Journal of Pain and Symptom Management. Russell K. Portenoy, editor. Elsevier Science, Inc., 655 Avenue of the Americas, New York, NY 10010; telephone: 1-800-437-4636; fax: 212-633-3680; e-mail: usinfo-f@elsevier.com.

Journal of Palliative Medicine. Charles von Gunten, editor-in-chief. Mary Ann Liebert, Inc., 2 Madison Avenue, Larchmont, NY 10538; telephone: 914-834-3100; fax: 914-834-3582; website: www.liebertpub.com.

Pain. Elsevier Science, Inc., 655 Avenue of the Americas, New York, NY 10010; telephone: 1-800-437-4636; fax: 212-633-3680; e-mail: usinfo-f@elsevier.com.

PATIENT EDUCATION MATERIALS FOR CLINICIANS

Aspen Reference Group. *Pain Management, Patient Education Manual.* Aspen Publishers, Inc., 200 Orchard Ridge Drive, Gaithersburg, MD 20878; telephone: 1-800-638-8437; website: www.aspenpub.com.

This loose-leaf manual (in binder form) is designed to help physicians provide customized patient education on managing pain. Updates are available yearly at an additional fee.

Palliative Care Patient and Family Counseling Manual. Aspen Publishers, Inc., 200 Orchard Ridge Drive, Gaithersburg, MD 20878; telephone: 1-800-638-8437; website: www.aspenpub.com.

This loose-leaf manual (in binder form) is designed to help physicians provide customized patient education on palliative care topics. Updates are available yearly at an additional fee.

Scriptographic Booklets. Channing L. Bete Co., Inc., 200 State Road, South Deerfield, MA 01373-0200; telephone: 1-800-628-7733; fax: 1-800-499-6464.

Booklets are available on a wide range of topics of interest to patients with cancer and their families. Subjects include (but are not limited to) pain management, advance medical directives, social work services, hospice under Medicare, home care, long-term care, grief, depression, adult and child bereavement, and dying.

CD-ROM

Completing a Life: An Interactive Multimedia CD-ROM for Patient and Family Education in End of Life Care. Information from www.completingalife.msu.edu.

VIDEOTAPES

Advances in the Use of Opioids in Pain Management. Purdue Frederick Company, Norwalk, CT 06850-3560.

Free videotape, produced in 1997. Also available is a monograph edited by pain management experts Richard Payne, Michael H. Levy, Stephen P. Long, and Winston C. V. Parris.

Alternative Medicine: Implications for Clinical Practice. Harvard MED-CME, P.O. Box 825, Boston, MA 02117-0825

Videotape of a three-day conference at Harvard Medical School and Beth Israel Hospital, directed by David Eisenberg, M.D., director of Beth Israel Hospital's Center for Alternative Medicine (14 videocassettes and a 370-page syllabus).

Before I Die: Medical Care and Personal Choices. PBS Home Video, 320 Braddock Place, Alexandria, VA 22314; telephone: 1-800-424-7963; fax: 703-739-5269.

Segmented version available from Crystal Coleman, telephone: 703-827-8771; fax: 703-827-0783; website: www.wnet.org/archive/bid.

Interested clinicians and educators can obtain a video of the entire 1997 broadcast or a special edition that is divided into segments for discussion purposes. Also available are copies of the Viewer's Guide and additional support materials to use as a study guide as part of an educational program on end-of-life issues.

Helping to Control Cancer Pain. Purdue Frederick Company, Norwalk, CT 06850-3560.

This 1993 video is available free of charge.

On the Edge of Being: When Doctors Confront Cancer. Developed by Cerenex pharmaceuticals, a Division of Glaxo, Inc.; telephone: 1-800-824-2896.

Provided free to physicians, this video is an excellent resource for seminar leaders who teach medical students, residents, or fellows about the experiences associated with cancer, cancer treatment, and helping patients who are dying. The physicians appearing in the video either had cancer, still have it, or had a loved one who died of cancer. They discuss a wide range of topics such as having cancer, experiencing the health care system as a patient, losing a child, and facing death. The episodes could also be edited and used individually. Running time about 45 minutes.

Spirituality and Healing in Medicine. Harvard MED-CME, P.O. Box 825, Boston, MA 02117-0825; telephone: 617-432-1525; fax: 617-432-1562.

A series of four videotapes of a conference on Spirituality and Healing in Medicine held at Harvard Medical School in 1995. Hindu, Buddhist, Jewish, Catholic, Islamic, Hispanic-Pentecostal, Christian Science, and Seventh-Day Adventist spiritual healing practices are discussed. A much shorter overview, Healing Words, Healing Practices, *is also available.*

WEBSITES/DATABASES (SEE ALSO PATIENT AND FAMILY BIBLIOGRAPHY)

American Medical Association. Caregiver Self-assessment Tool. www.ama-assn.org.

A caregiver self-assessment tool designed to help caregivers recognize their need for home health services. Clinicians can refer caregivers to this website to help them recognize how much stress they are experiencing, and encourage them to ask for help. The tool is available in English and Spanish.

American Society of Clinical Oncology. People Living with Cancer. www.plwc.org.

The website of the American Society of Clinical Oncology (ASCO) is designed for people living with cancer and their families and friends.

Bailey, F. Amos, Palliative Response. www.hospice.va.gov *and* www.hospice.va .gov/Amosbaileybook/index.htm.

These websites offer the full text of F. Amos Bailey's manual on palliative care, Palliative Response. *Dr. Bailey helped develop the innovative programs at Balm of Gilead hospice and wrote a clear, concise manual for hospice care.*

Cancer Information Network. www.cancernetwork.com.
CANCERLIT Topic Searches. www.cancer.gov/cancerinfo.
Cansearch (National Coalition for Cancer Survivorship). www.canceradvocacy .org.
Center to Advance Palliative Care. www.capcmssm.org.

The Center to Advance Palliative Care (CAPC) website is the resource for administrators and clinicians who wish to plan, fund, and sustain a hospital-based palliative care program. The website also lists the schedule of management training seminars offered by CAPC.

Cochrane Collaboration. http://hiru.mcmaster.ca/cochrane.

Reviews of research evidence, including pain and symptom management and care at the end of life.

Department of Health and Human Services, Healthfinder. www.healthfinder .gov.
Educating Physicians in End of Life Care. www.epec.net.

The Educating Physician in End of Life Care (EPEC) 14-module curriculum, developed and refined by the AMA, is downloadable free of charge for AMA members.

End of Life Palliative Care. www.eperc.mcw.edu.

The End of Life / Palliative Education Resource Center (EPERC)—created by the innovators at the Medical College of Wisconsin, led by Dr. David Weissman—is a comprehensive resource site for clinicians and educators. It includes peer-reviewed educational materials and the very valuable "Fast Facts": one-page items containing practical, useful nuggets of palliative care information and communication techniques. All the material is available at no charge. More information about the program at the Medical College of Wisconsin can be found at www.mcw.edu/pallmed.

Growth House. www.growthhouse.org/palliative.

This website has posted tools for organizations that wish to develop an outpatient palliative care program. The toolkit and blueprint from the Kaiser Permanente Program are provided, as are suggestions on how to modify the program to different organizational structures.

HealthAnswers. www.healthanswers.com.

This database, created in partnership with the American Academy of Family Physicians, contains information from the AAFP and from the American Academy of Pediatrics, the National Health Council, the National Library of Medicine, the U.S. Pharmacopoeia, the American Society on Aging, the National Alliance for Caregiving, and the National Association for Home Care. While this database also offers materials for the lay public, a number of features are of interest to physicians. For example a Health Professionals Only area, focusing on CME, contains video transcripts and graphics on a number of topics for which CME credit is available. MEDLINE and AIDS-LINE databases are also available, as are bulletin boards and listings of patient education materials that can be purchased.

Initiative to Improve Palliative Care. www.iipca.org.

This website for the Initiative to Improve Palliative Care among African Americans contains valuable educational programs and listings of upcoming offerings.

Johns Hopkins Center for Cancer Pain Research. www.hopkinskimmelcancer-center.org/specialtycenters/hop.cfm.

The Johns Hopkins Center for Cancer Pain Research provides its opioid conversion program on this site as a free software download.

Last Chapters Forum. www.lastchapters.org.

As stated in the Journal of Palliative Medicine *(vol. 6, p. 690, 2003), this website "offers a collection of inspiring stories and video interviews of people who are facing death or chronic illness." It also hosts The Last Chapters Forum, through which viewers can discuss their reactions to the stories.*

Pain.com.www.pain.com.

Sponsored by Dannemiller Memorial Educational Foundation, this site includes interactive professional forums and chat rooms; the World Wide Congress on Pain's Virtual Library; on-line CME modules and accreditation; a weekly advice column; and over 200 links to other health care sites.

PainLink.www.edc.org/PainLink.

Sponsored by the Mayday Fund, a New York City foundation dedicated to relieving unnecessary pain.

Pain Medicine and Palliative Care Department at Beth Israel Medical Center. www.stoppain.org.

This website has valuable resources for pain control.

Partners Against Pain. www.partnersagainstpain.com/pro/pro.html.

Professional Education section has a summary of the latest consensus statement prepared by the American Academy of Pain Medicine and the American Pain Society: The Use of Opioids for the Treatment of Chronic Pain.

PDQ Search Service. Telephone: 1-800-345-3300; fax: 1-800-380-1575; e-mail: pdqsearch@icic.nci.nih.gov.

Monday to Friday 9 a.m. to 6 p.m., EST.PDQ is a government-sponsored database that contains information about cancer prevention, early detection, treatment, and supportive care. If you do not want to search the database yourself, the search service provides answers to questions sent by mail, fax, or e-mail. They'll also respond by express mail if you cover the cost.

UB Center for Clinical Ethics and Humanities in Health Care. http://wings .buffalo.edu/faculty/research/bioethics/index.html.
University of Pennsylvania Center for Bioethics. www.bioethics.upenn.edu.
University of Wisconsin Pain and Policy Studies Group. www.medsch.wisc .edu./painpolicy.
www.cme-webcredits.org/COIN.html.

A valuable educational palliative care website that also offers CME options.

ORGANIZATIONS (SEE ALSO PATIENT AND FAMILY BIBLIOGRAPHY)

American Academy of Hospice and Palliative Medicine, 11250 Roger Bacon Drive, Suite 8, Reston, VA 20190-5202; telephone: 703-787-7718; fax: 703-435-4390; e-mail: aahpm@aahpm.org; website: www.aahpm.org.

A professional organization for physicians in many medical specialties dedicated to the advancement of hospice/palliative medicine, its practice, research, and education.

American Hospice Foundation. www.americanhospice.org.
American Pain Society, 5700 Old Orchard Road, First Floor, Skokie, IL 60077; telephone: 708-966-5595; website: www.ampainsoc.org.

Publishes Directory of Pain Management Facilities.

Hospice Foundation of America. www.hospicefoundation.org.
Hospice and Palliative Nurses Association. www.hpna.org.
Mayday Pain Resource Center, City of Hope National Medical Center, 1500 E. Duarte Road, Duarte, CA 91010; website: www.cityofhope.org/mayday/ Default.htm.
National Hospice and Palliative Care Organization. www.nhpco.org.
Pain Intervention Network, Janssen Pharmaceuticals (newsletter). Editor, Pain Intervention Network, RAR & Assoc., Inc., 180 S. Street, Murray Hill, NJ 07974.

Partners Against Pain, Purdue Frederick Company and Purdue Pharma. Purdue Frederick Company, Norwalk, CT 06850-3560; website: www .partnersagainstpain.com/index.html.

Patient education and other materials about the treatment of pain are available at no charge from the Purdue Frederick representative.

Patient and Family Bibliography

BOOKS

General Reference

Babcock, Elise NeeDell. *When Life Becomes Precious: A Guide for Loved Ones and Friends of Cancer Patients*. New York: Bantam Books, 1997.

Elise Babcock founded Cancer Counseling, Inc., which has provided free professional counseling to cancer patients and their families since 1982. She has been a counselor for over 20 years. In this highly readable book, she answers very commonly asked questions about how to communicate about cancer, and gives families and friends practical suggestions on what they can do to help and support not only the patient but the caregiver and other family members. It also contains a helpful listing of community resources.

Barnard, David, and Anna M. Towers, Patricia Boston, and Yanna Lambrinidou. *Crossing Over: Narratives of Palliative Care*. Oxford: Oxford University Press, 2000.

Billings, J. Andrew. *Outpatient Management of Advanced Cancer: Symptom Control, Support, and Hospice-in-the-Home*. Philadelphia: J. B. Lippincott, 1985.

An outstanding resource for families who want to understand more about symptom control and psychological and social support. This book presents a unique, insightful approach to the concerns of dying patients and their families. Extensively referenced. (Out of print.)

Buckman, Robert, in collaboration with the specialists at M.D. Anderson Cancer Center. *What You Really Need to Know about Cancer: A Comprehensive Guide for Patients and Their Families*. Baltimore: Johns Hopkins University Press, 1997.

Dr. Buckman is an experienced family physician and oncologist who has written several books on communication between people with cancer and their families, friends, and the physicians caring for them. This book is an excellent introduction to various types of cancer for people who do not have any medical background but who want to understand more about the disease and the treatments used.

Byock, Ira. *Dying Well: Peace and Possibilities at the End of Life*. New York: Riverhead Books, 1997.

Dr. Byock's inspirational book uses the narratives of patients and families he has cared for to explore the possibilities for growth even at the end of life.

Byock, Ira. *The Four Things That Matter Most: A Book about Living.* New York: Free Press, 2004.

Expanding on themes raised in Dying Well, *Dr. Byock offers a continued meditation on how families and patients can communicate the important things to each other when the patient's time is short.*

Cancer Care. *A Helping Hand: The Resource Guide for People with Cancer,* 2nd ed. Available from Cancer Care, Inc., 1180 Avenue of the Americas, New York, NY 10036-3602; telephone: 1-800-813-HOPE (4673) or 212-221-3300; e-mail: info©cancercare.org; website: www.cancercare.org.

A comprehensive and detailed listing of the growing number of services available across the country to people with cancer. In addition to the addresses, telephone and fax numbers, and e-mail addresses of hundreds of resources for people with cancer, each organizational listing contains a description of its mission and the services it provides.

Coleman, C. Norman. *Understanding Cancer: A Patient's Guide to Diagnosis, Prognosis, and Treatment.* Baltimore: Johns Hopkins University Press, 1998.

Dr. Coleman is professor and chairman of the Joint Center for Radiation Therapy in the Department of Radiation Oncology at Harvard Medical School. He seeks to help people with cancer prepare for encounters with physicians, understand the processes of diagnosis, and weigh the treatment options offered.

Corless, Inge B., Barbara B. Germino, and Mary A. Pittman. *A Challenge for Living: Dying, Death, and Bereavement.* Boston: Jones and Bartlett, 1995.

A compilation of essays by leaders in a variety of disciplines on the physical, psychosocial, and spiritual needs of the patient and the caregivers, as well as the needs of the bereaved. Each essay is referenced.

Doyle, Derek. *Caring for a Dying Relative: A Guide for Families.* Oxford: Oxford University Press, 1994.

A very clearly written, sensitive book from the director and consulting physician of St. Columba's Hospice in Edinburgh. It is useful for families not as a symptom management manual, but as a resource for how to deal with less tangible issues, such as visiting the cancer patient, truth telling, the place of food and drink, "unmentionable feelings," ethical issues, and "worrying events."

Finkbeiner, Ann K. *After the Death of a Child.* Baltimore: Johns Hopkins University Press, 1996.

The author, a science writer, lost her own son in a train accident when he was 18. After she had somewhat recovered, she wondered about the experiences of other parents who were similarly bereaved. She investigated thirty parents who had also lost children of various ages from a variety of causes and shares the results of her work in this book.

Gawande, A. *Complications: A Surgeon's Notes on an Imperfect Science.* New York: Picador, 2002.

A beautifully written, insightful work. It can be recommended also for clinicians.

Harpham, Wendy Schlessel. *When a Parent Has Cancer: A Guide to Caring for Your Children.* New York: HarperCollins, 1997.

*This is actually two books, one for children (*Becky and the Worry Cup*) and another that describes how to use the storybook for children of various ages. It has been highly recommended for any cancer patient who has concerns about how to discuss the cancer and the needs and fears it engenders in both the patient and the child.*

Houts, Peter S., ed. *Home Care Guide for Cancer.* Baltimore: Johns Hopkins University Press, 1996.

You can recommend this book to caregivers who need practical, step-by-step methods by which they can evaluate and manage the physical and psychosocial problems that they and the people they care for face.

Johnson, Judi, and Linda Klein. *I Can Cope: Staying Healthy with Cancer.* Minneapolis: Chronimed, 1994.

Judi and Linda developed the I Can Cope program, sponsored by the American Cancer Society. In the program, nurses and social workers guide cancer patients through the most common problems they face during and after treatment. This book will provide your patients with the core information delivered by the program, including information about cancer and its treatment and side effects, staying mentally healthy and active, communication issues, and resources available.

Levine, Margie. *Surviving Cancer.* New York: Broadway Books, 2001.

An incredibly useful narrative from a smart, strong, courageous woman who fought her cancer while maintaining her personal style and integrity every step of the way.

Lynn, J., and J. Harrold. *Handbook for Mortals: Guidance for People Facing Serious Illness.* New York: Oxford University Press, 1999.

Handbook for Mortals *is a straightforward, clearly written manual that I give to patients and families who are facing a terminal prognosis. It includes practical suggestions and seeks to empower families to get the information they need from their health providers. It is a valuable book also for nurses and physicians who are not familiar with the demands that caring for these patients place on them and on their families as they try to navigate the health care system and care for the patients at home.*

Remen, Rachel Naomi. *Kitchen Table Wisdom: Stories That Heal.* New York: Riverhead Books, 1996.

Remen, Rachel Naomi. *My Grandfather's Blessings: Stories of Strength, Refuge, and Belonging.* New York: Riverhead Books, 2000.

Rachel Remen is co-founder and medical director of the Commonweal Cancer Help Program. She has extensive experience in the clinical care of those who are suffering and facing life-threatening illnesses as well as in teaching undergraduate, graduate, and practicing physicians how to heal the pain of their own losses—and to become better physicians in the process. In these very readable, engaging books, she uses stories that teach by indirection and very powerfully convey her message.

Sankar, Andrea. *Dying at Home: A Family Guide for Caregiving,* revised and expanded edition. Baltimore: Johns Hopkins University Press, 1999.

Dr. Sankar, a medical anthropologist, was inspired to write this book by her work as a member of a home care team for two years and by her own experience caring for a dying relative at home. The stories she tells will be wonderfully helpful for families. They will recognize themselves in one or more of the families described, who relate how they dealt with the various problems that occurred while they cared for a dying relative at home.

ALTERNATIVE THERAPIES

Benson, Herbert, with Marg Stark. *Timeless Healing: The Power and Biology of Belief.* New York: Scribner (Simon & Schuster), 1996.

Cassileth, Barrie R. *The Alternative Medicine Handbook: The Complete Reference Guide to Alternative and Complementary Therapies.* New York: W. W. Norton, 1998.

Dr. Cassileth is an internationally known expert on alternative medicine and unorthodox therapies. This book is an extremely valuable reference tool for patients who seek these therapies, many of which can be used along with more traditional medical treatments.

BEREAVEMENT/GRIEF

Rando, Theresa A. *Grieving: How to Go on Living When Someone You Love Dies.* Lexington, Mass.: Lexington Books, 1988.

A comprehensive, useful book designed to help those who are mourning through the process of grieving. The author includes the specific problems faced by spouses, children, friends, and significant others. Includes both resource and reference lists.

ETHICS

Jonsen, A. R., M. Siegler, and W. W. Winslade. *Clinical Ethics,* 3rd ed. New York: McGraw-Hill, 1992.

PAIN

Cowles, Jane. *Pain Relief: How to Say No to Acute, Chronic & Cancer Pain!* New York: Mastermedia Limited, 1993.

Dr. Cowles is a medical journalist and patient's rights advocate who has written on a wide range of medical topics. She has had numerous experiences of inadequate pain control both for herself and her family and friends, even those suffering from cancer. After finishing this book, patients will have clear explanations for why this is so, guidelines that enable them to describe their problems to us more accurately, and lists of community and national resources on which they can call for additional help. The chapter on home care and home care resources is an unusual and especially useful one. Patients should be alert, however, to changes in addresses and phone numbers that may have occurred in the years since the book's publication.

Haylock, Pamela J., and Carol P. Curtiss. *Cancer Doesn't Have to Hurt: How to Conquer the Pain Caused by Cancer and Cancer Treatment.* Salt Lake City: Hunter House, 1997.

The authors are nurses who have worked with cancer patients for over twenty-five years. Their book would be useful for patients and families who want an overview of what is available to optimize relief of pain, including how it can be paid for. It also contains a list of resources for managing cancer pain.

Miaskowski C, Cleary J, Burney R, et al. *Guideline for the Management of Cancer Pain in Adults and Children.* APS Clinical Practice Guidelines Series, No. 3. Glenview, Ill.: American Pain Society, 2005. www.ampainsoc.org.

This landmark publication is a consensus document prepared by the leading national pain experts from numerous clinical fields, and includes pharmacologic and nonpharmacologic techniques.

Patt, Richard B., and Susan Lang. *You Don't Have to Suffer: A Complete Guide to Relieving Cancer Pain for Patients and Their Families.* New York: Oxford University Press, 1994.

You might recommend this book to patients who need more help understanding their pain or communicating to you how they feel, or who would like to use nonpharmacologic techniques to deal with their pain. It will also reinforce what you've told them about pain medications and their associated side effects.

RELIGIOUS TEACHINGS ON PAIN MANAGEMENT AND CARE OF THE DYING

Catechism of the Catholic Church. Pauline, St. Paul Books and Media, 1994.

The great matter of life and death. *Tricycle: The Buddhist Review,* Vol. 7, Fall. 1997.

Responsa of Rav Moshe Feinstein, Volume 1, Care of the Critically Ill, translated and annotated by Moshe Dovid Tendler. Hoboken, N.J.: KTAV Publishing House, 1996.

Rinpoche, S. *The Tibetan Book of Living and Dying*, P. Gaffney and A. Harvey, eds. New York: Harper San Francisco, 1993.

OTHER BOOKS OF GENERAL INTEREST

Albom, Mitch. *Tuesdays with Morrie: An Old Man, a Young Man, and Life's Greatest Lesson*. New York: Doubleday, 1997.

Mitch Albom writes a marvelous account of his "last course" with his former professor who is dying of Lou Gehrig's disease (amyotrophic lateral sclerosis). The reader joins this intelligent, sophisticated, and talented author on his unsentimental journey of self-discovery and deepening appreciation for previously unexamined aspects of life.

Anderson, Patrick. *Affairs in Order: A Complete Resource Guide to Death and Dying*. New York: Macmillan, 1991.

Barnett, Terry J. *Living Wills and More*. New York: John Wiley and Sons, 1992.

A guide for patients and their families who need more information on the legal requirements for ensuring that their wishes regarding medical care will be known, regardless of their medical condition.

Becker, Marilyn R. *Last Touch: Preparing for a Parent's Death*. Oakland, Calif.: New Harbinger Publications, 1992.

Ms. Becker, an M.S.W., offers this clearly written personal account of how she helped in her parents' final days, and how she coped with the experience.

Bone, R. C. *Reflections: A Guide to End of Life Issues for You and Your Family*. Available from National Kidney Cancer Association, telephone: 1-800-850-9132 or 847-332-1051; fax: 847-332-2978; website: www.nkca.org.

This free pamphlet, written by a physician who has since died of kidney cancer, is an excellent short introduction to a number of the important issues that dying people need to address.

Broyard, Anatole. *Intoxicated by My Illness*. New York: Fawcett Columbine, 1992.

Anatole Broyard, journalist and author, died of metastatic prostate cancer. This very moving, very lively collection of articles deals with a number of subjects of interest to patients as well as a discussion of other books about cancer. It also includes a short story that mirrors Broyard's experience as one of his parents died of cancer.

Buckman, Robert. *I Don't Know What to Say . . . How to Help Support Someone Who Is Dying*. Boston: Little Brown, 1989.

Dr. Buckman is an oncologist who has particular insight into how to communicate, even about subjects that are hard to discuss. His very practical suggestions will be of great benefit to friends and families of dying patients.

Chappell, Fred. *Farewell, I Am Bound to Leave You*. New York: Picador USA, 1996.

> *Fred Chappell is a master poet and storyteller. In this collection of short stories that reads like a novel, he retells the family tales told by a son-in-law to his son as they await the death of their much-beloved mother-in-law and grandmother. The first selection, The Clocks, and the end piece, The Voices, are surreal descriptions of the very real passing of a loved one.*

Chappell, Fred. *I Am One of You Forever.* Baton Rouge: Louisiana State University Press, 1985.

> *The Telegram, a chapter in this novel, describes a family's experience of loss upon learning of the death of a beloved friend.*

Dollinger, M., E. Rosenbaum, and G. Cable. *Everyone's Guide to Cancer Therapy.* Kansas City: Andrews and McNeal, 1991.

Dubler, Nancy, and David Nimmons. *Ethics on Call.* New York: Harmony Books, 1992.

> *A medical ethicist shows how to take charge of life and death choices.*

Kabat-Zinn, J. *Full Catastrophe Living: Using the Wisdom of Your Body and Mind to Face Stress, Pain, and Illness.* New York: Dell, 1990.

> *A complete, step-by-step guide describing the philosophy and the day-to-day program of the Stress Reduction Clinic founded by Dr. Kabat-Zinn at the University of Massachusetts Medical Center.*

Kübler-Ross, E. *On Death and Dying.* New York: Collier Books, Macmillan, 1969.

LeShan, Lawrence. *Cancer as a Turning Point: A Handbook for People with Cancer, Their Families, and Health Professionals,* revised edition. New York: Plume/Penguin, 1994.

> *Dr. LeShan is a psychotherapist with over thirty-five years of experience in working with cancer patients. His book may be useful for those of your patients who are interested in exploring their inner life; it includes a workbook full of exercises to help them do this.*

Nuland, Sherwin B. *How We Die: Reflections on Life's Final Chapter.* New York: Alfred A. Knopf, 1994.

> *You'll find Dr. Nuland's book especially valuable for those patients or families who have never seen anyone die and want to know what it will look like. The book contains much more than this and will be of interest to those who can deal with its graphic details.*

Peck, M. Scott. *Denial of the Soul: Spiritual and Medical Perspectives on Euthanasia and Mortality.* New York: Harmony Books, 1997.

> *M. Scott Peck, author of, among many other works,* The Road Less Traveled, *deals with the difficult subjects of emotional pain, euthanasia, and the importance of the soul. His is*

a thoughtful discussion that would be of interest to those engaged in the debate about physician-assisted suicide.

Quill, Timothy. *A Midwife through the Dying Process: Stories of Healing and Hard Choices at the End of Life.* Baltimore: Johns Hopkins University Press, 1996.

Dr. Quill shares with the reader many moving stories of the people he has cared for.

Rosenbaum, Ernest. *Living with Cancer.* St. Louis: Mosby; New York: New American Library, Plume Books, 1982.

An experienced, empathetic oncologist provides patients and their families with useful suggestions and very helpful insights.

Rosenblum, Daniel. *A Time to Heal, A Time to Help: Listening to People with Cancer.* New York: Free Press, Macmillan, 1993.

Tells the stories of some people with cancer and the issues the cancer raises in their lives.

Sulmasy, D. P. *The Healer's Calling: A Spirituality for Physicians and Other Health Care Professionals.* New York: Paulist Press, 1997.

Daniel Sulmasy is a philosopher, a health services researcher, a Franciscan Friar, and a medical oncologist. In this eloquent, thoughtful book he relates his "personal experience of being a man of faith engaged in the work of a health care professional" as a basis for our own self-explorations. Chapters include Spirituality and the Health Care Professional; Medicine, Love and the Art of Being Uncertain; The Wine of Fervent Zeal and the Oil of Compassion; God-Talk at the Bedside; Prayer and the Five Senses: A Physician's Meditation; Suffering, Spirituality, and Health Care; and Wounded Healers.

Verghese, A. *My Own Country.* New York: Simon & Schuster, 1994.

The odyssey of a young physician who chooses to care for patients with AIDS in the rural South; its impact on him and his family, his patients and their families.

Webb, Marilyn. *The Good Death: The New American Search to Reshape the End of Life.* New York: Bantam, 1997.

Marilyn Webb is an investigative journalist who spent six years exploring this topic. In this almost 500-page volume, she shares the stories of patients and families for whom death provided the opportunity for either growth or unremitting pain, and explains the many factors that contributed to such different outcomes. She outlines the components of a good experience, barriers to be overcome, and allies to seek along the way.

VIDEOS/MOVIES

Cancer Pain Control: Winning the Battle and *Cancer Pain Control: Controlling Your Cancer Pain*. Marshfield Video Network, 1000 North Oak Avenue, Marshfield, WI 54449.

Videos made in 1990 by the Wisconsin Cancer Pain Initiative.

A Guide to Pain Management in Advanced Prostate Cancer. Immunex Corporation, Seattle; telephone: 1-800-220-6302.

This 1997 video is produced by the sellers of Novantrone, a chemotherapy drug approved for patients with hormone-refractory prostate cancer. Patients may find this useful as it discusses a variety of approaches to pain management. As expected, it suggests how useful Novantrone may be, though it does include appropriate disclaimers that not all patients will benefit. Free copies are available along with patient booklets and a Health Care Professional Edition.

Nature videotapes to relieve stress (e.g., *Rafting through Canyons at Dawn*). Environmental Television Network, 440 East 79th Street, Suite 6C, New York, NY 10021-1437; telephone: 212-861-2385 or 1-800-752-5843; e-mail: envtv@concentric.net.

Running time 30 minutes each.

To Gillian on Her Thirty-seventh Birthday. Columbia Pictures.

This 1996 movie is a compelling, believable story of a bereaved husband and daughter who, a year later, after much pain, gain the insights and strength they need to accept their loss.

CD-ROMS

Completing a Life: An Interactive Multimedia CD-ROM for Patient and Family Education in End of Life Care. Information from www.completingalife.msu.edu.

Easing Cancer Pain. American Cancer Society, telephone: 1-800-723-0360; sample can be viewed at the Easing Cancer Pain website: www.commtechlab.msu.edu/sites/cancer-pain.

This interactive CD-ROM was designed by researchers at Michigan State University to help cancer patients and their families learn more about pain management. Viewers visit a "fireside retreat" from which they can choose paths that lead to information about assessment, barriers, treatment, and personal narratives told by cancer patients and their spouses and children.

WEBSITES/DATABASES

ABCD—Americans for Better Care of the Dying. www.abcd-caring.org.

American Cancer Society. www.cancer.org.

American Medical Association. Caregiver Self-assessment Tool. www.ama-assn
.org.

*A caregiver self-assessment tool designed to help caregivers recognize their need for home
health services. Clinicians can refer caregivers to this site to assist them in recognizing
how much stress they are experiencing, and encourage them to ask for help. The tool is
available in English and Spanish.*

American Society of Clinical Oncology. People Living with Cancer. www.plwc
.org.

ASCO's website is for people living with cancer, their families and friends.

Bailey, F. Amos, Palliative Response. www.hospice.va.gov *and* www.hospice.va
.gov/Amosbaileybook/index.htm.

These websites offer the full text of F. Amos Bailey's manual on palliative care, Palliative
Response. *Dr. Bailey helped develop the innovative programs at Balm of Gilead hospice
and wrote a clear, concise manual for hospice care.*

Candlelighters Childhood Cancer Foundation. www.candle.org.

*Information on written materials, over 400 peer support groups, and contacts for all
family members nationwide.*

Caregiver Survival Resources. www.caregiver911.com.

Catholic Health Association of the United States. www.chausa.org.

Center to Advance Palliative Care. http://capc.org/programs.

*This website has posted tools for organizations that wish to develop palliative care pro-
grams in the inpatient or outpatient setting.*

Counseling for Loss. www.counselingforloss.com.

Crisis, Grief & Healing Discussion. www.webhealing.com.

A Web page created by psychotherapist Tom Golden.

Dying Well. www.dyingwell.com.

Eldercare Web. www.elderweb.com.

Growth House. www.growthhouse.org/palliative.

*The best website for information on palliative and end-of-life care, with extensive links to
other websites. Includes professional forums, electronic versions of books, an electronic
bookstore, and information on hospice, palliative care, pain, and grief. Telephone number
for healthcare providers: 415-863-3045*

HealthAnswers. www.healthanswers.com.

This database was created in partnership with the American Academy of Family Physicians. It contains an online U.S. Pharmacopoeia drug reference and links to caregiving and patient support sites. The HealthAnswers Knowledge Base can be searched, like a CD-ROM, for information on an extensive variety of conditions.

Last Chapters Forum. www.lastchapters.org.

As stated in the Journal of Palliative Medicine *(vol. 6, p. 690, 2003), this website "offers a collection of inspiring stories and video interviews of people who are facing death or chronic illness." It also hosts The Last Chapters Forum, through which viewers can discuss their reactions to the stories. Partnership for Caring, Inc., telephone: 800-989-9455.*

Last Acts—Care and Caring at the End of Life. www.lastacts.org. Medicare Rights Center. www.medicarerights.org.

Provides free counseling services for Medicare beneficiaries who cannot afford private assistance.

National Alliance of Breast Cancer Organizations. www.nabco.org.
National Coalition for Cancer Survivorship. www.canceradvocacy.org.
National Family Caregivers Association. www.nfcacares.org.
OncoLink. www.oncolink.upenn.edu.
On-line Grief and Loss

To subscribe, send an e-mail message to rivendell@rivendell.org. In the body of the message, type: subscribe rivendell [your e-mail address].

Pain Medicine and Palliative Care at Beth Israel Medical Center, www.stoppain.org.

This website provides valuable clinical and educational resources for pain control, palliative care, and hospice. Telephone: 212-844-8970.

SeniorScape. www.seniorscape.com.

A valuable comprehensive educational site, including information on elder law, community resources for elders, senior health and nutrition, senior lobbying efforts, geriatric care, financial management in later years, and other topics.

ORGANIZATIONS

American Academy of Hospice and Palliative Medicine, 4700 W. Lake Ave., Glenview, IL 60025; telephone: 847-375-4712; website: www.aahpm.org.
American Brain Tumor Association, 2720 River Road, Suite 146, Des Plaines, IL 60018; telephone: 1-800-886-2282; website: http://hope.abta.org.
American Cancer Society, 1599 Clifton Road N.E., Atlanta, GA 30329 (National

Office); telephone: 1-800-227-2345 (call for phone number of local division); website: www.cancer.org.

American Foundation for Urologic Disease, 300 West Pratt Street, Suite 401, Baltimore, MD 21201-2463; website: www.afud.org.

For information on cancer of the prostate and bladder.

American Hospice Foundation, 2120 L Street NW, Suite 200, Washington, DC 20037; website: www.americanhospice.org.

American Society for Clinical Hypnosis, 140 N. Bloomingdale Road, Bloomingdale, IL 60108-1017; telephone: 630-980-4740; website: www.asch.net.

Bloch Cancer Foundation, Inc., 4410 Main Street, Kansas City, MO 64111; telephone: 816-932-8453; website: www.blochcancer.org.

Cancer Care, Inc., 1180 Avenue of the Americas, New York, NY 10036; telephone: 212-221-3300; website: www.cancercare.org.

See also Cancer Care Counseling Line, listed under Support Groups.

Cancer Information Service, National Cancer Institute, Office of Cancer Communications, Center Drive, Building 31, Room 10A10, Bethesda, MD 20892-2580; website: http://cis.nci.nih.gov.

Candlelighters Childhood Cancer Foundation, National Office, P.O. Box 498, Kensington, MD 20895-0498; website: www.candlelighters.org.

City of Hope Medical Center, 1500 East Duarte Road, Duarte, CA 91010-0269; telephone: 626-256-4673; website: www.cityofhope.org.

Compassionate Friends; telephone: 410-560-3358; website: www.compassionatefriends.org.

A self-help group for survivors of suicides.

Cure for Lymphoma Foundation, 215 Lexington Avenue, New York, NY 10016-6023; telephone: 212-213-9595; fax: 212-213-1987; e-mail: infocfl@aol.com; website: www.cfl.healthology.com.

Hospice Association of America, 228 7th Street SE, Washington, DC 20003; telephone: 202-546-5419; website: www.hospice-america.org.

Hospice Foundation of America, 2001 S Street NW, #300, Washington, DC 20009; telephone: 800-854-3402; website: www.hospicefoundation.org.

Hospice and Palliative Nurses Association, Penn Center West One, Suite 229, Pittsburgh, PA 15276; telephone: 412-787-9301; website: www.hpna.org.

International Myeloma Foundation, 12650 Riverside Drive, Suite 206, North Hollywood, CA 91607-3421; telephone: 800-452-2873; website: www.myeloma.org.

Leukemia and Lymphoma Society. telephone: 800-955-4572; website: www.leukemia.org.

Lymphoma Research Foundation of America, Inc., 8800 Venice Boulevard, Suite

207, Los Angeles, CA 90034; telephone: 310-204-7040.

National Brain Tumor Foundation, 22 Battery Street, Suite 612, San Francisco, CA 94111-5520; telephone: 415-834-9970; website: www.braintumor.org.

National Breast Cancer Coalition, 1101 17th Street NW, Suite 1300, Washington, DC 20036; telephone: 202-296-7477; website: www.natlbcc.org.

National Cancer Institute Cancer Information Service; telephone: 1-800-422-6227; fax: 301-402-5874 (CANCERFAX); website: www.cancer.gov.

National Cancer Institute Publications Ordering Service, P.O. Box 24128, Baltimore, MD 21227; telephone: 1-800-4CANCER (1-800-422-6237).

Easy to read booklets are available free of charge. Get Relief from Cancer Pain *and* Helping Yourself during Chemotherapy *are available in large print for those who are visually impaired.*

National Family Caregivers Association, 10400 Connecticut Avenue, Suite 500, Kensington, MD 20895; telephone: 1-800-896-3650; website: thefamilycaregiver.org.

National Hospice Organization, 1901 North Moore Street, Suite 901, Arlington, VA 22209; telephone: 1-800-658-8898; website: www.nhpco.org.

National Hospice and Palliative Care Organization. www.nhpco.org.

National Kidney Cancer Association, 1234 Sherman Avenue, Suite 203, Evanston, IL 60202; telephone: 800-850-9132; website: www.nkca.org.

National Ovarian Cancer Coalition, Inc., 500 NE Spanish River Boulevard, Suite 8, Boca Raton, FL 33431; telephone: 1-888-OVARIAN (1-888-682-7426); fax: 561-393-7275; e-mail: NOCC@ovarian.org; website: www.ovarian.org.

Wisconsin Cancer Pain Initiative, Cancer Pain Resource Center, Medical Science Center, Room 3671, 1300 University Avenue, Madison, WI 53706; telephone: 608-265-4013; fax: 608-265-4014; e-mail: wcpi@facstaff.wisc.edu; website: www.aacpi.uisc.edu/wcpi.

Pamphlets and videos for children and adults are available.

Y-ME, National Breast Cancer Organization, 212 West Van Buren, 4th Floor, Chicago, IL 60607; telephone: 1-800-221-2141; 24-hour Hot Line: 312-986-8228; website: www.y-me.org.

SUPPORT GROUPS

American Cancer Society, National Office, 1599 Clifton Road N.E., Atlanta, GA 30329; telephone: 1-800-227-2345; website: www.cancer.org.

Send for Guidelines on Support and Self Help Groups, *1995.*

Bone Marrow Transplant Family Support Network, P.O. Box 845, Avon, CT 06001; telephone: 1-800-826-9376; website: www.employerhealth.com.

Cancer Care, Inc., 1180 Avenue of the Americas, New York, NY 10036; telephone: 1-800-813-HOPE (4673) or 212-221-3300; website: www.cancercare.org.

An organization that offers free counseling and other services to cancer patients and their families. Staffed by social workers.

Cancer Care Counseling Line; telephone: 1-800-813-4673 (1-800-813-HOPE); Monday to Friday, 9 a.m. to 5 p.m. EST; e-mail: CancerCare@aol.com.

This is a free counseling line sponsored by Cancer Care, Inc., in which callers can receive one-to-one counseling from experienced oncology social workers, as well as referrals, free educational materials, and information on telephone support groups and educational seminars. All Cancer Care, Inc., services are free of charge.

Cancer Information Service; telephone: 1-800-4CANCER (1-800-422-6237); TTY: 1-800-332-8615.

This is the National Cancer Institute's national telephone service; staff answer questions in English and Spanish and distribute NCI materials.

CHEMOcare, Cleveland Clinic Foundation, sponsored by Ortho Biotech. www .chemocare.com.

Cancer patients are paired with a volunteer who has had the same type of cancer.

Hospice Education Institute, 3 Unity Square, P.O. Box 98, Machiasport, ME 04655-0098; telephone: 800-331-1620 or 207-255-8800; website: www.hospice-world.org.

The Hospice Education Institute provides information and education and referrals to local providers of hospice and palliative care.

Mary-Helen Mautner Project for Lesbians with Cancer, 1707 L Street NW, Suite 1060, Washington, DC 20036; telephone: 202-332-5536 (voice/TTY); fax: 202-265-6854; website: www.mautnerproject.org.

National Women's Health Network, 514 10th Street NW, Suite 400, Washington, DC 20004; telephone: 202-347-1140; website: www.womenshealthnetwork .org.

Office of Minority Health Resource Center, U.S. Department of Health and Human Services, P.O. Box 37337, Washington, DC 20013-7337; telephone: 800-444-6472; www.omhrc.org.

Provides information on health resources at federal, state, and local levels.

US TOO! International, Inc., 930 North York Road, Suite 50, Hinsdale, IL 60521; telephone: 1-800-80 US TOO (1-800-808-7866); www.ustoo.com.

Provides prostate cancer education and support.

The Wellness Community, 919 18th Street NW, Suite 54, Washington, DC 20006; telephone: 202-659-9709 or 888-793-9355; website: www.thewellnesscommunity.org.

Index

*Page numbers in **boldface** type refer to practice points (in boxes in text).*